D1032602

FUTURE OF EMERGENCY CARE

EMERGENCY MEDICAL SERVICES AT THE CROSSROADS

Committee on the Future of Emergency Care
in the United States Health System

Board on Health Care Services

INSTITUTE OF MEDICINE
OF THE NATIONAL ACADEMIES

THE NATIONAL ACADEMIES PRESS
Washington, D.C.
www.nap.edu

THE NATIONAL ACADEMIES PRESS   500 Fifth Street, N.W.   Washington, DC 20001

NOTICE: The project that is the subject of this report was approved by the Governing Board of the National Research Council, whose members are drawn from the councils of the National Academy of Sciences, the National Academy of Engineering, and the Institute of Medicine. The members of the committee responsible for the report were chosen for their special competences and with regard for appropriate balance.

This study was supported by Contract No. 282-99-0045 between the National Academy of Sciences and the U.S. Department of Health and Human Services' Agency for Healthcare Research and Quality (AHRQ); Contract No. B03-06 between the National Academy of Sciences and the Josiah Macy, Jr. Foundation; and Contract No. HHSH25056047 between the National Academy of Sciences and the U.S. Department of Health and Human Services' Health Resources and Services Administration (HRSA) and Centers for Disease Control and Prevention (CDC), and the U.S. Department of Transportation's National Highway Traffic Safety Administration (NHTSA). Any opinions, findings, conclusions, or recommendations expressed in this publication are those of the author(s) and do not necessarily reflect the view of the organizations or agencies that provided support for this project.

Library of Congress Cataloging-in-Publication Data

Emergency medical services at the crossroads / Committee on the Future of Emergency Care in the United States Health System, Board on Health Care Services.
    p. ; cm. — (Future of emergency care series)
Includes bibliographical references.
ISBN-13: 978-0-309-10174-5 (hardback)
ISBN-10: 0-309-10174-3 (hardback)
1. Emergency medical services. 2. Disaster medicine. I. Institute of Medicine (U.S.). Committee on the Future of Emergency Care in the United States Health System. II. Series.
    [DNLM: 1. Emergency Medical Services—United States. 2. Emergency Medical Services—trends—United States. 3. Emergency Treatment—United States. 4. Health Care Reform—United States. WX 215 E53509 2007]
RA645.5.E4488 2007
362.18—dc22

                                                                2007002810

Additional copies of this report are available from the National Academies Press, 500 Fifth Street, N.W., Lockbox 285, Washington, DC 20055; (800) 624-6242 or (202) 334-3313 (in the Washington metropolitan area); Internet, http://www.nap.edu.

For more information about the Institute of Medicine, visit the IOM home page at: **www.iom.edu.**

The serpent has been a symbol of long life, healing, and knowledge among almost all cultures and religions since the beginning of recorded history. The serpent adopted as a logotype by the Institute of Medicine is a relief carving from ancient Greece, now held by the Staatliche Museen in Berlin.

"Knowing is not enough; we must apply.
Willing is not enough; we must do."
—Goethe

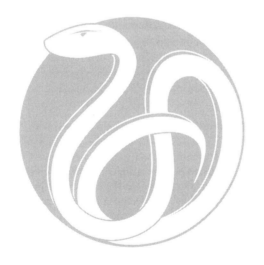

INSTITUTE OF MEDICINE
OF THE NATIONAL ACADEMIES

Advising the Nation. Improving Health.

THE NATIONAL ACADEMIES
Advisers to the Nation on Science, Engineering, and Medicine

The **National Academy of Sciences** is a private, nonprofit, self-perpetuating society of distinguished scholars engaged in scientific and engineering research, dedicated to the furtherance of science and technology and to their use for the general welfare. Upon the authority of the charter granted to it by the Congress in 1863, the Academy has a mandate that requires it to advise the federal government on scientific and technical matters. Dr. Ralph J. Cicerone is president of the National Academy of Sciences.

The **National Academy of Engineering** was established in 1964, under the charter of the National Academy of Sciences, as a parallel organization of outstanding engineers. It is autonomous in its administration and in the selection of its members, sharing with the National Academy of Sciences the responsibility for advising the federal government. The National Academy of Engineering also sponsors engineering programs aimed at meeting national needs, encourages education and research, and recognizes the superior achievements of engineers. Dr. Wm. A. Wulf is president of the National Academy of Engineering.

The **Institute of Medicine** was established in 1970 by the National Academy of Sciences to secure the services of eminent members of appropriate professions in the examination of policy matters pertaining to the health of the public. The Institute acts under the responsibility given to the National Academy of Sciences by its congressional charter to be an adviser to the federal government and, upon its own initiative, to identify issues of medical care, research, and education. Dr. Harvey V. Fineberg is president of the Institute of Medicine.

The **National Research Council** was organized by the National Academy of Sciences in 1916 to associate the broad community of science and technology with the Academy's purposes of furthering knowledge and advising the federal government. Functioning in accordance with general policies determined by the Academy, the Council has become the principal operating agency of both the National Academy of Sciences and the National Academy of Engineering in providing services to the government, the public, and the scientific and engineering communities. The Council is administered jointly by both Academies and the Institute of Medicine. Dr. Ralph J. Cicerone and Dr. Wm. A. Wulf are chair and vice chair, respectively, of the National Research Council.

www.national-academies.org

COMMITTEE ON THE FUTURE OF EMERGENCY CARE IN THE UNITED STATES HEALTH SYSTEM

GAIL L. WARDEN *(Chair)*, President Emeritus, Henry Ford Health System, Detroit, Michigan

STUART H. ALTMAN, Sol C. Chaikin Professor of National Health Policy, Heller School of Social Policy, Brandeis University, Waltham, Massachusetts

BRENT R. ASPLIN, Associate Professor of Emergency Medicine, University of Minnesota and Department Head, Regions Hospital Emergency Department, St. Paul

THOMAS F. BABOR, Chair, Department of Community Medicine and Health Care, University of Connecticut Health Center, Farmington

ROBERT R. BASS, Immediate Past President, National Association of State EMS Officials and Executive Director, Maryland Institute for Emergency Medical Services Systems, Baltimore

BENJAMIN K. CHU, Regional President, Southern California, Kaiser Foundation Health Plan and Hospital, Pasadena

A. BRENT EASTMAN, Chief Medical Officer, N. Paul Whittier Chair of Trauma, ScrippsHealth, San Diego, California

GEORGE L. FOLTIN, Director, Center for Pediatric Emergency Medicine, Associate Professor of Pediatrics and Emergency Medicine, New York University School of Medicine, Bellevue Hospital Center, New York

SHIRLEY GAMBLE, Chief Operating Officer, United Way Capital Area, Austin, Texas

DARRELL J. GASKIN, Associate Professor, Department of Health Policy and Management, Johns Hopkins Bloomberg School of Public Health, Baltimore, Maryland

ROBERT C. GATES, Project Director, Medical Services for Indigents, Health Care Agency, Santa Ana, California

MARIANNE GAUSCHE-HILL, Clinical Professor of Medicine and Director, Prehospital Care, Harbor-UCLA Medical Center, Torrance, California

JOHN D. HALAMKA, Chief Information Officer, Beth Israel Deaconess Medical Center, Boston, Massachusetts

MARY M. JAGIM, Internal Consultant for Emergency Preparedness Planning, MeritCare Health System, Fargo, North Dakota

ARTHUR L. KELLERMANN, Professor and Chair, Department of Emergency Medicine and Director, Center for Injury Control, Emory University School of Medicine, Atlanta, Georgia

WILLIAM N. KELLEY, Professor of Medicine, Biochemistry & Biophysics, University of Pennsylvania School of Medicine, Philadelphia

v

Reviewers

This report has been reviewed in draft form by individuals chosen for their diverse perspectives and technical expertise, in accordance with procedures approved by the National Research Council's Report Review Committee. The purpose of this independent review is to provide candid and critical comments that will assist the institution in making its published report as sound as possible and to ensure that the report meets institutional standards for objectivity, evidence, and responsiveness to the study charge. The review comments and draft manuscript remain confidential to protect the integrity of the deliberative process. We wish to thank the following individuals for their review of this report:

DENIS A. CORTESE, Mayo Clinic, Rochester, Minnesota
THEODORE R. DELBRIDGE, Department of Emergency Medicine, Brody School of Medicine at East Carolina University, Greenville, North Carolina
DIA GAINOR, Emergency Medical Services Bureau, Idaho Department of Health and Welfare, Boise
RONALD MAIO, Department of Emergency Medicine and University of Michigan Injury Research Center, University of Michigan, Ann Arbor
GREGG MARGOLIS, National Registry of Emergency Medical Technicians, Columbus, Ohio
RICARDO MARTINEZ, The Schumacher Group, Kennesaw, Georgia
MURRAY N. ROSS, Health Policy Analysis and Research, Kaiser Permanente Institute for Health Policy, Oakland, California

JOHN SACRA, Medical Control Board, Emergency Medical Services
Authority, Tulsa, Oklahoma
JAMES W. VARNUM, Mary Hitchcock Memorial Hospital and
Dartmouth-Hitchcock Alliance, Lebanon, New Hampshire

Although the reviewers listed above have provided many constructive
comments and suggestions, they were not asked to endorse the conclusions
or recommendations nor did they see the final draft of the report before its
release. The review of this report was overseen by **Enriqueta C. Bond,** Bur-
roughs Wellcome Fund, and **Fernando Guerra,** San Antonio Metropolitan
Health District. Appointed by the National Research Council and Institute
of Medicine, they were responsible for making certain that an independent
examination of this report was carried out in accordance with institutional
procedures and that all review comments were carefully considered. Responsibility for the final content of this report rests entirely with the authoring
committee and the institution.

Foreword

The state of emergency care affects every American. When illness or injury strikes, Americans count on the emergency care system to respond with timely and high-quality care. Yet today, the emergency and trauma care that Americans receive can fall short of what they expect and deserve.

Emergency care is a window on health care, revealing both what is right and what is wrong with the care delivery system. Americans increasingly rely on hospital emergency departments because of the skilled specialists and advanced technologies they offer. At the same time, the increasing use of the emergency care system represents failures of the larger health care system—the growing numbers of uninsured Americans, the limited alternatives available in many communities, and the inadequate preventive care and chronic care management received by many. The resulting demands on the system can degrade the quality of emergency care and hinder the ability to provide urgent and lifesaving care to seriously ill and injured patients wherever and whenever they need it.

The Committee on the Future of Emergency Care in the United States Health System, ably chaired by Gail Warden, set out to examine the emergency care system in the United States; explore its strengths, limitations, and future challenges; describe a desired vision of the system; and recommend strategies for achieving that vision. The committee's efforts build on past contributions of the National Academies, including the landmark National Research Council report *Accidental Death and Disability: The Neglected Disease of Modern Society* in 1966, *Injury in America: A Continuing Health Problem* in 1985, and *Emergency Medical Services for Children* in 1993.

The committee's task in the present study was to examine the full scope of emergency care, from 9-1-1 and medical dispatch to hospital-based emergency and trauma care. The three reports produced by the committee—*Hospital-Based Emergency Care: At the Breaking Point, Emergency Medical Services at the Crossroads,* and *Emergency Care for Children: Growing Pains*—provide three different perspectives on the emergency care system. The series as a whole unites the often fragmented prehospital and hospital-based systems under a common vision for the future of emergency care.

As the committee prepared its reports, federal and state policy makers were turning their attention to the possibility of an avian influenza pandemic. Americans are asking whether we as a nation are prepared for such an event. The emergency care system is on the front lines of surveillance and treatment. The more secure and stable our emergency care system is, the better prepared we will be to handle any possible outbreak. In this light, the recommendations presented in these reports take on increased urgency. The guidance they offer can assist all of the stakeholders in emergency care—the public, policy makers, providers, and educators—to chart the future of emergency care in the United States.

Harvey V. Fineberg, M.D., Ph.D.
President, Institute of Medicine
June 2006

Preface

Emergency care has made important advances in recent decades: emergency 9-1-1 service now links virtually all ill and injured Americans to immediate medical response; organized trauma systems transport patients to advanced, lifesaving care within minutes; and advances in resuscitation and lifesaving procedures yield outcomes unheard of just two decades ago. Yet just under the surface, a growing national crisis in emergency care is brewing. Emergency departments (EDs) are frequently overloaded, with patients sometimes lining hallways and waiting hours and even days to be admitted to inpatient beds. Ambulance diversion, in which overcrowded EDs close their doors to incoming ambulances, has become a common, even daily problem in many cities. Patients with severe trauma or illness are often brought to the ED only to find that the specialists needed to treat them are unavailable. The transport of patients to available emergency care facilities is often fragmented and disorganized, and the quality of emergency medical services (EMS) is highly inconsistent from one town, city, or region to the next. In some areas, the system's task of dealing with emergencies is compounded by an additional task: providing nonemergent care for many of the 45 million uninsured Americans. Furthermore, the system is ill prepared to handle large-scale emergencies, whether a natural disaster, an influenza pandemic, or an act of terrorism.

This crisis is multifaceted and impacts every aspect of emergency care—from prehospital EMS to hospital-based emergency and trauma care. The American public places its faith in the ability of the emergency care system to respond appropriately whenever and wherever a serious illness or injury occurs. But while the public is largely unaware of the crisis, it is real and growing.

The Institute of Medicine's Committee on the Future of Emergency Care in the United States Health System was convened in September 2003 to examine the emergency care system in the United States, to create a vision for the future of the system, and to make recommendations for helping the nation achieve that vision. The committee's findings and recommendations are presented in the three reports in the *Future of Emergency Care* series:

- *Hospital-Based Emergency Care: At the Breaking Point* explores the changing role of the hospital ED and describes the national epidemic of overcrowded EDs and trauma centers. The range of issues addressed includes uncompensated emergency and trauma care, the availability of specialists, medical liability exposure, management of patient flow, hospital disaster preparedness, and support for emergency and trauma research.

- *Emergency Medical Services at the Crossroads* describes the development of EMS over the last four decades and the fragmented system that exists today. It explores a range of issues that affect the delivery of prehospital EMS, including communications systems; coordination of the regional flow of patients to hospitals and trauma centers; reimbursement of EMS; national training and credentialing standards; innovations in triage, treatment, and transport; integration of all components of EMS into disaster preparedness, planning, and response actions; and the lack of clinical evidence to support much of the care that is delivered.

- *Emergency Care for Children: Growing Pains* describes the special challenges of emergency care for children and considers the progress that has been made in this area in the 20 years since the establishment of the federal Emergency Medical Services for Children (EMS-C) program. It addresses how issues affecting the emergency care system generally have an even greater impact on the outcomes of critically ill and injured children. The topics addressed include the state of pediatric readiness, pediatric training and standards of care in emergency care, pediatric medication issues, disaster preparedness for children, and pediatric research and data collection.

THE IMPORTANCE AND SCOPE OF EMERGENCY CARE

Each year in the United States approximately 114 million visits to EDs occur, and 16 million of these patients arrive by ambulance. In 2002, 43 percent of all hospital admissions in the United States entered through the ED. The emergency care system deals with an extraordinary range of patients, from febrile infants, to business executives with chest pain, to elderly patients who have fallen.

EDs are an impressive public health success story in terms of access to care. Americans of all walks of life know where the nearest ED is and understand that it is available 24 hours a day, 7 days a week. Trauma systems also represent an impressive achievement. They are a critical component of the emergency care system since approximately 35 percent of ED visits are injury-related, and injuries are the number one killer of people between the ages of 1 and 44. Yet the development of trauma systems has been inconsistent across states and regions.

In addition to its traditional role of providing urgent and lifesaving care, the emergency care system has become the "safety net of the safety net," providing primary care services to millions of Americans who are uninsured or otherwise lack access to other community services. Hospital EDs and trauma centers are the only providers required by federal law to accept, evaluate, and stabilize all who present for care, regardless of their ability to pay. An unintended but predictable consequence of this legal duty is a system that is overloaded and underfunded to carry out its mission. This situation can hinder access to emergency care for insured and uninsured alike, and compromise the quality of care provided to all. Further, EDs have become the preferred setting for many patients and an important adjunct to community physicians' practices. Indeed, the recent growth in ED use has been driven by patients with private health insurance. In addition to these responsibilities, emergency care providers have been tasked with the enormous challenge of preparing for a wide range of emergencies, from bioterrorism to natural disasters and pandemic disease. While balancing all of these tasks is difficult for every organization providing emergency care, it is an even greater challenge for small, rural providers with limited resources.

Improved Emergency Medical Services: A Public Health Imperative

Since the Institute of Medicine (IOM) embarked on this study, concern about a possible avian influenza pandemic has led to worldwide assessment of preparedness for such an event. Reflecting this concern, a national summit on pandemic influenza preparedness was convened by Department of Health and Human Services Secretary Michael O. Leavitt on December 5, 2005, in Washington D.C., and has been followed by statewide summits throughout the country. At these meetings, many of the deficiencies noted by the IOM's Committee on the Future of Emergency Care in the United States Health System have been identified as weaknesses in the nation's ability to respond to large-scale emergency situations, whether disease outbreaks, naturally occurring disasters, or

continued

acts of terrorism. During any such event, local hospitals and emergency departments will be on the front lines. Yet of the millions of dollars going into preparedness efforts, a tiny fraction has made its way to medical preparedness, and much of that has focused on one of the least likely threats—bioterrorism. The result is that few hospital and EMS professionals have had even minimal disaster preparedness training; even fewer have access to personal protective equipment; hospitals, many already stretched to the limit, lack the ability to absorb any significant surge in casualties; and supplies of critical hospital equipment, such as decontamination showers, negative pressure rooms, ventilators, and intensive care unit beds, are wholly inadequate. A system struggling to meet the day-to-day needs of the public will not have the capacity to deal with a sustained surge of patients.

FRAMEWORK FOR THIS STUDY

This year marks the fortieth anniversary of the publication of the landmark National Academy of Sciences/National Research Council report *Accidental Death and Disability: The Neglected Disease of Modern Society*. That report described an epidemic of automobile-related and other injuries, and harshly criticized the deplorable state of trauma care nationwide. The report prompted a public outcry, and stimulated a flood of public and private initiatives to enhance highway safety and improve the medical response to injuries. Efforts included the development of trauma and prehospital EMS systems, creation of the specialty in emergency medicine, and establishment of federal programs to enhance the emergency care infrastructure and build a research base. To many, the 1966 report marked the birth of the modern emergency care system.

Since then, the National Academies and the Institute of Medicine (IOM) have produced a number of reports examining various aspects of the emergency care system. The 1985 report *Injury in America: A Continuing Health Problem* called for expanded research into the epidemiology and treatment of injury, and led to the development of the National Center for Injury Prevention and Control within the Centers for Disease Control and Prevention. The 1993 report *Emergency Medical Services for Children* exposed the limited capacity of the emergency care system to address the needs of children, and contributed to the expansion of the EMS-C program within the Department of Health and Human Services. It has been 10 years, however, since the IOM examined any aspect of emergency care in depth. Furthermore, no National Academies report has ever examined the full range of issues surrounding emergency care in the United States.

That is what this committee set out to do. The objectives of the study were to (1) examine the emergency care system in the United States; (2) explore its strengths, limitations, and future challenges; (3) describe a desired vision for the system; and (4) recommend strategies for achieving this vision.

STUDY DESIGN

The IOM Committee on the Future of Emergency Care in the United States Health System was formed in September 2003. In May 2004, the committee was expanded to comprise a main committee of 25 members and three subcommittees. A total of 40 main and subcommittee members, representing a broad range of expertise in health care and public policy, participated in the study. Between 2003 and 2006, the main committee and subcommittees met 19 times; heard public testimony from nearly 60 speakers; commissioned 11 research papers; conducted site visits; and gathered information from hundreds of experts, stakeholder groups, and interested individuals.

The magnitude of the effort reflects the scope and complexity of emergency care itself, which encompasses a broad continuum of services that includes prevention and bystander care; emergency calls to 9-1-1; dispatch of emergency personnel to the scene of injury or illness; triage, treatment, and transport of patients by ambulance and air medical services; hospital-based emergency and trauma care; subspecialty care by on-call specialists; and subsequent inpatient care. Emergency care's complexity can be also traced to the multiple locations, diverse professionals, and cultural differences that span this continuum of services. EMS, for example, is unlike any other field of medicine—over one-third of its professional workforce consists of volunteers. Further, EMS has one foot in the public safety realm and one foot in medical care, with nearly half of all such services being housed within fire departments. Hospital-based emergency care is also delivered by an extraordinarily diverse staff—emergency physicians, trauma surgeons, critical care specialists, and the many surgical and medical subspecialists who provide services on an on-call basis, as well as specially trained nurses, pharmacists, physician assistants, nurse practitioners, and others.

The division into a main committee and three subcommittees made it possible to break down this enormous effort into several discrete components. At the same time, the committee sought to examine emergency care as a comprehensive system, recognizing the interdependency of its component parts. To this end, the study process was highly integrated. The main committee and three subcommittees were designed to provide for substantial overlap, interaction, and cross-fertilization of expertise. The committee concluded that nothing will change without cooperative and visionary leadership at many levels and a concerted national effort among the principal stakeholders—federal, state, and local officials; hospital leadership; physicians, nurses, and other clinicians; and the public.

The committee hopes that the reports in the *Future of Emergency Care* series will stimulate increased attention to and reform of the emergency care system in the United States. I wish to express my appreciation to the members of the committee and subcommittees and the many panelists who provided input at the meetings held for this study, and to the IOM staff for their time, effort, and commitment to the development of these important reports.

Gail L. Warden
Chair

Acknowledgments

The *Future of Emergency Care* series benefited from the contributions of many individuals and organizations. The committee and Institute of Medicine (IOM) staff take this opportunity to recognize and thank those who helped in the development of the reports in the series.

A large number of individuals assembled materials that helped the committee develop the evidence base for its analyses. The committee appreciates the contributions of experts from a variety of organizations and disciplines who gave presentations during committee meetings or authored papers that provided information incorporated into the series of reports. The full list of presenters is provided in Appendix C. Authors of commissioned papers are listed in Appendix D.

Committee members and IOM staff conducted a number of site visits throughout the course of the study to gain a better understanding of certain aspects of the emergency care system. We appreciate the willingness of staff from the following organizations to meet with us and respond to questions: Beth Israel Deaconess Medical Center, Boston Medical Center, Children's National Medical Center, Grady Memorial Hospital, Johns Hopkins Hospital, Maryland Institute for Emergency Medical Services Systems, Maryland State Police Aviation Division, Richmond Ambulance Association, and Washington Hospital Center.

We would also like to express appreciation to the many individuals who shared their expertise and resources on a wide range of issues: Karen Benson-Huck, Linda Fagnani, Carol Haraden, Lenworth Jacobs, Tom Judge, Nadine Levick, Ellen MacKenzie, Dawn Mancuso, Rick Murray, Ed

Racht, Dom Ruscio, Carol Spizziri, Caroline Steinberg, Rosemary Stevens, Peter Vicellio, and Mike Williams.

This study received funding from the Josiah Macy, Jr. Foundation, the National Highway Traffic Safety Administration (NHTSA), and three agencies within the Department of Health and Human Services: the Agency for Healthcare Research and Quality (AHRQ), the Centers for Disease Control and Prevention (CDC), and the Health Resources and Services Administration (HRSA). We would like to thank the staff from those organizations who provided us with information, documents, and insights throughout the project, including Drew Dawson, Laurie Flaherty, Susan McHenry, Gamunu Wijetunge, and David Bryson of NHTSA; Dan Kavanaugh, Christina Turgel, and David Heppel of HRSA; Robin Weinick and Pam Owens of AHRQ; Rick Hunt and Bob Bailey from CDC's National Center for Injury Prevention and Control; and many other helpful members of the staffs of those organizations.

Important research and writing contributions were made by Molly Hicks of Keene Mill Consulting, LLC. Karen Boyd, a Christine Mirzayan Science and Technology Fellow of the National Academies, and two student interns, Carla Bezold and Neesha Desai, developed background papers. Also, our thanks to Rona Briere, who edited the reports, and to Alisa Decatur, who prepared them for publication.

Contents

EMERGENCY MEDICAL SERVICES AT THE CROSSROADS

Summary

Emergency medical services (EMS) is a critical component of the nation's emergency and trauma care system. Hundreds of thousands of EMS personnel provide more than 16 million medical transports each year. These personnel deal with an extraordinary range of conditions and severity on a daily basis—from mild fevers to massive head traumas. The work they do is challenging, stressful, at times dangerous, and often highly rewarding.

EMS encompasses the initial stages of the emergency care continuum. It includes emergency calls to 9-1-1; dispatch of emergency personnel to the scene of an illness or trauma; and triage, treatment, and transport of patients by ambulance and air medical service. The speed and quality of emergency medical services are critical factors in a patient's ultimate outcome. For patients who cannot breathe, are in hemorrhagic shock, or are in cardiac arrest, the decisions made and actions taken by EMS personnel may determine the outcome as much as the subsequent hospital-based care—and may mean the difference between life and death.

DEVELOPMENT OF THE EMS SYSTEM

The modern EMS system in the United States developed only within the past 50 years, yet its progress has been dramatic. In the 1950s, EMS provided little more than first aid, and it was not uncommon for the local ambulance service to comprise a mortician and a hearse. In the late 1950s, researchers demonstrated the effectiveness of mouth-to-mouth ventilation, and in 1960 cardiopulmonary resuscitation (CPR) was shown to be effective in restoring breathing and circulation. These clinical advances led to the

1

realization that rapid response of trained community members to emergency situations could significantly improve patient outcomes. Over time, local communities began to develop more sophisticated EMS capacity, although there was significant variation nationwide. Increased recognition of the importance of EMS in the 1970s led to strong federal leadership and funding that resulted in considerable advances, including the nationwide adoption of the 9-1-1 system, the development of a professional corps of emergency medical technicians (EMTs), and the establishment of more organized local EMS systems.

Federal funding for EMS, however, declined abruptly in the early 1980s. Since then, the push to develop more organized systems of EMS delivery has diminished, and EMS systems have been left to develop haphazardly across the United States. There is now enormous variability in the design of EMS systems among states and local areas. Nearly half of these systems are fire-based, meaning that EMS care is organized and delivered through the local fire department. Other systems are operated by municipal or county governments or may be delivered by private companies, including for-profit ambulance providers and hospital-based systems. Adding to this diversity, there are more than 6,000 9-1-1 call centers across the country, each run differently by police, fire, county or city government, or other entities.

Given the wide variation in EMS system models, there is broad speculation about which systems perform best and why. However, there is little evidence to support alternative models. For the most part, systems are left to their own devices to develop the arrangement that appears to work best for them.

Fire-based systems across the United States are in transition. The number of fires is decreasing while the number of EMS calls is increasing, raising questions about system design and resource allocation. An estimated 80 percent of fire service calls are now EMS related. While there is little evidence to guide localities in designing their EMS systems, there is even less information on how well any system performs and how to measure that performance.

A key objective of any EMS system is to ensure that each patient is directed to the most appropriate setting based on his or her condition. Coordination of the regional flow of patients is an essential tool in ensuring the quality of prehospital care, and also plays an important role in addressing systemwide issues related to hospital and trauma center crowding. Regional coordination requires that many elements within the regional system—community hospitals, trauma centers, and particularly prehospital EMS—work together effectively to achieve this common goal. Yet only a handful of systems around the country coordinate transport effectively. There is often very little information sharing between hospitals and EMS regarding emergency and trauma center patient loads or the availability of emergency department (ED) beds, operating suites, equipment, trauma surgeons, and critical specialists—information that could be used to balance the patient load among EDs and trauma centers in a region. The benefits of better regional coordination of patients have been demonstrated, and the technologies needed to facilitate such approaches currently exist.

Strengths of the Current System

EMS care has made important advances in recent years. Emergency 9-1-1 services now link virtually all ill and injured Americans to immediate medical response; through organized trauma systems, patients are transported to advanced, lifesaving care within minutes; and advances in resuscitation and lifesaving procedures yield outcomes unheard of a decade ago. Automatic crash notification technology, while still nascent, allows for immediate emergency notification of crashes in which vehicle air bags have deployed. And medical equipment, including air ambulance service, has extended the care available to emergency patients, for example, by bringing rural residents within closer range of emergency and trauma care facilities.

Systemic Problems

Despite the advances made in EMS, sizable challenges remain. At the federal policy level, government leadership in emergency care is fragmented and inconsistent. As it is currently organized, responsibility for prehospital and hospital-based emergency and trauma care is scattered across multiple agencies and departments. Similar divisions are evident at the state and local levels. In addition, the current delivery system suffers in a number of key areas:

- **Insufficient coordination**—EMS care is highly fragmented, and often there is poor coordination among providers. Multiple EMS agencies—some volunteer, some paid, some fire-based, others hospital or privately operated—frequently serve within a single population center and do not act cohesively. Agencies in adjacent jurisdictions often are unable to communicate with each other. In many cases, EMS and other public safety agencies cannot talk to one another because they operate with incompatible communications equipment or on different frequencies. Coordination of transport within regions is limited, with the result that the management of the regional flow of patients is poor, and patients may not be transported to facilities that are optimal and ready to receive them. Communications and handoffs between EMS and hospital personnel are frequently ineffective and omit important clinical information.

• **Disparities in response times**—The speed with which ambulances respond to emergency calls is highly variable. In some cases this variability has to do with geography. In dense population centers, for example, the distances ambulances must travel are small, but traffic and other problems can cause delays, while rural areas involve longer travel times and sometimes difficult terrain. Determining the most effective geographic deployment of limited resources is an intrinsic problem in EMS. But speed of response is also affected by the organization and management of EMS systems, the communications and coordination between 9-1-1 dispatch and EMS responders, and the priority placed on response time given the resources available.

• **Uncertain quality of care**—Very little is known about the quality of care delivered by EMS. The reason for this lack of knowledge is that there are no nationally agreed-upon measures of EMS quality and virtually no accountability for the performance of EMS systems. While most Americans assume that their communities are served by competent EMS systems, the public has no idea whether this is true, and no way to know.

• **Lack of readiness for disasters**—Although EMS personnel are among the first to respond in the event of a disaster, they are the least prepared component of community response teams. Most EMS personnel have received little or no disaster response training for terrorist attacks, natural disasters, or other public health emergencies. Despite the massive amounts of federal funding devoted to homeland security, only a tiny proportion of those funds has been directed to medical response. Furthermore, EMS representation in disaster planning at the federal level has been highly limited.

• **Divided professional identity**—EMS is a unique profession, one that straddles both medical care and public safety. Among public safety agencies, however, EMS is often regarded as a secondary service, with police and fire taking more prominent roles; within medicine, EMS personnel often lack the respect accorded other professionals, such as physicians and nurses. Despite significant investments in education and training, salaries for EMS personnel are often well below those for comparable positions, such as police officers, firefighters, and nurses. In addition, there is a cultural divide among EMS, public safety, and medical care workers that contributes to the fragmentation of these services.

• **Limited evidence base**—The evidence base for many practices routinely used in EMS is limited. Strategies for EMS have often been adapted from settings that differ substantially from the prehospital environment; consequently, their value in the field is questionable, and some may even be harmful. For example, field intubation of children, still widely practiced, has been found to do more harm than good in many situations. While some recent research has added to the EMS evidence base, a host of critical clinical questions remain unanswered because of limited federal research support, as well as inherent difficulties associated with prehospital research due to its sporadic nature and the difficulty of obtaining informed consent for the research.

The committee addresses these problems through a series of recommendations that encompass a wide range of strategic and operational issues, from workforce training, to additional investment in research, to the development of national standards for EMS system performance.

CHARGE TO THE COMMITTEE

The Committee on the Future of Emergency Care in the United States Health System was formed by the Institute of Medicine (IOM) in September 2003 to examine the emergency care system in the United States; explore its strengths, limitations, and future challenges; describe a desired vision of the system; and recommend strategies for achieving that vision. The committee was also tasked with taking a focused look at the state of hospital-based emergency care, prehospital emergency care, and pediatric emergency care. This report, one of a series of three, is focused on the committee's findings and recommendations with respect to prehospital EMS.

ACHIEVING THE VISION OF
A 21ST-CENTURY EMERGENCY CARE SYSTEM

While today's emergency care system offers significantly more medical capability than was available in years past, it continues to suffer from severe fragmentation, an absence of systemwide coordination and planning, and a lack of accountability. To overcome these challenges and chart a new direction for emergency care, the committee envisions a system in which all communities will be served by well-planned and highly coordinated emergency care services that are accountable for their performance.

In this new system, dispatchers, EMS personnel, medical providers, public safety officers, and public health officials will be fully interconnected and united in an effort to ensure that each patient receives the most appropriate care, at the optimal location, with the minimum delay. From the patient's point of view, delivery of services for every type of emergency will be seamless. The delivery of all services will be evidence-based, and innovations will be rapidly adopted and adapted to each community's needs. Ambulance diversions—instances where crowded hospitals essentially close their doors to new ambulance patients—will never occur, except in the most extreme situations. Standby capacity appropriate to each community based on its disaster risks will be embedded in the system. The performance of the system will be transparent, and the public will be actively engaged in its operation through prevention, bystander training, and monitoring of system performance.

While these objectives involve substantial, systemwide change, they are achievable. Early progress toward the goal of more integrated, coordinated, regionalized emergency care systems has become derailed over the last 25 years. Efforts have stalled because of deeply entrenched political interests and cultural attitudes, as well as funding cutbacks and practical impediments to change. These obstacles remain today, and they represent the primary challenges to achieving the committee's vision. However, the problems are becoming more apparent, and this provides a catalyst for change. The committee calls for concerted, cooperative efforts at multiple levels of government and the private sector to finally break through and achieve the goals outlined above. Presented below are the committee's findings and recommendations for achieving its vision of a 21st-century emergency care system.

Federal Lead Agency

Responsibility for all aspects of emergency care is currently dispersed among many federal agencies within the Department of Health and Human Services, Department of Transportation, and Department of Homeland Security. This situation reflects the unique history and the inherent nature of emergency care. As described above, unlike other sectors of the medical provider community, EMS has one foot planted firmly in the public safety community, along with police, fire, and emergency management. In addition, the early development of the modern EMS system grew out of concerns regarding the epidemic of highway deaths in the 1960s. Thus while EMS is a medical discipline, the National Highway Traffic Safety Administration became its first federal home, and it has remained the informal lead agency for EMS ever since. The need for a formal lead agency for emergency care has been promoted for years, and was highlighted in the 1996 report of the National Highway Traffic Safety Administration *Emergency Medical Services Agenda for the Future*. In 2005, the Safe, Accountable, Flexible, Efficient Transportation Equity Act: A Legacy for Users (SAFETEA-LU) gave statutory authority to what had been an informal planning group, the Federal Interagency Committee on EMS (FICEMS). While this group holds promise for improving coordination across federal emergency care agencies, the committee sees it as a valuable complement to but not a substitute for a lead agency, as some have suggested it should be.

The committee believes a true federal lead agency is required if its vision of a coordinated, regionalized, and accountable emergency care system is to be fully realized. It therefore recommends that **Congress establish a lead agency for emergency and trauma care within 2 years of the release of this** report. This lead agency should be housed in the Department of Health and Human Services, and should have primary programmatic responsibility for the full continuum of emergency medical services and emergency and trauma care for adults and children, including medical 9-1-1 and emergency medical dispatch, prehospital emergency medical services (both ground and air), hospital-based emergency and trauma care, and medical-related disaster preparedness. Congress should establish a working group to make recommendations regarding the structure, funding, and responsibilities of the new agency, and design and monitor the transition to its assumption of the responsibilities outlined above. The working group should include representatives from federal and state agencies and professional disciplines involved in emergency and trauma care (3.5).[1]

This lead agency would be designed to create a large, combined federal presence to increase the visibility of emergency and trauma care within the government and to the public; coordinate programs to eliminate overlaps and gaps in funding; create unified accountability for the performance of the emergency care system; and bring together multiple professional groups and cultures for interaction and collaboration that would model and reinforce the integration of services envisioned by the committee. As an established planning group with representation from the appropriate agencies, FICEMS could act as a credible forum for monitoring and advising the working group during the transition.

System Finance

While the proposed lead agency would help rationalize the federal grant payments allocated to the emergency care system, these grants make up a small share of total payments to EMS providers. Payments for EMS are made primarily through public and private insurance reimbursements and local subsidies. A large percentage of EMS transports are for elderly patients, making Medicare a particularly important payer.

EMS costs include the direct costs of each emergency response, as well as the readiness costs associated with maintaining the capability to respond quickly, 24 hours a day, 7 days a week—costs that are not adequately reimbursed by Medicare. In addition, by paying only when a patient is transported, Medicare limits the flexibility of EMS in providing the most appropriate care for each patient. The committee recommends that the Centers for Medicare and Medicaid Services convene an ad hoc working group with expertise in emergency care, trauma, and emergency medical services

---

[1] The committee's recommendations are numbered according to the chapter of the main report in which they appear. Thus, for example, recommendation 2.1 is the first recommendation in Chapter 2.

systems to evaluate the reimbursement of emergency medical services and make recommendations with regard to including readiness costs and permitting payment without transport (3.7).

Regionalization

Because not all hospitals within a community have the personnel and resources to support the delivery of high-level emergency care, critically ill and injured patients should be directed specifically to facilities that have such capabilities. That is the goal of regionalization. There is substantial evidence that the use of regionalization of services to direct such patients to designated hospitals with greater experience and resources improves outcomes and reduces costs across a range of high-risk conditions and procedures. Thus the committee supports further regionalization of emergency care services. However, use of this approach requires that prehospital providers, as well as patients and caregivers, be clear on which facilities have the necessary resources. Just as trauma centers are categorized according to their capabilities (i.e., level I–level IV/V), a standard national approach to the categorization of EDs that reflects their capabilities is needed so that the categories will be clearly understood by providers and the public across all states and regions of the country. To that end, the committee recommends that **the Department of Health and Human Services and the National Highway Traffic Safety Administration, in partnership with professional organizations, convene a panel of individuals with multidisciplinary expertise to develop evidence-based categorization systems for emergency medical services, emergency departments, and trauma centers based on adult and pediatric service capabilities (3.1).**

This information, in turn, could be used to develop protocols that would guide EMS personnel in the transport of patients. More research and discussion are needed, however, to determine under what circumstances patients should be brought to the closest hospital for stabilization and transfer as opposed to being transported directly to the facility offering the highest level of care, even if that facility is farther away. Therefore, the committee also recommends that **the National Highway Traffic Safety Administration, in partnership with professional organizations, convene a panel of individuals with multidisciplinary expertise to develop evidence-based model prehospital care protocols for the treatment, triage, and transport of patients (3.2).** These transport protocols should also reflect the state of readiness of facilities within a region at a given point in time, including real-time, concurrent information on the availability of hospital resources and specialty care.

National Standards for Training and Credentialing

The education and training requirements for EMTs and paramedics differ substantially from one state to the next, and consequently, not all EMS personnel are equally prepared. For example, while the National Standard Curricula developed by the federal government call for paramedics to receive 1,000–1,200 hours of didactic training, states vary in their requirements from as little as 270 hours to as much as 2,000 hours in the classroom. The range of responsibilities assigned to EMTs and paramedics, known as their scope of practice, varies significantly across the states as well. National efforts to promote greater uniformity have been progressing in recent years, but significant variation remains.

The National EMS Scope of Practice Model Task Force has created a national model to aid states in developing and refining their scope-of-practice parameters and licensure requirements for EMS personnel. The committee supports this effort and recommends that **state governments adopt a common scope of practice for emergency medical services personnel, with state licensing reciprocity (4.1)**. In addition, to support greater professionalism and consistency among and between the states, the committee recommends that **states accept national certification as a prerequisite for state licensure and local credentialing of emergency medical services providers (4.3)**. Further, to improve EMS education nationally, the committee recommends that **states require national accreditation of paramedic education programs (4.2)**. The federal government should provide technical assistance and possibly financial support to state governments to help with this transition.

Medical Direction

Substantial variation also exists nationwide in the way medical oversight and review are conducted; in many localities, physicians with little or no training and experience in out-of-hospital medical care provide this service. The committee believes that physicians who provide medical direction for EMS systems should meet standardized minimum requirements for training and certification that reflect their responsibilities. The specialty of emergency medicine currently offers 1- and 2-year fellowships in EMS to residency-trained emergency physicians, but there is no recognized subspecialty of EMS. Therefore, the committee recommends that **the American Board of Emergency Medicine create a subspecialty certification in emergency medical services (4.4)**.

Coordination

Dispatch, EMS, ED and trauma care providers, public safety, and public health should be fully interconnected and united in an effort to ensure that each patient receives the most appropriate care, at the optimal location, with the minimum delay. Yet coordination among 9-1-1 dispatch, prehospital EMS, air medical providers, and hospital and trauma centers is frequently lacking. Moreover, EMS personnel arriving at the scene of an incident often do not know what to expect regarding the number of injured or their condition. EMS personnel are frequently unaware which hospital EDs are on diversion and which are ready to receive the type of patient they are transporting. In addition, deployment of air medical services often is not well coordinated. While air medical providers are not permitted to self-dispatch, a lack of coordination at the ground EMS and dispatch level sometimes results in multiple air ambulances arriving at the scene of a crash even when all are not needed. Similarly, police, fire, and EMS personnel and equipment often overcrowd a crash scene because of insufficient coordination regarding the appropriate response.

Many of these problems are magnified when incidents cross jurisdictional lines. Significant problems are often encountered near municipal, county, and state border areas. In cases where a street delineates the boundary between two municipal or county jurisdictions, responsibility for care—as well as the protocols and procedures employed—may depend on the side of the street on which the incident occurred.

Communications and Data Systems

Communication between EMS and other health care and public safety providers remains highly limited. Antiquated and incompatible voice communication systems often result in a lack of coordination among emergency personnel as they respond to incidents. Many EMS systems rely on voice communication equipment that was purchased in the 1970s with federal financial assistance and has never been upgraded. Similarly, technologies that enable direct transmission of clinical information to hospitals prior to the arrival of an ambulance have not been uniformly adopted. Consequently, there is a growing gap between the types of EMS data and information systems that are available and those that are commonly used in the field.

These problems are compounded by the significant variation in EMS operational structures at the local and regional levels. EMS agencies may be operated by local governments, by fire departments, by private companies, or through other arrangements. This makes communications and data integration difficult, even among EMS providers within a given local area. Communication among EMS, public safety, public health, and other hospital providers is even more problematic given the technical challenges associated with developing interoperable networks. As a result of these challenges and the need for improved coordination discussed above, the committee recommends that **hospitals, trauma centers, emergency medical services agencies, public safety departments, emergency management offices, and public health agencies develop integrated and interoperable communications and data systems (5.2)**.

In addition, as the development of a National Health Information Infrastructure moves forward in the United States, representatives of prehospital emergency care should be involved at every level. The initial focus of this effort was on hospitals, ambulatory care providers, pharmacies, and other, more visible components of the health care system. Given the role played by prehospital EMS providers in providing essential and often lifesaving treatment to patients, however, their omission from this initiative has been a significant oversight. Therefore, the committee recommends that **the Department of Health and Human Services fully involve prehospital emergency medical services leadership in discussions about the design, deployment, and financing of the National Health Information Infrastructure (5.3)**.

Air Medical Services

The number of air medical providers has grown substantially since they first emerged in the 1970s. Today there are an estimated 650–700 medical helicopters operating in the United States, up from approximately 230 in 1990. These air ambulance operations have served thousands of critically ill or injured persons over the past several decades. However, questions remain regarding the clinical efficacy and appropriateness of sophisticated air ambulance care, as well as its cost-effectiveness, given that the cost can be more than five times greater than that of ground ambulance service. In addition, in recent years there has been a significant increase in fatal crashes involving air ambulances, resulting in heightened safety concerns. While the Federal Aviation Administration is responsible for safety inspections, helicopter licensure, and air traffic control, the committee recommends that **states assume regulatory oversight of the medical aspects of air medical services, including communications, dispatch, and transport protocols (5.1)**.

Accountability

Accountability has failed to take hold in emergency care to date because responsibility for the services provided is dispersed across many different components of the system, so it is difficult even for policy makers to determine where system breakdowns occur and how they can subsequently be addressed. To build accountability into the system, the committee recommends that **the Department of Health and Human Services convene a panel of individuals with emergency and trauma care expertise to develop evidence-based indicators of emergency care system performance (3.3)**.

Because of the need for an independent, national process that involves the broad participation of every component of emergency care, the federal government should play a lead role in promoting and funding the development of these performance indicators. The indicators developed should include structure and process measures, but evolve toward outcome measures over time. These performance measures should be nationally standardized so that statewide and national comparisons can be made. Measures should evaluate the performance of individual components of the system, as well as the performance of the system as a whole. Measures should also be sensitive to the interdependence among the various components. For example, EMS response times may be related to EDs going on diversion.

Using the measures developed through such a national, evidence-based, multidisciplinary effort, performance data should be collected at regular intervals from all hospitals and EMS agencies in a community. Public dissemination of performance data is crucial to driving the needed changes in the delivery of emergency care services. Because of the potential sensitivity of performance data, the data should initially be reported in the aggregate rather than at the level of individual provider agencies. However, individual agencies should have full access to their own data so they can understand and improve their performance, as well as their contribution to the overall system.

Disaster Preparedness

Promoting an emergency and trauma care system that works well on a day-to-day basis is fundamental to establishing a system that will work well in the event of a disaster. But the frequency of ambulance diversions and extended off-load times for ambulance patients indicate that the current system is not well prepared for such events. Moreover, EMS and trauma systems have to a large extent been overlooked in disaster preparedness planning at both the state and federal levels. Although they represent a third of the nation's first responders, EMS providers received only 4 percent of the $3.38 billion distributed by the Department of Homeland Security for emergency preparedness in 2002 and 2003, and only 5 percent of the Bioterrorism Hospital Preparedness Grant administered by the Department of Health and Human Services. The committee recommends that **the Department of Health and Human Services, the Department of Transportation, the Department of Homeland Security, and the states elevate emergency and trauma care to a position of parity with other public safety entities in disaster planning and operations (6.1).**

While significant federal funding is available to states and localities for disaster preparedness, emergency care in general has not been able to secure a meaningful share of these funds because they have been folded into other public safety functions that consider emergency medical care a low priority. To address the serious deficits in health-related disaster preparedness, **Congress should substantially increase funding for emergency medical services–related disaster preparedness through dedicated funding streams (6.2).**

In addition, there must be a coordinated and well-funded national effort to ensure effective training in disaster preparedness that involves both professional and continuing education. The committee recommends that **the professional training, continuing education, and credentialing and certification programs for all the relevant professional categories of emergency medical services personnel incorporate disaster preparedness into their curricula and require the maintenance of competency in these skills (6.3).** Doing so would ensure that emergency personnel would remain current in needed disaster skills and would bolster preparedness efforts.

Research

The National Institutes of Health and other agencies that have supported emergency and trauma care research have devoted relatively small amounts of funding to prehospital EMS, and the funding that has been made available has not been spent in a coordinated fashion. To address this issue, the committee recommends that **the Secretary of the Department of Health and Human Services conduct a study to examine the gaps and opportunities in emergency and trauma care research, and recommend a strategy for the optimal organization and funding of the research effort (7.3).** Moreover, to address the sizable gaps in the knowledge base supporting EMS, the committee recommends that **federal agencies that fund emergency and trauma care research target additional funding at prehospital emergency medical services research, with an emphasis on systems and outcomes research (7.1).**

Achieving the Vision

As noted above, there is substantial variation among emergency and trauma care systems in states and regions across the country. Differences exist along a number of dimensions, such as the level of development of trauma systems; the effectiveness of state EMS offices and regional EMS councils; and the degree of coordination among fire departments, EMS, hospitals, trauma centers, and emergency management. Thus no single approach to enhancing emergency care systems will achieve the goals outlined above. Instead, a number of different avenues should be explored and evaluated to determine what types of systems are best able to achieve these goals. The committee therefore recommends that **Congress establish a demonstration program, administered by the Health Resources and Services**

Administration, to promote coordinated, regionalized, and accountable emergency and trauma care systems throughout the country, and appropriate $88 million over 5 years to this program (3.4). Grants should be targeted at states, which could develop projects at the state, regional, or local level; cross-state collaborative proposals would also be encouraged. Over time, and over a number of controlled initiatives, such a process should lead to important insights about what strategies work under different conditions. These insights would provide best-practice models that could be widely adopted to advance the nation toward the committee's vision for efficient, high-quality emergency care.

EMS is now at a crossroads. In the 40 years since the publication of the landmark National Academies report *Accidental Death and Disability: The Neglected Disease of Modern Society*, much progress has been made in improving the nation's EMS capabilities. But in some important ways, the quality of the delivery of those services has declined. This report documents both strengths and limitations of the current prehospital EMS system. The committee's overall conclusion, however, is that today the system is more fragmented than ever, and the lack of effective coordination and accountability stands in the way of further progress and improved quality of care. The opportunity now exists to move toward a more integrated and accountable EMS system through fundamental, systemic changes. Failing to seize this opportunity and continuing on the current path risks further entrenchment of the fragmentation that stands in the way of system improvement and higher-quality care.

1

Introduction

Emergency medical services (EMS) plays a vital role in the nation's emergency and trauma care system, providing response and medical transport for millions of sick and injured Americans each year. Recent estimates indicate that more than 15,000 EMS systems and upwards of 800,000 EMS personnel (emergency medical technicians [EMTs] and paramedics) respond to more than 16 million transport calls annually (Mears, 2004; McCaig and Burt, 2005; Lindstrom, 2006). Through these encounters, prehospital EMS care is delivered directly to patients, in the locations where help is needed.

Prehospital EMS encompasses a range of related activities, including 9-1-1 dispatch, response to the scene by ambulance, treatment and triage by EMS personnel, and transport to a care facility via ground and/or air ambulance. Importantly, it also includes medical direction provided through preestablished medical protocols or a direct link to a hospital or physician. EMS may encompass multiple levels of medical response, depending on how the system is configured in a community. These may include EMS call takers and emergency medical dispatchers working in a 9-1-1 call center; first responders (often fire or police units); basic life support (BLS) and/or advanced life support (ALS) ground ambulances staffed by individuals with different levels of training, depending on the requirements of the state; and air medical EMS units, which are usually staffed by paramedics or critical care nurses, but may sometimes carry a physician. EMS represents the first stage in a full continuum of emergency care that also includes hospital emergency departments (EDs), trauma systems/centers, inpatient critical care services, and interfacility transport.

STRENGTHS OF THE CURRENT SYSTEM

The EMS system has a number of notable strengths. Prehospital EMS is far more sophisticated and far more capable than it was 40 years ago. The 9-1-1 emergency notification system is available to virtually all Americans and is regarded as highly responsive and reliable. The system enables rapid response to medical emergencies and facilitates crucial lifesaving care. In addition, the broad availability of cell phones has expanded 9-1-1 access to emergency and trauma scenes where no help was available before. The development of automatic crash notification technology, now becoming more widely available, has further improved emergency response, providing immediate and increasingly detailed crash information to dispatchers automatically, even before anyone on scene places a call.

In general, Americans have access to rapid ambulance response in emergency situations. While there are many glaring exceptions, first responders in urban and suburban areas are generally able to arrive on scene within minutes of notification, with ambulance crews close behind. Moreover, with greater emphasis now being placed on bystander care and prearrival instructions provided by dispatchers, care to patients can be initiated even more rapidly. In addition, air ambulance operations allow more advanced medical capacity to be delivered to patients directly and can often reduce transport times to medical facilities. In areas where trauma systems have developed, EMS and trauma providers are interdependent, working closely within an established protocol to help ensure that patients are transported to the most appropriate facility as quickly as possible.

EMS personnel form the backbone of the prehospital care system despite working under conditions that are stressful and at times dangerous. Many of them provide their services on a volunteer basis. The sophisticated equipment now at the disposal of many EMS providers, such as automated external defibrillators (AEDs) and 12-lead electrocardiographs (ECGs), as well as more effective medications, allow them to provide a much broader array of services than was available in years past.

PATIENT DEMOGRAPHICS

Of the 113.9 million ED visits that occurred in 2003, an estimated 14 percent were made by patients who arrived by ambulance. The most frequent complaints included chest pains, shortness of breath, stomach pain, injury from a motor vehicle crash or some type of accident, convulsions, and general weakness. The majority of visits were for illness (59.3 percent), whereas 40.7 percent were for injury, poisoning, or adverse effects of medical treatment (Burt et al., 2006). Prehospital cardiac arrests occur at a rate of 250,000 per year or more than 650 per day across the country, and these cases are frequently handled by EMS providers (Zheng et al., 2001). While only 14 percent of ED visitors arrived by ambulance in 2003, 40 percent of hospital admissions from the ED in that year were transport patients. In general, transport patients have more complex medical conditions and require more care than walk-in patients. In 2003, an average of 6.5 different diagnostic tests and services were ordered or performed for transport cases—about 40 percent higher than the average for nontransport cases.

While transport patients tend to have more severe conditions than walk-in patients, a significant percentage of those treated by EMS personnel do not have life-threatening problems. Often these patients contact 9-1-1 because they are experiencing acute onset of conditions that cause alarming symptoms, and frequently substantial pain and anxiety. Over the last several years, EMS providers and researchers have acknowledged this situation and have had much greater interest in determining how best to care for these patients (Maio et al., 2002; Alonso-Serra et al., 2003).

A high proportion of transport patients are seniors. In 2003, less than 4 percent of children under age 15 were brought in to the ED by ambulance, but more than 40 percent of those aged 75 or older were transport patients (see Table 1-1). Because children make up a relatively small percentage of transports, it is a challenge to ensure that EMS personnel have the skills and equipment required to address their needs (e.g., properly sized equipment and knowledge of appropriate care procedures). However, the sizable number of elderly transport patients also presents significant challenges, in terms of both patient care (e.g., complications from chronic illness) and reimbursement (i.e., a greater percentage of payments made through Medicare, which does not cover all costs). With the aging of the baby boomers, even greater percentages of seniors are projected to require ambulance transport in the coming years.

TABLE 1-1 Proportion of Emergency Department Visits Made by Walk-in Versus Transport Patients, by Patient Age (United States, 2003)

Age	Number of ED Visits (in thousands)	Walk-ins (%)	Transports via Ambulance (%)
All Ages	113,903	79.1	14.2
Under 15	24,733	88.2	3.8
15–24	17,731	83.8	9.5
25–44	32,906	82.6	11.3
45–64	20,992	76.5	17.3
65–74	7,153	66.3	27.5
75+	10,389	52.8	40.9

NOTE: The percentages above do not tabulate to 100 percent. The remainder of ED arrivals occurred via public service or unknown means.
SOURCE: McCaig and Burt, 2005.

AN EVOLVING AND EMERGING CRISIS

Many experts date the development of modern EMS systems in the United States back to the publication of the landmark report *Accidental Death and Disability: The Neglected Disease of Modern Society* (NAS and NRC, 1966). Following the publication of this report and subsequent congressional action, EMS systems began to develop rapidly across the country. However, this momentum was lost in 1981 when direct federal funding for the planning and development of EMS systems ended and was replaced by block grants to states. Over the past 25 years, EMS systems have developed haphazardly nationwide, regulated by state EMS offices that have been highly inconsistent in their level of sophistication and control. The result has been a fragmented and sometimes balkanized network of underfunded EMS systems that often lack strong quality controls, cannot or do not collect data to evaluate and improve system performance, fail to communicate effectively within and across jurisdictions, allocate limited resources inefficiently, and lack effective strategies and resources for recruiting and retaining personnel.

A significant lack of funding and infrastructure for EMS research has sharply limited studies of the safety and efficacy of many common EMS practices. Pressing questions remain regarding a number of central issues, such as the value of ALS services, the safety and efficacy of many common EMS procedures, the optimal approach to managing multisystem trauma, and the cost-effectiveness of public-access defibrillation programs. Barriers to data collection, a lack of standardized terms, and a limited pool of researchers trained and interested in EMS all pose significant challenges to research in the field. As a result, the prehospital emergency care system provides a stark example of how standards of care and clinical protocols can take root despite an almost total lack of evidence to support their use.

Because of this lack of supporting evidence, EMS systems often must operate blindly in addressing such questions as how available EMS personnel should be deployed, what services should be provided in the out-of-hospital setting, and what approach to organizing the EMS system is best. Multiple models of EMS organization have evolved over time, including fire department–based systems, hospital-based systems, and other public and private models. However, there is little research to demonstrate whether any one of these approaches is more effective than the others.

Within the last several years, complex problems facing the emergency care system have come into public view. Press coverage has highlighted instances of slow EMS response times, ambulance diversions, trauma center closures, and ground and air crashes during patient transport. This heightened public awareness of problems that have been building over time has made clear the need for a comprehensive review of the U.S. emergency care system. Although emergency care represents a vital component of the U.S.

health system, to date no such study of the system has been conducted. The events of September 11, 2001, and more recent disasters, such as Hurricane Katrina and the subway bombings in London and Madrid, have further raised awareness of the need for this type of study.

An assessment of the emergency care system in the United States is a logical extension of previous work conducted by the National Academy of Sciences (NAS), the National Research Council (NRC), and the Institute of Medicine (IOM). In addition to *Accidental Death and Disability*, other reports, such as *Roles and Resources of Federal Agencies in Support of Comprehensive Emergency Medical Services* (NAS and NRC, 1972) and *Emergency Medical Services at Midpassage* (NAS and NRC, 1978), have had a major impact in shaping the development of the emergency care system.

More recently, several IOM studies on injury and disability have emphasized the need for skilled emergency care to limit the adverse consequences of illness and injury (IOM, 1985). Additionally, the IOM produced a study of EMS systems for children (IOM, 1993) that generated unprecedented attention to the subject and has led to many improvements in the delivery of pediatric emergency care.

One way to assess the overall quality of EMS is to consider the six quality aims defined by the IOM in its seminal report *Crossing the Quality Chasm: A New Health System for the 21st Century* (IOM, 2001): health care should be safe, effective, patient-centered, timely, efficient, and equitable (see Box 1-1). While the evidence is limited, there are strong indications that the current EMS system fails the American public in significant ways along all of these dimensions of quality care.

Safety

Prehospital emergency care services are delivered in an uncertain, stressful environment where the need for haste and other potential distractions produce threats to patient care and safety. In addition, shift work and around-the-clock coverage contribute to fatigue among EMS providers (Fairbanks, 2004). Error rates for such procedures as endotracheal intubation are high, especially compared with the same procedures performed in a hospital setting (Katz and Falk, 2001; Wang et al., 2003; Jones et al., 2004).

In addition to these concerns regarding patient safety, there are concerns about the safety of EMS personnel. Working conditions for these personnel are physically demanding and often dangerous. Injury rates for EMS workers are high; back injuries are especially common, as are other "sprains, strains, and tears" (Maguire et al., 2005). EMS personnel are frequently exposed to the threat of violence and other unpredictable and

---

BOX 1-1
The Six Quality Aims of the
Institute of Medicine's *Quality Chasm* Report

Health care should be:

- **Safe**—avoiding injuries to patients from the care that is intended to help them.
- **Effective**—providing services based on scientific knowledge to all who could benefit and refraining from providing services to those not likely to benefit.
- **Patient-centered**—providing care that is respectful of and responsive to individual patient preferences, needs, and values and ensuring that patient values guide all clinical decisions.
- **Timely**—reducing waits and sometimes harmful delays for both those who receive and those who give care.
- **Efficient**—avoiding waste, including waste of equipment, supplies, ideas, and energy.
- **Equitable**—providing care that does not vary in quality because of personal characteristics such as gender, ethnicity, geographic location, and socioeconomic status.

SOURCE: IOM, 2001, pp. 5–6.

---

uncontrolled situations (Franks et al., 2004). Moreover, they can be exposed to potentially infectious bodily fluids and airborne pathogens. In addition to these dangers, crashes involving ground ambulances are a major concern; according to the Centers for Disease Control and Prevention (CDC), 300 fatal crashes involving ambulances occurred in the United States between 1991 and 2000 (CDC, 2003).

Effectiveness

As noted above, there is very limited evidence about the effectiveness of many EMS interventions. Although there have been a small number of landmark studies in EMS, for the most part the knowledge base is quite limited. As a result, patients cannot be certain that they will receive the best possible care in their encounters with the EMS system. Questions related to core aspects of current clinical EMS practice remain unresolved, and EMS personnel must often rely on their best judgment in the absence of evidence. Not infrequently, treatments with established effectiveness and safety profiles in hospital- or office-based settings are implemented in the out-of-hospital setting without adequate examination of patient outcomes (Gausche-Hill, 2000; Gausche et al., 2000).

Another example is the debate over whether EMS personnel should perform ALS procedures in the field, or rapid transport to definitive care is best (Wright and Klein, 2001). EMS responders who provide stabilization before the patient arrives at a critical care unit are sometimes subject to criticism because of a strongly held belief among many physicians that out-of-hospital stabilization only delays definitive treatment without adding value. However, there is little evidence that the prevailing "scoop and run" paradigm of EMS is optimal (Orr et al., 2006) except in certain circumstances, such as reducing time to reperfusion for heart attack patients (Waters et al., 2004).

In addition to the significant gaps in knowledge regarding appropriate treatments, there are important gaps in recording patient outcomes. Many cities do not track outcomes, so the performance of their EMS systems cannot be evaluated or benchmarked against that of the systems of other cities. The limited evidence that is available shows wide variation nationwide. For example, results of investigative research by *USA Today* indicate that the percentage of people suffering ventricular fibrillation who survive and are later discharged from the hospital with good brain function ranges from 3 to 45 percent depending on the municipality (Davis, 2003). This broad variation illustrates the tremendous challenge involved in making the EMS system overall more effective.

Recent EMS research has been able to contribute to the knowledge base regarding appropriate and effective EMS care. For example, the Ontario Prehospital Advanced Life Support study demonstrated that an optimized EMS system with rapid defibrillation capabilities may not benefit from the addition of ALS interventions. In addition, the Public Access Defibrillation trial found that providing AEDs in the community, along with adequate CPR training, can improve survival from cardiac arrest due to ventricular fibrillation. Studies have also shown that CPR involving only chest compressions can be effective, and a number of large U.S. cities have changed the way their 9-1-1 dispatchers provide CPR prearrival instructions as a result.

Patient-Centeredness

EMS systems are geared toward meeting the needs of patients with specific acute conditions, such as heart attack, stroke, and injuries resulting from automobile crashes and other types of accidents. However, they are not always well equipped to meet the needs of special populations or of patients with less acute medical conditions. For example, language barriers pose significant problems, both for EMS personnel arriving on scene and for 9-1-1 communicators and emergency medical dispatchers. As a result, patients may be unable to convey their situation adequately to these emergency responders. In addition, EMS providers often struggle to address the challenges presented by severely obese patients (Greenwood, 2004). Standard-issue equipment may be incapable of bearing the weight of these patients, and responses may require multiple personnel.

Children present special challenges to EMS personnel as well. Studies indicate that many prehospital providers are less comfortable caring for pediatric patients, particularly infants, than for adult patients. For example, paramedics have reported being very comfortable about terminating CPR on adults, but very uncomfortable about doing so on children (Hall et al., 2004). A study that looked at job satisfaction among paramedics found that they view pediatric calls as among the most stressful because of the low volume of such cases they typically encounter (Federiuk et al., 1993). For these and other special populations, EMS systems often struggle to provide adequate care.

In addition, while EMS systems are frequently organized to address major traumas and serious medical emergencies, the overwhelming majority of EMS patients have relatively minor complaints. Focusing on this broader spectrum of complaints could make the system more patient-centered.

Timeliness

Response times vary widely depending on the location where an incident occurs. Across the large, sparsely populated terrain of rural areas, EMS response times—from the medically instigating event to arrival at the hospital—are significantly increased compared with those in urban areas. These prolonged response times occur at each step in EMS activation and response, including time to EMS notification, time from EMS notification to arrival at the scene, and time from EMS arrival on the scene to hospital arrival.

Even across cities, however, there are substantial differences in EMS response times (Davis et al., 2003). As a result, a person who suffers a traumatic injury or acute illness in one city may be far more likely to die than the same person in another city. One important factor contributing to slow response times in some areas is the frequency of ED crowding and ambulance diversion. When EDs are crowded, as is frequently the case, EMS personnel wait with the transported patient until space becomes available in the ED. This wait reduces the time during which the ambulance could be servicing the community, thus increasing response times. When hospitals go on diversion status, ambulances may have to drive longer distances and take patients to less appropriate facilities. Again, definitive patient care is delayed. It is estimated that 501,000 ambulances were diverted in 2003 (Burt et al., 2006).

Efficiency

The health sector in general and emergency and trauma care services in particular lag behind other industries in adopting engineering principles and information technologies that can improve process management, lower costs, and enhance quality. Inefficiency in EMS care takes various forms:

- Little is known about the cost-effectiveness of EMS interventions. As with EMS research in general, sparse information exists to help guide the field in this area. Reimbursement policies and federal regulations also contribute to inefficiencies. In many cases, providers are not reimbursed unless they transport a patient to the ED, even though it may be more efficient and just as effective to treat the patient on site.
- Services are often poorly coordinated. In some situations, for example, multiple vehicles respond to a single small event. Significant problems are often encountered near municipal, county, and state border areas. When a street delineates the boundary between two city or county jurisdictions, responsibility for care—as well as the protocols and procedures employed—depends on the side of the street on which the incident occurred.
- The Emergency Medical Treatment and Active Labor Act may require that certain EMS agencies perform a medical screening exam when in fact a patient should be transported immediately to a trauma center for definitive care.
- Outdated and poorly planned technologies also contribute to inefficiencies. For example, many of the 9-1-1 calls placed today are from cellular phones, but dispatchers often lack the capability to trace the location of such callers. In the event of a disaster, most EMS communications systems are not compatible with those of other responders, such as police and fire departments.

Equity

Disparities in access to EMS systems are evident, particularly between urban and rural communities. For example, there are still small pockets of the country that do not offer even basic 9-1-1 coverage, and these are located exclusively in rural or frontier areas. Moreover, only 45 percent of counties nationwide have the more advanced 9-1-1 systems that can track the location of cellular callers, even though this information can be vitally important in responding to various emergency situations.

Ground and air ambulance coverage is also uneven across the country.

Because of the reduced call volume in rural areas, fewer ground ambulances are available to cover the wide expanses involved. In addition, the *Atlas and Database of Air Medical Services* indicates that many rural areas still do not have sufficient access to air ambulance providers. Given the inherent difficulty of providing timely care in remote areas, crash fatalities in these locales are more frequent. In 2001, 61 percent of all crash fatalities occurred along rural roads, even though only 39 percent of vehicle-miles were traveled in such areas (Flanigan et al., 2005).

OVERVIEW OF THE STUDY

The IOM's study of the Future of Emergency Care in the United States Health System was initiated in September 2003. Support for the study was provided by the Josiah Macy, Jr. Foundation, the National Highway Traffic Safety Administration (NHTSA), the Health Resources and Services Administration (HRSA), the Agency for Healthcare Research and Quality (AHRQ), and CDC. Given the broad scope of the effort, the work was divided among a main committee and three subcommittees (see Figure 1-1).

The main committee provided primary direction for the study and was responsible for investigating the systemwide issues that span the continuum of emergency care in the United States. The 13-member subcommittee on hospital-based emergency care was created to examine issues specific to the ED setting, including workforce supply, patient flow, use of information technologies, and disaster preparedness and surge capacity. The 11-member subcommittee on prehospital EMS was created to assess the current organization, delivery, and financing of EMS and EMS systems and to advance NHTSA's *Emergency Medical Services Agenda for the Future* (NHTSA, 1996). Finally, the 11-member subcommittee on pediatric emer-

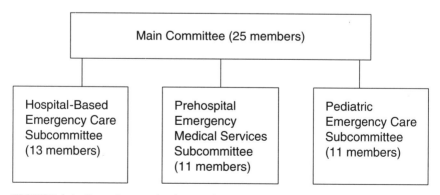

FIGURE 1-1 Committee and subcommittee structure.

gency care was created to examine the unique issues associated with the provision of emergency services to children and adolescents.

A total of 40 individuals served across all four committees (see Appendix A).[1] Subcommittee members were responsible for developing recommendations in their respective areas for presentation to the main committee, which had sign-off authority on all of the study recommendations. The subcommittees worked collaboratively, and considerable cross-fertilization occurred among them and their members.

The main committee and subcommittees each met separately four times between February 2004 and October 2005; a combined meeting for all members was held in March 2005. The study also benefited from the contributions of a wide range of experts who made presentations to the committee, wrote commissioned papers, and met with the committee members and/or IOM project staff on an informal basis. A report was produced in each of the three areas addressed by the subcommittees. The charge to the EMS subcommittee, which guided the development of the present report, is shown in Box 1-2.

KEY TERMS AND DEFINITIONS

To ensure clarity and consistency, the following terminology is used throughout this study's three reports. *Emergency medical services*, or *EMS*, denotes prehospital and out-of-hospital emergency medical services, including 9-1-1 and dispatch, emergency medical response, field triage and stabilization, and transport by ambulance or helicopter to a hospital and between facilities. *EMS system* refers to the organized delivery system for EMS within a specified geographic area—local, regional, state, or national—as indicated by the context.

Emergency care is broader than EMS and encompasses the full continuum of services involved in emergency medical care, including EMS, hospital-based ED and trauma care, specialty care, bystander care, and injury prevention. *Emergency care system* refers to the organized delivery system for emergency care within a specified geographic area.

Trauma care is the care received by a victim of trauma in any setting, while a *trauma center* is a hospital specifically designated to provide trauma care; some trauma care is provided in settings other than a trauma center. *Trauma system* refers to the organized delivery system for trauma care at the local, regional, state, or national level. Because trauma care is a component of emergency care, it is always assumed to be encompassed by the

---

[1]One committee member, Henri R. Manasse, Jr., resigned from the original 41-member body during the course of the study.

BOX 1-2
Charge to the EMS Subcommittee

The overall objectives of this study are to: (1) examine the emergency care system in the United States; (2) explore its strengths, limitations, and future challenges; (3) describe a desired vision of the emergency care system; and (4) recommend strategies required to achieve that vision. Within this context, the Subcommittee on Prehospital Emergency Medical Services (EMS) will examine prehospital EMS and include an assessment of the current organization, delivery, and financing of EMS and EMS systems, and assess progress toward the *Emergency Medical Services Agenda for the Future.* The subcommittee will consider a wide range of issues, including:

- The evolving role of EMS as an integral component of the overall health care system, including dispatch, medical direction, and integration with trauma systems, pediatric EMS, public health, prevention, and emergency department overcrowding;
- EMS system planning, preparedness, and coordination at the federal, state, and local levels;
- EMS funding and infrastructure investment, including equipment, communications, new technologies, and progress toward the development of interoperable EMS information systems;
- EMS workforce trends and professional education; and
- EMS research priorities and funding.

terms *hospital-based* or *inpatient emergency care, emergency care system,* and *regional emergency care system.*

The term *region* is used throughout the report to mean a broad geographic area, typically larger than a municipality and smaller than a state. However, a region in some cases encompasses an area that overlaps two states.

ORGANIZATION OF THIS REPORT

Chapter 2 highlights important developments in the history of EMS and describes the current state of the industry. It reviews the EMS delivery models now in operation nationwide and details the key challenges to the delivery of high-quality EMS care that meets the six aims outlined in Box 1-1. The chapter examines the gains achieved through previous reform efforts, as well as some of the key barriers to their full adoption.

Chapter 3 charts a new direction for the future of emergency care, one in which all communities are served by well-planned and highly coordinated emergency care systems that are accountable for their performance. The chapter establishes a vision in which the various components of the emergency and trauma care system are connected through improved communications networks and organized through a regionalized system of care. A national demonstration program is proposed in which states and communities would be able to create and test new models for the delivery of emergency and trauma care services.

Chapter 4 examines the EMS workforce, including EMTs and paramedics, volunteers, emergency medical dispatchers, and EMS physician medical directors. The chapter details the current education and training standards for EMS personnel and proposes the establishment of a national certification requirement. It also proposes the transition to a common scope of practice across states. In addition, the chapter addresses issues surrounding recruitment and retention of EMS personnel, including worker safety and pay.

Chapter 5 examines an array of issues relating to infrastructure and technologies employed by the EMS system, including 9-1-1, enhanced 9-1-1, and next-generation 9-1-1 capabilities; automatic crash notification systems; equipment-related issues, such as ambulance design and safety; and air medical capacity and operations. The chapter also describes the technology upgrades required to achieve the goal of interoperable communications among various public safety responders (EMS, fire, police), between EMS and medical facilities (including voice and video communications and electronic health records), and throughout the EMS system overall.

Chapter 6 reviews the steps needed to develop an emergency care system capable of meeting the challenge of a major terrorist event, unintentional man-made disaster, natural disaster, or other public health crisis. The chapter demonstrates that having an emergency care system that functions efficiently and effectively on a daily basis is fundamental to having a system that is ready to handle larger public health and public safety crises. In addition, the chapter describes EMS equipment and training needs, including greater distribution of personal protective equipment and development of more effective communications systems, as well as improved hospital surge capacity.

Chapter 7 examines the research required to support improvements in EMS. It reviews the need for data collection and outcome assessments and the mechanisms required to generate these data. In addition, the chapter describes enhanced research strategies, such as multicenter collaborations and support for talented investigators. The chapter also describes current data work now being conducted (e.g., the National EMS Information System [NEMSIS]) and steps required to change the regulatory environment (i.e., the Health Insurance Portability and Accountability Act) to make outcome assessments possible.

Finally, following the chapters are a number of appendixes:

• Appendix A contains a chart listing all committee and subcommittee members.
• Appendix B provides biographical information on members of the main committee and the Subcommittee on Prehospital EMS.
• Appendix C lists the presentations made during public sessions of the committee meetings.
• Appendix D lists the research papers commissioned by the committee.
• Appendix E contains the recommendations from all three reports in the *Future of Emergency Care* series and indicates the entities with primary responsibility for implementation of each recommendation.

REFERENCES

Alonso-Serra HM, Wesley K, National Association of EMS Physicians Standards and Clinical Practices Committee. 2003. Prehospital pain management. *Prehospital Emergency Care* 7(4):482–488.

Burt CW, McCaig LF, Valverde RH. 2006. *Analysis of Ambulance Transports and Diversions among U.S. Emergency Departments*. Hyattsville, MD: National Center for Health Statistics.

CDC (Centers for Disease Control and Prevention). 2003. Ambulance crash-related injuries among emergency medical services workers—United States, 1991–2002. *Morbidity & Mortality Weekly Report* 52(8):154–156.

Davis R. 2003, July. Many lives are lost across USA because emergency services fail. *USA Today*. P. 1A.

Davis R, Coddington R, West J. 2003. *The State of Emergency Medical Services across the USA: How 50 Major Cities Stack Up*. [Online]. Available: http://www.usatoday.com/graphics/life/gra/ems/flash.htm [accessed January 1, 2006].

Fairbanks T. 2004. *Human Factors & Patient Safety in Emergency Medical Services*. Science Forum on Patient Safety and Human Factors Research.

Federiuk CS, O'Brien K, Jui J, Schmidt TA. 1993. Job satisfaction of paramedics: The effects of gender and type of agency of employment. *Annals of Emergency Medicine* 22(4):657–662.

Flanigan M, Blatt A, Lombardo L, Mancuso D, Miller M, Wiles D, Pirson H, Hwang J, Thill J, Majka K. 2005. Assessment of air medical coverage using the atlas and database of air medical services and correlations with reduced highway fatality rates. *Air Medical Journal* 24(4):151–163.

Franks PE, Kocher N, Chapman S. 2004. *Emergency Medical Technicians and Paramedics in California University of California*. San Francisco, CA: San Francisco Center for the Health Professions.

Gausche M, Lewis RJ, Stratton SJ, Haynes BE, Gunter CS, Goodrich SM, Poore PD, McCollough MD, Henderson DP, Pratt FD, Seidel JS. 2000. Effect of out-of-hospital pediatric endotracheal intubation on survival and neurologic outcome: A controlled clinical trial. *Journal of the American Medical Association* 283(6):783–790.

Gausche-Hill M. 2000. Pediatric continuing education for out-of-hospital providers: Is it time to mandate review of pediatric knowledge and skills? *Annals of Emergency Medicine* 36(1):72–74.

Greenwood MD. 2004. Weighty matters: Transporting obese patients. *Journal of Emergency Medical Services* 33(10).

Hall WL II, Myers JH, Pepe PE, Larkin GL, Sirbaugh PE, Persse DE. 2004. The perspective of paramedics about on-scene termination of resuscitation efforts for pediatric patients. *Resuscitation* 60(2):175–187.

IOM (Institute of Medicine). 1985. *Injury in America: A Continuing Health Problem.* Washington, DC: National Academy Press.

IOM. 1993. *Emergency Medical Services for Children.* Washington, DC: National Academy Press.

IOM. 2001. *Crossing the Quality Chasm: A New Health System for the 21st Century.* Washington, DC: National Academy Press.

Jones JH, Murphy MP, Dickson RL, Somerville GG, Brizendine EJ. 2004. Emergency physician-verified out-of-hospital intubation: Miss rates by paramedics. *Academic Emergency Medicine* 11(6):707–709.

Katz SH, Falk JL. 2001. Misplaced endotracheal tubes by paramedics in an urban emergency medical services system. *Annals of Emergency Medicine* 37(1):32–37.

Lindstrom AM. 2006. 2006 JEMS platinum resource guide. *Journal of Emergency Medical Services* 31(1):42–56, 101.

Maguire BJ, Hunting KL, Guidotti TL, Smith GS. 2005. Occupational injuries among emergency medical services personnel. *Prehospital Emergency Care* 9(4):405–411.

Maio RF, Garrison HG, Spaite DW, Desmond JS, Gregor MA, Stiell IG, Cayten CG, Chew JL Jr, Mackenzie EJ, Miller DR, O'Malley PJ. 2002. Emergency Medical Services Outcomes Project (EMSOP) IV: Pain measurement in out-of-hospital outcomes research. *Annals of Emergency Medicine* 40(2):172–179.

McCaig LF, Burt CW. 2005. *National Hospital Ambulatory Medical Care Survey: 2003 Emergency Department Summary.* Hyattsville, MD: National Center for Health Statistics.

Mears G. 2004. *2003 Survey and Analysis of EMS Scope of Practice and Practice Settings Impacting EMS Services in Rural America: Executive Brief and Recommendations.* Chapel Hill, NC: University of North Carolina at Chapel Hill Department of Emergency Medicine.

NAS, NRC (National Academy of Sciences, National Research Council). 1966. *Accidental Death and Disability: The Neglected Disease of Modern Society.* Washington, DC: NAS.

NAS, NRC. 1972. *Roles and Resources of Federal Agencies in Support of Comprehensive Emergency Medical Services.* Washington, DC: NAS.

NAS, NRC. 1978. *Emergency Medical Services at Midpassage.* Washington, DC: NAS.

NHTSA (National Highway Traffic Safety Administration). 1996. *Emergency Medical Services Agenda for the Future.* Washington, DC: U.S. Department of Transportation.

Orr RA, Han YY, Roth K. 2006. Pediatric transport: Shifting the paradigm to improve patient outcome. In: Fuhrman B, Zimmerman J, eds. *Pediatric Critical Care* (3rd edition). Philadelphia, PA: Mosby, Elsevier Science Health. Pp. 141–150.

Wang HE, Kupas DF, Paris PM, Bates RR, Costantino JP, Yealy DM. 2003. Multivariate predictors of failed prehospital endotracheal intubation. *Academic Emergency Medicine* 10(7):717–724.

Waters RE II, Singh KP, Roe MT, Lotfi M, Sketch MH Jr, Mahaffey KW, Newby LK, Alexander JH, Harrington RA, Califf RM, Granger CB. 2004. Rationale and strategies for implementing community-based transfer protocols for primary percutaneous coronary intervention for acute ST-segment elevation myocardial infarction. *Journal of the American College of Cardiology* 43(12):2153–2159.

Wright JL, Klein BL. 2001. Regionalized pediatric trauma systems. *Clinical Pediatric Emergency Medicine* 2:3–12.

Zheng ZJ, Croft JB, Giles WH, Mensah GA. 2001. Sudden cardiac death in the United States, 1989 to 1998. *Circulation* 104(18):2158–2163.

2

History and Current State of EMS

Across the country, emergency medical services (EMS) agencies face numerous challenges with regard to their funding, management, workforce, infrastructure, and research base. Though the modern EMS system was instituted and funded in large part by the federal government through the Highway Safety Act of 1966 and the EMS Act of 1973, federal support for EMS agencies declined precipitously in the early 1980s. Since that time, states and localities have taken more prominent roles in financing and designing EMS programs. The result has been considerable fragmentation of EMS care and wide variability in the type of care that is offered from state to state and region to region. This chapter traces the development of the modern EMS system and describes the current state of EMS at the federal, state, and local levels.

A BRIEF HISTORY OF EMS

EMS dates back centuries and has seen rapid advances during times of war. At least as far back as the Greek and Roman eras, chariots were used to remove injured soldiers from the battlefield. In the late 15th century, Ferdinand and Isabella of Spain commissioned surgical and medical supplies to be provided to troops in special tents called *ambulancias*. During the French Revolution in 1794, Baron Dominique-Jean Larrey recognized that leaving wounded soldiers on the battlefield for days without treatment dramatically increased morbidity and mortality, weakening the fighting strength of the army. He instituted a system in which trained medical personnel initiated treatment and transported the wounded to field hospitals (Pozner et al., 2004).

This model was emulated by Americans during the Civil War. General Jonathan Letterman, a Union military surgeon, created the first organized system in the United States to treat and transport injured patients. Based on this experience, the first civilian-run, hospital-based ambulance service began in Cincinnati in 1865. The first municipally based EMS began in New York City in 1869 (NHTSA, 1996).

In 1910, the American Red Cross began providing first-aid training programs across the country, initiating an organized effort to improve civilian bystander care. During World Wars I and II, further advances were made in EMS, although typically these were not replicated in the civilian setting until much later (Pozner et al., 2004). Following World War II, city EMS activities were for the most part run by municipal hospitals and fire departments. In smaller communities, funeral home hearses often served as ambulances because they were the only vehicle capable of transporting patients quickly in stretchers. With the advent of federal involvement in EMS in the early 1970s and the articulation of standards at the state and regional levels, these EMS providers were gradually replaced by others, including third-service providers, fire departments, rescue squads, and private ambulances (NHTSA, 1996).

By the late 1950s, prehospital emergency care in the United States was still little more than first aid (IOM, 1993). Around that time, however, advances in medical care began to spur the rapid development of modern EMS. While the first recorded use of mouth-to-mouth ventilation had been in 1732, it was not until 1958 that Dr. Peter Safar demonstrated it to be superior to other modes of manual ventilation. In 1960, cardiopulmonary resuscitation (CPR) was shown to be efficacious. These two clinical advances led to the realization that rapid response of trained community members to cardiac emergencies could improve outcomes. The introduction of CPR and the development of portable external defibrillators in the 1960s provided the foundation for advanced cardiac life support (ACLS) that fueled much of the development of EMS systems in subsequent years.

In 1965, the President's Committee for Traffic Safety published the report *Health, Medical Care and Transportation of the Injured*. The report recommended a national program to reduce highway deaths and injuries. The following year, the National Academy of Sciences (NAS) and National Research Council (NRC) released *Accidental Death and Disability: The Neglected Disease of Modern Society* (NAS/NRC, 1966). That report emphasized that the health care system needed to address injuries, which at the time were the leading cause of death for those aged 1–37. It noted that in most cases, ambulances were inappropriately designed, ill-equipped, and often staffed with inadequately trained personnel. For example, the report called attention to the fact that at least 50 percent of ambulance services nationwide were being provided by morticians. The report contained a total of 29 recommendations, 11 of which applied directly to prehospital EMS (Delbridge et al., 1998). These included recommendations to (1) develop federal standards for ambulances (design, construction, equipment, supplies, personnel training and supervision); (2) adopt state ambulance regulations; (3) ensure provision of ambulance services applicable to the conditions of the local government; (4) initiate pilot programs to evaluate automotive and helicopter ambulance services in sparsely populated areas; (5) assign radio channels and equipment suitable for voice communications between ambulances and emergency departments (EDs) and other health-related agencies; and (6) develop a single nationwide telephone number for summoning an ambulance. The report also laid out a vision for the establishment of trauma systems as we know them today.

In addition to the momentum that had been provided by the President's Commission, support for the NAS/NRC report was fueled by surgeons with military experience in Korea and World War II who recognized that the trauma care available to soldiers overseas was better than the care available in local communities. In 1966, Congress passed the Highway Safety Act, which led to the formation of the National Highway Traffic Safety Administration (NHTSA) within the Department of Transportation (DOT). NHTSA was given authority to fund improvements in EMS. Among those improvements, NHTSA developed a national EMS education curriculum and model state EMS legislation. NHTSA's 70-hour basic EMT curriculum became the first standard EMT training in the United States. The department developed more extensive advanced life support (ALS) training several years later. Also as part of the 1966 act, DOT offered grant funding to states with the goal of improving the provision of EMS.

1970s: Rapid Expansion of Regional EMS Systems

In the early 1970s, additional research and policy planning focused on the unmet needs of EMS. In 1972, the NAS/NRC released another report on EMS entitled *Roles and Resources of Federal Agencies in Support of Comprehensive Emergency Medical Services* (NAS and NRC, 1972). The report expressed concern that the federal effort to upgrade EMS had not kept pace with what was needed. It urged integration of all federal EMS efforts into the Department of Health, Education and Welfare (DHEW, which later became the Department of Health and Human Services [DHHS]). The report also stated that the focal point for local EMS should be at the state rather than the federal level, and that all efforts should be coordinated through regional programs.

In 1973, Congress enacted the EMS Systems Act, which created a new grant program to further the development of regional EMS systems. The intent of the law was to improve and coordinate care throughout the country through the creation of a categorical grant program run by the new Division of Emergency Medical Services within DHEW. This program became a decisive factor in the nationwide development of regional EMS systems. Millions of dollars were earmarked for EMS training, equipment, and research. In total, more than $300 million was appropriated for EMS feasibility studies, planning, operations, expansion and improvement, and research. (In 2004 dollars, this investment equates to $1.3 billion.) Also, in 1974 The Robert Wood Johnson Foundation appropriated $15 million to fund 44 regional EMS projects ($64 million in 2004 dollars). To this day, this remains the largest private grant for EMS system development ever awarded.

An important feature of the grant program was its emphasis on the need for effective planning at the state, regional, and local levels to ensure coordination of prehospital and hospital emergency care. Across the country, state EMS offices began to emerge. With the federal support, states established a total of about 300 EMS regions—most covering several counties—each eligible to receive up to 5 years of funding (NHTSA, 1996). The law also identified 15 essential elements that should be included in an EMS system: manpower, training, communications, transportation, facilities, critical care units, public safety agencies, consumer participation, access to care, patient transfer, coordinated patient record keeping, public information and education, review and evaluation, disaster plan, and mutual aid. The EMS Systems Act helped guide the development of models of service delivery; informed system functions such as medical direction, triage protocols, communication, and quality assurance; and set the tone of the EMS system's interaction with the larger health care and public health systems. While the act identified ideal components of an EMS system from the federal government's perspective, however, the organization of systems on the ground, including their scope of practice and overall structure, was fundamentally driven by local needs, characteristics, and concerns. A patchwork quilt of systems began to emerge.

A 1978 report by the NAS/NRC, *Emergency Medical Services at Midpassage*, expressed criticism of DHEW and focused on the coordination problem between DOT and DHEW at the federal level (NAS and NRC, 1978). The report criticized the conflicting education standards developed by the two departments and recommended more research and evaluation of EMS system development. By 1981, an agreement between DOT and DHEW to coordinate efforts had been canceled, and the EMS program and DHEW grants had been eliminated.

1980s: Withdrawal of Federal Support and Leadership in EMS

In 1981, the Omnibus Budget Reconciliation Act (OBRA) eliminated the categorical federal funding to states established by the 1973 EMS Systems Act in favor of block grants to states for preventive health and health services. This change shifted responsibility for EMS from the federal to the state level. Once states had greater discretion regarding the use of funds, most chose to spend the money in areas of need other than EMS. Thus the immediate impact of the shift to block grants was a sharp decrease in total funding for EMS (U.S. Congress, Office of Technology Assessment, 1989). Moreover, states were left to develop their systems in greater isolation. Some increased their involvement in EMS, but others chose to cede more authority to cities and counties. Political, geographic, and fiscal disparities contributed to fragmented and diverse development of EMS systems at the local level. In addition, a lack of objective scientific evidence regarding the best models for EMS organization and delivery left many systems in the dark regarding appropriate steps to take.

The structure provided to local EMS systems by state governments varied. Lead state EMS agencies remained in all states, but with varying degrees of authority and funding. Maryland, for example, chose to maintain an active role and retained significant authority at the state level. The Maryland Institute for Emergency Medical Services Systems was established in 1972 and continued to take a strong leadership role in subsequent years. The state elected to provide emergency air and ground transportation as a public service and created a sophisticated trauma system that designates trauma centers on the basis of compliance with standards and demonstrated need (IOM, 1993).

By contrast, California and many other states elected to take a less active role. By default as much as by design, regional and county EMS systems took the lead in designing and managing their EMS programs. California state government maintained responsibility for such issues as investigating EMS system complaints and setting EMS training standards, but otherwise had a diminished role in the overall direction of EMS systems. During the 1980s, some states maintained vestiges of the regional systems that were developed in the 1970s, but other systems were fractured along smaller and smaller local lines. The result was even greater diversity among systems.

In the early to mid-1980s, the role of voluntary national EMS organizations increased. These included the National Association of State EMS Officials (NASEMSO, formerly the National Association of State EMS Directors [NASEMSD]), the National Association of Emergency Medical Technicians (NAEMT), the National Association of EMS Physicians (NAEMSP), the American College of Surgeons Committee on Trauma (ACS COT), and the American College of Emergency Physicians (ACEP) EMS Committee. In 1984, the Emergency Medical Services for Children (EMS-C) program was established at the Health Resources and Services Administration (HRSA) within DHHS.

In 1985, the NRC report *Injury in America: A Continuing Health Problem* described the limited progress that had been made in addressing the problem of accidental death and disability (IOM, 1985). The report described the need for a federal agency to focus on injuries as a public health problem. In response, an injury program was established at the Centers for Disease Control and Prevention (CDC) that approached injury prevention and control from a public health perspective. This program was later elevated to the status of a center at CDC—the National Center for Injury Prevention and Control (NCIPC).

During this period, rural EMS development lagged behind. The loss of federal funding and the limited financial resources available in states with large rural populations exacerbated this problem. In 1989, the Office of Technology Assessment released a report detailing the challenges faced by rural EMS (U.S. Congress, Office of Technology Assessment, 1989) (see the discussion of rural EMS below).

NHTSA implemented a statewide EMS technical assessment program in 1988. During these assessments, statewide EMS systems are evaluated on the basis of 10 essential components: regulation and policy, resource management, human resources and training, transportation, facilities, communications, public information and education, medical direction, trauma systems, and evaluation.

1990s to the Present: EMS—Looking Toward the Future

In 1995, through the urging of then NHTSA Administrator Ricardo Martinez, NHTSA and HRSA commissioned a strategic plan for the future EMS system. The resulting report, *Emergency Medical Services Agenda for the Future* (NHTSA, 1996), outlined a vision of an EMS system that is integrated with the health care system, proactive in providing community health, and adequately funded and accessible (see Table 2-1).

TABLE 2-1 New Vision for the Role of Emergency Medical Services

EMS Today (1996)	EMS Tomorrow
Isolated from other health services	Integrated with the health care system
Reacts to acute illness and injury	*Acts* to promote community health
Financed for service to individuals	Funded for service to the community
Access through fixed-point phone	Supports fixed and mobile phones

SOURCE: Martinez, 1998.

In 1997, NHTSA gathered members of the EMS community to develop an implementation guide for making the recommendations in *Agenda for the Future* a reality. The implementation guide focused on three strategies: improving linkages between EMS and other components of the health care system, creating a strong infrastructure, and developing new tools and resources to improve the effectiveness of EMS.

Agenda for the Future, now a decade old, has been effective in drawing attention to EMS and placing a spotlight on the vital role played by EMS within the emergency and trauma care system. Several of the goals it set forth, however, have not yet been realized. Its vision, such as placing a focus on the care provided to entire communities rather than individuals and thinking proactively rather than reactively, still represents a significant conceptual leap for most EMS systems. The types of changes envisioned by the *Agenda* are discussed in the relevant context in the chapters that follow.

More recently, in 2001, the U.S. General Accounting Office (GAO) released a comprehensive study of local EMS system needs and of the state regulatory agencies responsible for improving EMS outcomes. The report characterized the needs as substantial and wide-ranging, and grouped the problems identified under four categories: personnel, training, equipment, and medical direction. The report noted that the extent of local needs was difficult to determine since little standard and quantifiable information exists for use in comparing performance across systems. The report also noted that most of the available information is localized and anecdotal (GAO, 2001b).

The terrorist attacks of September 11, 2001, focused attention on the heroism of public safety personnel (fire, police, and EMS), but also exposed many of the technical and logistical challenges that confront the nation's public safety systems. Communications capabilities were shown to be grossly deficient among the units that responded to the World Trade Center attacks, and a lack of interoperability and inadequate communications with rescuers within the towers probably contributed to the deaths of many rescue personnel (National Commission on Terrorist Attacks upon the United States, 2004). In the aftermath of the disaster, the federal government took a number of steps to improve response capabilities, including development of the National Response Plan and the National Incident Management System (NIMS) (discussed in Chapter 6).

Boxes 2-1 and 2-2 detail the development and recent experience of EMS systems in two U.S. cities.

THE TROUBLED STATE OF EMS

EMS operates at the intersection of health care, public health, and public safety and therefore has overlapping roles and responsibilities (see

---

BOX 2-1
Seattle, Washington

Thirty years ago, Seattle had no organized EMS system and no paramedics. Several progressive individuals developed the concept that firefighters could be taught some of the medical skills that were normally reserved for physicians acting within a hospital. The goal was to provide these services at the earliest point of illness or injury. In 1970, the Seattle Fire Department, in cooperation with a small group of physicians at Harborview Medical Center and the University of Washington, trained the first class of firefighters as paramedics. With strong community support supplemented by grants from the National Highway Traffic Safety Administration, paramedic programs flourished in subsequent years. Research, much of it conducted within the Seattle "Medic One" EMS system, has shown that paramedics can provide high-quality care to patients outside of the hospital.

The prehospital emergency medical care system pioneered in Seattle has become famous around the world and remains a model that many others attempt to emulate. Further, Seattle has taken its unique approach to its citizens. In 1998, the Washington State Legislature enacted a law to facilitate the implementation of and compliance with a citizen defibrillation program. This city leads the nation in providing early care for victims of cardiac arrest as a result of the active involvement and training of civilians within the community. Citizens in Seattle are trained to recognize when a fellow citizen needs medical care, activate the 9-1-1 system, and help the victim until the EMS unit arrives. Seattle's Medic One system exemplifies what can be achieved with political leadership, strong and sustained physician medical direction, community support, and data-driven decision making.

Figure 2-1). Often, local EMS systems are not well integrated with any of these groups and therefore receive inadequate support from each of them. As a result, EMS has a foot in many doors, but no clear home.

Prehospital EMS faces a number of special challenges. First and foremost, EMS systems throughout the country are often highly fragmented. Although they are frequently required to work side by side, turf wars between EMS and fire personnel are not uncommon (Davis, 2003a, 2004). In addition, as noted above, the events of September 11, 2001, demonstrated that public safety agencies (including fire, police, emergency management, and EMS) often use incompatible equipment and are unable to communicate with each other during emergencies. Many of these problems are magnified when incidents cross jurisdictional lines. Significant problems are often encountered near municipal, county, and state borders. Where a street delineates the boundary between two city or county jurisdictions, responsibility for care—as well as the protocols and procedures employed—depends on the side of the street on which the incident occurred. One county in Michigan has 18 different EMS systems with a range of service models and protocols. In addition, EMS providers have found that coordinating services across state lines is particularly challenging.

In addition, coordination between EMS and hospitals is often inadequate. While hospital ED staff often provide direct, on-line medical direction to EMS personnel during transport, time pressures, competing demands, and a lack of trust can at times hinder these interactions. In addition, cultural differences between EMS and hospital staff can impede the exchange of information. Upon arrival at the hospital, busy ED staff who are strug-

---

BOX 2-2
San Francisco, California

Prior to 1997, San Francisco's EMS system fell under the jurisdiction of the public health department, with the fire department providing first-responder support. During the late 1990s and early 2000s, a seven-phase merger process was initiated to place EMS under the jurisdiction of the fire department. However, this process experienced difficulties from the beginning and later resulted in a partial separation.

The merger called for the cross-training of EMS personnel and fire-fighters, the placement of paramedics on city fire trucks, and institution of a "one and one" response program, with ambulances staffed by one paramedic and one EMT. However, the cross-training of firefighters as paramedics was delayed because of lengthy union negotiations. EMS workload constraints delayed EMTs' fire-suppression cross-training. This in turn delayed the changes in personnel configuration. In addition, a requirement that EMS personnel work 24-hour shifts rankled paramedics and raised concerns about the impact on patient care. These and other issues revealed a clash between the firefighting and EMS cultures and raised questions about the advisability of the merger. An audit later determined that, despite the increased resources devoted by the fire department to EMS during the first 4 years of the merger, average response times had increased (City and County of San Francisco, Office of the Budget Analyst, 2002). The city later instituted a new plan in which a lower-paid group of paramedics and EMTs was hired and located outside of fire stations, partially ending the merger attempt.

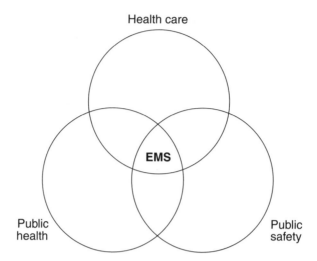

FIGURE 2-1 The overlapping roles and responsibilities of EMS.
SOURCE: NHTSA, 1996.

gling to manage a very crowded ED often greet arriving EMS units with, at best, a lack of enthusiasm. As a result, clinically important information is sometimes lost in patient handoffs between EMS and hospital staff.

Second, there is little doubt that ED crowding has had a very adverse impact on prehospital care. When an ED is crowded, ED staff may be unable to find the physical space needed to off-load patients. Under these circumstances, EMS units may be stuck in the ED for prolonged periods of time, leaving them out of service for other emergency calls. In addition, ED diversion has become commonplace in many major cities, further hindering the performance of EMS. In major metropolitan areas, it is not uncommon for all of the city's trauma centers to request ambulance diversion at the same time. When hospital EDs go on diversion status, ambulances may have to drive longer distances and take patients to less appropriate facilities (GAO, 2003). Fully 45 percent of EDs reported going on diversion at some point in 2003, and the problem was especially pronounced in urban areas. Overall, it is estimated that 501,000 ambulances were diverted during that year (Burt et al., 2006).

Although it is likely that ambulance diversions endanger patients, there are no data directly linking ambulance diversions with higher mortality rates. No agency has sponsored a systematic study to examine this question, and fears of legal liability inhibit candid disclosure of adverse events (IOM, 2000). However, a study by the Joint Commission on Accreditation of Healthcare Organizations (JCAHO, 2002) revealed that more than half of all "sentinel" ED events—defined as "an unexpected occurrence involving death or serious physical or psychological injury, or risk thereof"—were caused by delayed treatment. While this study was not centered on ambulance diversion, its findings are consistent with the argument that delays in treatment resulting from diversion can have deleterious effects on patients.

Third, the cost of maintaining an EMS system in a state of readiness is extremely high, and it is rarely compensated. The EMS reimbursement model used by the Centers for Medicare and Medicaid Services (CMS) and emulated by many payers reimburses on the basis of transport to a medical facility. This model ignores the increasingly sophisticated care provided by EMS personnel, as well as the growing proportion of elderly patients with multiple chronic conditions who frequently utilize EMS. Medicaid typically pays a fixed rate—as low as $25 in some states—for an EMS transport, regardless of the complexity of the case or the resources utilized. The fact that payers generally withhold reimbursement in cases where transport is not provided is a major impediment to the implementation of processes that allow EMS to "treat and release," to transport patients directly to a dialysis unit or another appropriate site, or to terminate unsuccessful cardiac resuscitation in the field. In addition, many systems of all types provide both 9-1-1 call services and medical transportation. To make up for funding shortfalls, these systems often offset the cost of the former services with revenues from the latter.

EMS is widely viewed as an essential public service, but it has not been supported through effective federal and state leadership and sustainable funding strategies. Unlike other such services—electricity, highways, airports, and telephone service, for example—all of which were created and are actively maintained through major national infrastructure investments, access to timely and high-quality emergency and trauma care has largely been relegated to local and state initiatives. As a result, EMS care remains extremely uneven across the United States. Even when EMS is located within a publicly funded agency such as the fire service, it may receive a disproportionately small amount of fire service funding (including grants and line item disbursements), despite the fact that a large majority of calls to fire departments are medical in nature.

Fourth, EMS agencies face a number of personnel challenges. The training of EMTs and paramedics is uneven across the United States, and as a result, EMS professionals exhibit a wide range of skill levels. There are currently no national requirements for training, certification, or licensure, nor is there required national accreditation of schools that provide EMS training. In addition, recruitment and retention are significant challenges for EMS systems. The work of prehospital providers can be challenging and dangerous. EMS personnel face potential violence from patients; risks due to bloodborne and airborne pathogens; and dangers from ambulance crashes, which increasingly result in provider fatalities (Franks et al., 2004). In addition, many EMS professionals are frustrated by low pay—the average salary for EMTs is about $18,000 and for paramedics is $34,000 (Brown et al., 2003)—and limited career growth opportunities, especially relative to firefighters and other public servants with whom they work side by side. Worse, they are often treated as second-class citizens by those same colleagues, by the systems in which they work, and by the state and federal institutions that fund and support the services they provide. As a result of these and other challenges, recently surveyed EMS agencies and administrators ranked recruitment and retention as the number one issue they face (EMS Insider, 2005).

Perhaps most disturbing is how little is known about what does and does not work in prehospital emergency care. There is little or no scientific evidence to support many widely employed EMS clinical procedures and system design features. The value and proper application of common clinical practices, such as rapid sequence intubation (Murray et al., 2000; Gausche et al., 2000; Davis et al., 2003; Wang et al., 2004) and cardiac resuscitation (Keim et al., 2004), remain unresolved. Field triage models that are widely considered to be out of date are still in use today. Evidence on the value of delivery models, such as tiered levels of response, intensity of on-line medical direction, type of EMS system (e.g., fire-based, volunteer), and deployment of paramedics, is either nonexistent or inconclusive.

The lack of available data on prehospital care not only discourages research on the effectiveness of prehospital interventions, but also hinders the development of process and outcome measures for evaluating the performance of the system. In fact, policy makers and the public have very little information on how well local EMS systems function and how care varies across jurisdictions.

Rural areas face a different set of problems, principally involving a scarcity of resources. EMS and trauma services are dispersed across wide distances, and recruitment and retention of EMTs and paramedics is a pervasive problem. In rural areas, volunteers make up the majority of the EMS workforce (National Registry of Emergency Medical Technicians, 2003). EMS is the only component of the U.S. medical system that has a significant volunteer component, but in many rural communities, younger residents are leaving as the remaining population becomes more elderly. As a result, the pool of potential volunteers is dwindling as their average age and the demands on their time increase. The closure or restructuring of many rural hospital facilities has further increased the demand on rural EMS agencies by creating an environment that requires long-distance, time-consuming, and high-risk interfacility transfers. The final section of this chapter provides a detailed discussion of rural EMS.

EMS is the first line of defense in responding to the medical needs of the public in the event of a disaster, yet EMS personnel are often the least prepared and most poorly equipped of all public safety personnel. According to New York University's Center for Catastrophe Preparedness and Response, more than half of EMTs and paramedics have received less than 1 hour of training in dealing with biological and chemical agents and explosives since the September 11 terrorist attacks, and 20 percent have received no such training. Fewer than 33 percent of EMTs and paramedics have participated in a drill during the past year simulating a radiological, biological, or chemical attack. And in 25 states, half or fewer EMTs and paramedics have adequate personal protective equipment to respond to a biological or chemical attack (Center for Catastrophe Preparedness and Response NYU, 2005). These findings call into question the readiness of the current EMS system to deal with potential disasters.

FEDERAL OVERSIGHT AND FUNDING

The federal government is extremely fragmented in its approach to regulating EMS. A host of departments, divisions, and agencies at the federal level play a role in various aspects of EMS, but none is officially designated as the lead agency. With the passage of the Highway Safety Act in 1966, EMS found its unofficial home within NHTSA in DOT. At the time, a principal focus of the government's effort in EMS was on reducing the number of deaths and disabilities caused by crashes on the nation's motorways, so this placement within DOT seemed appropriate.

As described above, NHTSA's Office of EMS has been able to provide significant leadership in the field over the past several decades. Indeed, since the early 1970s, NHTSA is the only federal agency that has consistently focused on improving the overall EMS system (AEMS, 2005a). However, NHTSA's Office of EMS is a small program within a very large federal department that is devoted to transportation. Obscured as it often is within the vast federal bureaucracy, EMS is sometimes overlooked and at times virtually forgotten. This is evidenced by the fact that to date, EMS has received only a small percentage of homeland security funds allocated by the federal government. Although EMS providers represent a third of the nation's first responders and have a key mission in treating the casualties of a terrorist strike, they received only 4 percent of the $3.38 billion allocated by the Department of Homeland Security for enhancing emergency preparedness in 2002 and 2003 (Center for Catastrophe Preparedness and Response NYU, 2005).

While NHTSA has served as the informal lead agency for EMS within the federal government, a number of other federal agencies also have a stake in EMS. DHHS houses several programs within HRSA, including the EMS-C program and the Trauma and EMS Program (although both of these programs have been targeted for elimination in recent federal budgets). HRSA also administers the Office of Rural Health Policy. CMS is responsible for Medicare and Medicaid reimbursement for emergency services, which makes up a significant portion of EMS revenues. CDC's NCIPC plays an important role in trauma and prevention research that is closely allied with emergency services. The National Institutes of Health (NIH) funds emergency- and trauma-related research. The Department of Homeland Security's Preparedness Directorate supports emergency preparedness programs through the Chief Medical Officer, the U.S. Fire Administration, the Office of Grants and Training, and other agencies.

In an effort to coordinate the efforts of these various components of the federal bureaucracy, Congress established a Federal Interagency Committee on Emergency Medical Services (FICEMS) in 2005. This group was formed to ensure coordination among the federal agencies involved with state, local, or regional EMS and 9-1-1 systems and to identify ways of streamlining the process through which federal agencies provide support to these systems (see Chapter 3).

Federal Funding of EMS

Today, financial support for EMS is provided by the various departments and agencies that have jurisdiction over EMS. An array of federal grant programs provide limited amounts of funding to states, localities, and EMS providers (see Table 2-2 for examples). Typically, EMS receives a very small percentage of the funds devoted to larger programs.

Within DHHS, both HRSA and CDC fund EMS. HRSA operates a number of EMS-related programs, including trauma and EMS (funded at $3.5 million in fiscal year 2005), rural outreach grants ($39 million), hospital flex grants ($39 million), a poison control program ($23 million), and the EMS-C program ($23 million). As noted, however, recent budget proposals would eliminate several of these programs, including trauma and EMS, EMS-C, and the poison control program. By far the largest of the HRSA programs is the Hospital Bioterrorism Preparedness program ($495 million). This program aims to improve the capacity of hospitals, EDs, health centers, EMS systems, and poison control centers to respond to acts of terrorism and other public health emergencies. As detailed in Chapter 6, however, a very small percentage of these funds is directed to EMS.

CDC operates two large EMS-related programs. The Preventive Health and Health Services block grant ($131 million) provides states with resources to address priority health concerns in their communities. States are also charged with designing prevention and health promotion programs that address the national health objectives contained in Healthy People

TABLE 2-2 EMS-Related Fiscal Year 2005 Federal Funding

	2005 Enacted Millions of Dollars
Labor HHS & Education Bill	
Health and Human Services	
HRSA	
Rural EMS Training and Equipment	0.5
Rural and Community Access to AEDs	9
Hospital BT Preparedness	495
Trauma/EMS	3
EMS for Children	20
Traumatic Brain Injury	9
Rural Outreach Grants	39
Rural Hospital Flex Grants	39
Poison Control	23
CDC	
Prevention Block Grant	131
Injury Prevention (NCIPC)	138
Transportation, Treasury Bill	
NHTSA	
EMS Division	4
EMS State Grants	0
Homeland Security Bill	
Office of Domestic Preparedness	
State and Local Programs:	
State Homeland Security Grant Program:	1,100
Law enforcement terrorism prevention grants	400
Urban Area Security Initiative:	
High-threat, high-density urban area	885
Targeted infrastructure protection	0
Buffer Zone Protection Program	0
Port security grants	150
Rail and transit security	150
Trucking security grants	5
Intercity bus security grants	10
Commercial equipment direct assistance program	50
National Programs:	
National domestic preparedness consortium	135
National exercise program	52
Technical assistance	30
Metropolitan Medical Response System	30
Demonstration training grants	30
Continuing training grants	25
Citizen Corps	15
Evaluations and assessments	14
Rural domestic preparedness consortium	5

continued

TABLE 2-2 Continued

	2005 Enacted Millions of Dollars
Firefighter Assistance Grants	
Fire department staffing assistance grants:	
Grants	650
Staffing for Adequate Fire and Emergency Response (SAFER) Act	65
Emergency Management Performance Grants	180
Total Office of Domestic Preparedness	3,985

NOTE: AED = automated external defibrillator; BT = bioterrorism; NCIPC = National Center for Injury Prevention and Control.
SOURCE: AEMS, 2005b.

2010. These include increasing the proportion of adults who are aware of the early warning signs of a heart attack and the importance of accessing emergency care by calling 9-1-1 (GAO, 2001b). CDC also runs NCIPC, which works to reduce morbidity, disability, mortality, and costs associated with injuries (funded at $138 million in fiscal year 2005). Overall, however, a small percentage of the funds allotted to these CDC programs is devoted specifically to EMS.

The Department of Homeland Security's Office of Domestic Preparedness awarded nearly $4 billion in federal funding in fiscal year 2005 under its first-responder grant programs—the Firefighter Assistance Grants program ($895 million) and the State and Local Programs fund ($3.1 billion). The latter included $885 million for high-threat, high-density urban areas; $150 million each for port security and rail and transit security; and $135 million for the national domestic preparedness consortium. As detailed in Chapter 6, however, non-EMS first responders were the primary recipients of these funds.

Federal Reimbursement for EMS Services

In addition to small portions of the federal funding detailed above, EMS systems across the country receive federal funds through reimbursements from the Medicare program. Because the elderly are heavy users of EMS, Medicare represents a very large percentage of billings and collections in a typical EMS agency. Those aged 65 and older are 4.4 times more likely to use EMS than younger individuals, and they represent a growing segment of the population. Since Medicare payments have traditionally been used to cross-subsidize Medicaid and uninsured EMS users, Medicare represents an even larger percentage of total patient revenues for EMS agencies (Overton,

2002). An example from the Richmond Ambulance Authority is shown in Figure 2-2. In that system, Medicare represents 40 percent of billings, but 55 percent of revenues.

The Medicare program recently completed a 5-year transition to a new fee schedule. Under the old reimbursement system, EMS agencies received two payments per transport. The primary payment was a cost-based, fee-for-service rate that reimbursed EMS for the service provided. The secondary payment was reimbursement for the number of miles the ambulance traveled. Under that system, ambulance services were concerned primarily with reporting their charges and mileage. The new system keeps the mileage reimbursement but abandons the cost-based payment and replaces it with a prospective payment system, similar to the system in place for outpatient health services (Overton, 2002). EMS was the last Medicare Part B provider to transition from a fee-for-service to a prospective payment system. Under the new system, ALS transports are reimbursed at a higher rate than basic life support (BLS) transports, and higher payments are provided for transport in rural areas to reflect the typically long travel times to and from hospitals (MedPAC, 2003).

Overall, the new fee schedule significantly reduces Medicare payments to EMS providers. Two years into the transition to the new system, data indicated that Medicare reimbursements were approximately 45 percent below the national cost average for transport, leading to a $600 million shortfall for services provided to Medicare beneficiaries. As a result, local EMS systems may now need greater subsidization from local governments or may be forced to reduce costs through personnel cuts, reductions in

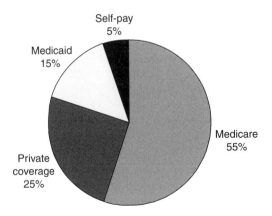

FIGURE 2-2 EMS patient revenues, Richmond, Virginia.
SOURCE: Overton, 2002.

capital expenditures, or other means. These dynamics illustrate the tension among federal, state, and local governments regarding the locus of responsibility for funding EMS systems across the country.

Medicare payments have significantly shaped the provision of EMS nationwide, as evidenced in several areas, including the availability of responders, the therapeutic interventions provided, treat and release practices, and transport and transfer policies (NASEMSD, 2005). For example, EMS systems relying on Medicare and other third-party payers for significant revenue must generally provide patient transportation to be reimbursed for their services. While the primary determinants of EMS costs relate to maintaining readiness capacity, the primary determinant of payment for services is patient transport. Thus in an urban area that receives a large number of 9-1-1 calls, the cost of readiness is spread over a large number of users, keeping the cost per transport relatively low, whereas in rural areas, the lower volume of emergency calls in relation to the high overhead of maintaining a prepared staff results in very high costs per transport. Although many rural EMS squads rely on volunteers rather than paid EMS personnel to reduce these costs, doing so results in a less stable system.

Federal Regulation of EMS

The current organization and delivery of emergency and trauma care is shaped largely by federal and state legislation. The legal and regulatory framework provides many protections and benefits, but also presents obstacles to achieving efficient and high-quality care delivery.

Emergency Medical Treatment and Active Labor Act (EMTALA)

EMTALA represents one example of how the federal government's fragmented regulatory structure has resulted in confusion for EMS providers and potential harm to emergency patients. This law, passed in 1986, requires hospitals that participate in the Medicare program to provide a medical screening exam and stabilize all patients that come to the hospital for care before they are discharged or transferred to another hospital. EMTALA was intended to protect access to emergency care by preventing private hospitals from turning away needy emergency patients who are uninsured or underinsured or precipitously transferring these patients to the closest public hospital, a practice known as "dumping" (GAO, 2001a).

Over time, the law has progressively expanded, and it now covers patients seen anywhere on hospital property, which includes ambulances owned and operated by the hospital (Wanerman, 2002; Elting and Toddy, 2003). As a result, hospitals may be required to provide medical screening exams to patients arriving in a hospital-owned ambulance even if the patient requires immediate care at a regional trauma center because the local hospital does not have the personnel or equipment required to respond effectively to the patient's critical medical needs. This situation also arises in cases where a ground and an air ambulance are attempting to rendezvous at a hospital's helipad so that the patient can be transported quickly to a trauma center. Providers in the field have experienced confusion as to whether a screening exam is mandated in this case.

The expansion of EMTALA to include transports by hospital-owned ambulances created a barrier to regional coordination. The goal of regional coordination is to ensure that patients receive the optimal care, and a key component of that task is ensuring that avoidable and costly delays are eliminated. However, EMTALA may require that patients receive initial care at a less-than-optimal facility, creating avoidable delays in the provision of needed care.

This problem is compounded by the fact that no one agency is responsible for making regulatory decisions regarding EMTALA, and as a consequence, federal rules on this issue are not clear. The Office of the Inspector General (OIG) has produced advisories on EMTALA, including a letter of opinion stating that ambulances may take patients directly to hospitals that are appropriate for the patient's condition (including trauma centers) in cases where there are "regional protocols" in place (DHHS, 2003). However, the OIG is not a rule-making entity and is not responsible for enforcement. CMS's enforcement of EMTALA has been shown to be highly variable among regions (GAO, 2001a). Consequently, providers across the country are uncertain as to whether EMTALA requires that a medical screening exam be conducted even when a patient requires immediate care at a trauma facility, and there is no simple or straightforward way to have this issue clarified. Various people involved in making the decision at the local level, including the hospital administrator, the hospital's attorney, the state EMS office, and others, may all have a different point of view. As a result, providers are making decisions that may compromise care based on their own reading of this complex regulatory environment.

Health Insurance Portability and Accountability Act (HIPAA)

The federal regulatory environment has also created confusion with HIPAA. Enacted to regulate the transmission of electronic health data among providers and payers and to protect the privacy of patient health information, HIPAA often presents challenges for providers seeking to share health information with other providers, potentially compromising both patient care and provider protections; it also creates difficulties for investigators seeking to obtain research data. There are exceptions to HIPAA that recognize the unique characteristics of emergency and trauma care, such as the urgency of care and the potential inability of patients in distress to provide consent (Lewis et al., 2001); however, HIPAA continues to pose a number of impediments to EMS.

The regulatory environment at the federal level does not provide clear assurances regarding HIPAA rules for dispatch centers and radio communications, resulting in guesswork at the local level. EMS represents a small segment of the health care continuum and received little attention during the development of the HIPAA regulations, but the cost of HIPAA compliance for EMS providers is substantial.

Based on their interpretation of current federal rules and their fear of liability, some hospitals believe HIPAA excludes outside agencies from participating in multidisciplinary quality assurance projects. As a result, trauma morbidity and mortality conferences convened by hospitals may exclude EMS personnel. This happens despite the fact that EMS personnel are responsible for transporting patients to the hospital, often have salient information about events on the scene, and may benefit from learning what happened after patients reached the hospital.

HIPAA has created additional barriers to information sharing between hospitals and EMS agencies. For example, EMS agencies may want to assess patient outcomes following hospital transport; however, patient-specific outcome data often are not shared. EMS personnel may also seek to determine whether a particular patient transported to the hospital is suffering from an air- or bloodborne pathogen or some other malady that may compromise the safety of the transporting EMS personnel. But hospitals are often unwilling to share this information with EMS agencies for fear of violating HIPAA regulations, even in cases where such information sharing may be allowable.

For researchers investigating patient outcomes resulting from out-of-hospital interventions such as cardiac resuscitation, it is necessary to obtain outcome information from each of the facilities in which patients were treated. Out-of-hospital and ED records must be linked with hospital records, vital statistics, and coroner's records when appropriate. The patient identifiers required to perform such linkages are subject to the confidentiality provisions of the HIPAA legislation, making gathering these data difficult in an environment where EMS-related research is already lacking.

EMS OVERSIGHT AT THE STATE LEVEL

In most states, state law governs the scope, authority, and operation of local EMS systems. Each state has a lead EMS agency that is typically a part of the state health department, but in some states may be part of the public safety department or an independent agency. The mission, funding, and size of EMS agencies vary considerably from state to state. For example, a survey conducted by NASEMSO found that the number of full-time positions within state EMS agencies varied from a low of 4 to a high of 90. Most states have an EMS medical director, though many do not. Table 2-3 shows the range of functions that EMS agencies provide.

State EMS agencies regulate and oversee local and regional EMS systems and personnel. They typically license and certify EMS personnel and ambulance providers and establish testing and training requirements. Some may also be responsible for approving statewide EMS plans, allocating federal EMS resources, and monitoring performance (GAO, 2001b). States have begun to take a more proactive role in trauma planning, with 35 states having formal trauma systems. One key function of many EMS agencies is data collection. However, only about half of state EMS offices have the capabilities to provide information on how many EMS responses occur in their state (Mears, 2004).

In regulating local and regional EMS systems, many state EMS offices are placed in the difficult position of being both an advocate/technical advisor and a regulator. This dual role can create internal conflicts. For example, state EMS offices are often responsible for both ensuring an adequate supply of EMS personnel and regulating those personnel. If an EMS office seeks to increase the educational requirements for EMS personnel, it may also create the type of workforce shortage it is working to avoid. For this reason, other professions separate the regulatory and advocacy roles (Shimberg and Roederer, 1994; Schmitt and Shimberg, 1996).

TABLE 2-3 State EMS Agency Functions

Function	States Performing (%)
Complaint Investigation	100
EMS Training Standards	96
EMS System Planning	94
Disciplinary Action of Personnel	90
EMS Personnel Credentialing	90
State EMS Data Collection	88
Air Ambulance Credentialing	84
Ambulance Inspections	84
Ambulance Credentialing	82
Disaster Planning	78
Local EMS Technical Assistance	74
Trauma System Management	72
Local EMS Data Collection	68
Medical Director Education	62
Funding for Local EMS Operations	34
Communications Operations	18

SOURCE: Mears, 2004.

Some states provide direct funding for EMS, which may be derived from vehicle or driver licensing fees, motor vehicle violations, or other taxes. However, EMS funding is subject to cutbacks in tight fiscal environments. Approximately 87 percent of funds for state EMS office budgets comes from in-state revenues. The remaining 13 percent that comes from the federal government includes grants from multiple agencies with diverse priorities. There is currently no single, comprehensive federal vision for the development of the EMS system nationwide. NASEMSO maintains that this situation may have contributed to the lack of sustained and meaningful development in many areas identified in *Emergency Medcical Services Agenda for the Future* (NASEMSD, 2005).

State Medicaid agencies are responsible for developing Medicaid reimbursement policies for EMS. It is estimated that for most EMS agencies, Medicaid patients represent 20–40 percent of all EMS patients. The proportion of users covered by Medicaid tends to be higher in rural areas. The way EMS services are reimbursed can vary greatly from state to state; however, Medicaid reimbursement rates are almost universally low. As noted earlier, the majority of states use a fee-for-service payment system and a mileage rate for Medicaid reimbursement; five states pay EMS a "reasonable charge," an amount that the state has decided is reasonable for the public to pay (Kaiser Commission on Medicaid and the Uninsured, 2003). Medicaid reimbursement is typically based on transportation rather than service provided. Thus, for example, EMS agencies in Virginia receive $75 for transporting a patient 0–5 miles to a hospital, regardless of whether the patient was transported by BLS or ALS providers and regardless of the severity of the patient's condition or the services rendered. In most states, payment is not provided unless the EMS agency actually transports the patient.

NHTSA provides some technical assistance to state EMS agencies through statewide assessments. For the assessments and reassessments, NHTSA serves as a facilitator by assembling a team of experts in EMS development and implementation to work with and advise the state. The state EMS office provides NHTSA and the assessment team with background information on the EMS system, and the technical assistance team develops a findings report. A mid-1990s review of EMS assessments revealed "widespread fundamental problems in most areas," but the lack of quality management programs was a common theme across systems. The review found that the majority of states did not have quality improvement programs for evaluating patient care, methods for assessing current levels of system resources, or mechanisms for identifying necessary system improvements (NHTSA Technical Assistance Program, 2000). The technical assistance provided to state EMS agencies is critical. All of these agencies face complex structural and operational issues that include system design, reimbursement strategies, quality management, performance improvement, and business remodeling. EMS administrators are typically career EMS personnel; many have little formal training in organizational management, and there are no standardized courses for providing them with this training (Mears, 2004).

MODELS OF ORGANIZATION AND SERVICE DELIVERY AT THE LOCAL LEVEL

Across the United States today, EMS systems are fundamentally local in nature (GAO, 2001b). Counties and municipalities play central roles in deciding how their systems will be structured and how they will adapt to changes in the environment (e.g., changes in Medicare payment rates or added liability concerns). They determine the organization of the delivery system, the structure of EMS response times, the development of finance mechanisms, and the management of other system components. As a result of this local control, EMS systems across the country are extremely variable and fragmented. This diversity of systems can be viewed as a strength in that it promotes local self-determination and tailors systems to the needs and expectations of local residents. However, it is also a profound weakness, especially in cases where local standards of care fall below generally accepted standards and patients suffer as a result. Across cities, for example, the percentage of people suffering ventricular fibrillation who survive and are later discharged from the hospital with good brain function ranges from 3 to 45 percent (Davis, 2003a). EMS response times overall vary substantially, and many cities do not collect the data necessary to track their performance.

Emergency Dispatch Centers

Today, virtually all Americans (99 percent) have access to 9-1-1 service (National Emergency Number Association, 2004). However, the apparent uniformity of the 9-1-1 system is misleading: the system is actually locally based and operated, and its structure varies widely across the country. There currently exist more than 6,000 public safety answering points (PSAPs), or 9-1-1 call centers, nationwide. These include both primary PSAPs, which field all types of 9-1-1 calls (police, fire, and EMS), and secondary PSAPs, which handle service-specific calls, such as medical emergencies. These emergency call centers are operated primarily by public safety agencies, as well as city and county communications centers, hospitals, and others (see Figure 2-3). Over time, it may become necessary to reduce the large number of call centers, especially in the context of disaster preparedness efforts, which dictate a more streamlined emergency call structure in response to catastrophic events.

In 2004, 9-1-1 call centers fielded approximately 200 million emergency calls, including medical, police, fire, and other calls. In some cases, medical

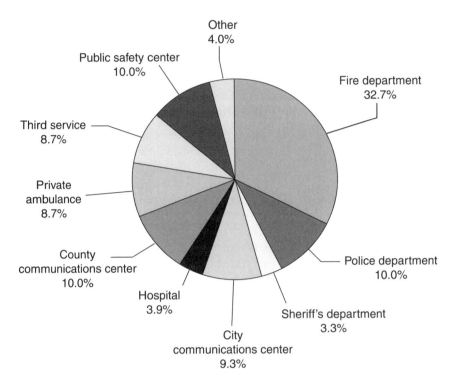

FIGURE 2-3 Agency responsible for dispatch in the 200 most populous cities.
SOURCE: Monosky, 2004.

calls are received by primary call centers and then routed to secondary calls centers with dedicated medical dispatch. In other cases, all calls are handled at the primary call center. When different types of calls are handled by different call centers, the potential for "call switching" and miscommunication is dramatically increased.

Not only do 9-1-1 dispatchers determine the appropriate level of response, but they also often provide prearrival instructions to the caller. The prototype for this process was dispatcher-assisted CPR, pioneered by Eisenberg and colleagues in King County, Washington, and subsequently validated by an independent research team in Memphis. The list of conditions amenable to prearrival instructions was quickly expanded to include, for example, childbirth, seizures, and trauma/bleeding.

Prearrival instructions are designed to enable the caller to provide assistance when certain emergency conditions are present, to protect the patient and caller from potential hazards, and to protect the patient from well-meaning bystanders who could provide assistance that might do more harm than good (Hauert, 1990). The level of prearrival assistance from the dispatcher can vary from simple advice, such as "call a doctor," to instructions for performing CPR. Instructions are typically available to the dispatcher on flip cards.

EMS Systems

A survey of EMS systems conducted in 2003 by NASEMSD and HRSA's Office of Rural Health Policy indicated that there were 15,691 credentialed EMS systems in the United States (Mears, 2004). However, the survey also indicated that the definition of an EMS system varies from state to state, making accurate tabulations nearly impossible. Among the systems identified by the survey, 45 percent were fire department–based, 6.5 percent were hospital-based, and 48.5 percent were labeled as neither (see Figure 2-4). The total number of ALS and BLS transport vehicles reported was 24,570. More recent data from the American Ambulance Association (AAA) indicate that there are 12,254 ambulance services operating in the United States (a figure that includes private for-profit and not-for-profit, hospital-based, volunteer, and fire department–based services), and a total of 23,575 ground ambulance vehicles (AAA, 2006).

While no statistics are available to provide greater detail about EMS system types nationwide, the *Journal of Emergency Medical Services* conducts an annual survey of the 200 largest metropolitan areas in the United

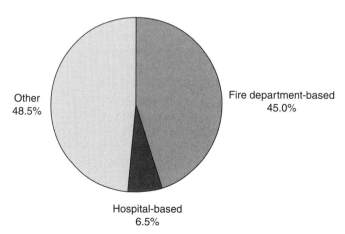

FIGURE 2-4 Types of EMS systems.
SOURCE: Mears, 2004.

TABLE 2-4 Reported Provider Types

Provider Type	Percentage (Number)
First Responders (n = 163)	
Fire Department	89.0 (145)
Other	7.4 (12)
None	3.7 (6)
Transport Providers (n =163)	
Private Organization	36.2 (59)
For-Profit	31.3 (51)
Not-for-Profit	4.9 (8)
Fire Department	31.9 (52)
Single-Role	4.9 (8)
Dual-Role	27.0 (44)
Third Service	8.6 (14)
Hospital	7.4 (12)
Other	4.9 (8)
Public–Private Partnership	4.3 (7)
Public Utility Model	3.7 (6)
Public Safety	1.2 (2)
Volunteer	1.2 (2)

SOURCE: Williams, 2005.

States and is able to provide statistics for these areas (Williams, 2005) (see Table 2-4). The figures shown do not reflect smaller cities or rural areas. Results of the 2006 survey indicate that 36 percent of ambulance systems in these large metropolitan areas are private (either for-profit or not-for-profit), 32 percent are fire department–based, and just under 10 percent are third-service and hospital-based. However, an overwhelming number of first responders are fire department–based (89 percent).

Fire Department–Based EMS Systems

As is evident from the Mears (2004) survey, a strong plurality of EMS systems nationwide is fire department–based. The number of services has steadily increased over the past several decades as fire chiefs have recognized the central role of EMS in firefighting operations. EMS is an element of the response and service delivery of approximately 80 percent of fire departments in America (U.S. Fire Administration, 2005).

At an operational level, a fire department–based EMS system is one in which EMS is part of the fire department and ambulances are housed in or operate out of fire stations, with integrated dispatch. The integration of fire and EMS varies with each department. Some departments utilize personnel whose sole function is to provide EMS, while others utilize dual-role personnel who function as both firefighters and EMS providers. Some fire departments offer a full range of EMS, including BLS and ALS response and transport, while others limit their role to providing first-responder BLS or ALS care without transport.

Fire departments have chief officers who oversee operations and provide leadership at multiple levels. The chief of the department is usually a firefighter and, increasingly, may also have an EMS background, although frequently this is not the case. The organization and leadership of EMS within fire departments vary considerably. Some departments divide EMS and firefighting into separate divisions, while others integrate the two services under general operations. All fire departments that provide ALS must have a physician medical director, whether paid or volunteer; those that provide only BLS services may not.

Fire departments are financed primarily through public funds. Some departments bill for EMS, but collection rates vary. Collections are especially low in urban areas. Many small-town and rural fire departments in the United States, especially the latter, are volunteer, but the number of volunteer firefighters appears to be declining (see the discussion in Chapter 4).

In most jurisdictions, EMS calls now exceed fire-related calls by a wide margin. According to the National Fire Protection Association (2005), 80 percent of national fire service calls are EMS-related. This trend is likely to persist as fire prevention techniques continue to improve and as the aging of the U.S. population adds to the projected number of EMS calls.

One advantage of having an integrated fire and EMS system is structural efficiency. Firehouses are traditionally well positioned to serve the local population in most areas of the country. These physical structures can provide a strategic location for the EMS units they house, as well as a place for EMS personnel to rest between calls. Fire departments also provide the administrative infrastructure necessary to manage personnel, provide training, and purchase and maintain equipment and supplies.

But there are also disadvantages to fire-based EMS systems. A series of articles in *USA Today* documented the cultural divide, discussed earlier, that can exist between EMS and fire personnel (Davis, 2003b). Generally, the orientation of EMS personnel centers on providing medical care, whereas that of firefighters centers on conducting rescue operations and battling fires. As a result, there is some difference between the types of individual who become EMTs and firefighters (Davis, 2003a). These personnel often do not work together in a coordinated fashion.

In many cities, such as Washington, D.C., and Los Angeles, EMS is under the leadership of the fire department, which tends to consider fire suppression its principal mission, with medical services assuming a secondary role (Davis, 2003a). As a result, priority is given to fire suppression when it comes to training and budget allocations. In many cases, firefighters are paid more than EMS personnel and have separate unions and command structures, even when based within the same fire department. Medical directors who are hired to supervise fire department–based emergency medical response may be viewed as outsiders, and may defer to the fire chiefs on the way resources should be deployed. Over the past decade, many EMS systems have become integrated with the fire service, although there is significant variation with respect to the level of integration.

Hospital-Based EMS Systems

Hospital-based EMS systems may provide stand-alone EMS coverage to a community or may operate in conjunction with a fire department. Typically, a hospital-based service is located at a community hospital and dispatched through a public safety communications system (9-1-1) or routed through a secondary call center that receives dispatches from a 9-1-1 center. Hospital-based systems function as private entities and typically bill for their services.

An advantage of a hospital-based system is that EMS personnel may benefit from the closer relationship between the ED and the hospital and may be better able to maintain professional skills through greater opportunities to observe ED procedures. Hospital-based systems also benefit from the reputation of the hospital with which they are affiliated and may be recognized by members of the community.

A challenge for hospital-based systems is potential competition among services and the need for better coordination of system resources. Since hospital-based ambulances bill for services and provide transport to their base hospital, there is an inherent competition for patients. For example, ambulance companies may seek to advertise their services, providing their own phone number and encouraging people to call them instead of 9-1-1. This may also occur with private ambulance services.

Another challenge in larger communities that use a number of hospital-based systems is optimizing system resources. Hospitals are not always located proportionally to populations or areas of greatest need. Further, depending on state regulations, hospitals may not be required to increase the number of available ambulances if EMS call volumes increase.

Private Systems

In some areas, local governments run their ambulance service by contracting with a private entity—either a local EMS operation or a national company. In these instances, private ambulance companies contract their services to local governments to provide 9-1-1 transports, including personnel, equipment, and vehicles. The contracts may or may not require medical oversight. The private firms compete for contracts, typically every several years. Some of these private firms are publicly owned stock-issuing corporations. For-profit providers now operate throughout most of the country.

Private EMS systems face some of the same challenges as fire department–based EMS systems. Some cities have found them to be a more economical alternative than expanding fire departments to provide EMS. However, their profit orientation also makes it more likely that EMS will suffer when contract disputes occur with the municipal agency.

There are several different models for private systems. First, under a level-of-effort model, a local government develops a contract with a private firm for a certain number of ambulances and other resources. The contractor is not held to specific performance standards, but must simply provide the contracted services. Under a performance-based model, the contractor is expected to meet specific performance standards to fulfill the contract. Finally, under a high-performance model, the contract creates a business relationship that tightly aligns the interests of the contractor with public needs. The contractor may be responsible for patient billing and may own some long-term infrastructure items, such as ambulances and medical communications systems. Additionally, an independent body is responsible for performance, medical oversight, and financial oversight; rate regulation; licensing; and market allocation (AAA, 2004).

One difficulty in evaluating the pros and cons of any service model (whether locally or nationally) is the dearth of objective process and outcome data for comparing one model of service delivery or even one ambulance company with another. As a result, local governments frequently rely on crude measures, such as numbers of personnel, numbers of ambulances operating per unit of time, EMS fractile response times by urgency of call, and patient complaints. These are poor proxies for quality of care and outcome-based measures of system performance.

Municipal Services

At the local level, municipal and county governments often deliberate between contracting out to a private EMS company and developing and operating an EMS unit themselves. In many cases, the locality chooses the latter option. This involves purchasing or leasing ambulance units, hiring EMS personnel to provide direct services and administrative personnel to run the program, and stocking ambulances with necessary medical and communications equipment. Some of these operations bill private insurers for services, while others rely solely on direct funding from the city or county.

In Kansas City, Missouri, fire department personnel serve as first responders, but transport is handled through a public utility model. This model entails a quasigovernmental authority with overall responsibility for EMS transport that owns all the equipment, including ambulances, and carries out billing and other logistical functions, but contracts with a private company for human resources. Kansas City was one of the first major cities to offer EMS transport using this model.

EMS System Staffing: Career- and Volunteer-Based

In career-based EMS systems, providers are paid to staff the ambulance units and have preassigned shifts. Benefits of such a system are thought to include greater standardization in the quality of patient care through employer oversight, mandated training, and quality assurance and improvement. Many states and communities, however, still rely heavily on volunteers to provide ambulance coverage; in particular, volunteer personnel have traditionally been the lifeblood of rural EMS agencies. Volunteers may also have preassigned shifts but generally are not paid for their time, although recent research suggests that a fairly large percentage of volunteers receive financial compensation for their EMS activity (Margolis and Studnek, 2006). Equipment and vehicles are frequently maintained using donations or public funds. Oversight of volunteer systems is sometimes provided by the municipal or county agency responsible for EMS, if one exists. The benefits of a volunteer system include the significant cost savings from not having to pay personnel. However, the challenge is maintaining a response system that consistently meets the public demand for quality services.

Most experts agree that there appears to be a national trend toward decreasing volunteerism and an increase in EMS personnel seeking paid careers. During the early stages of EMS, it was not uncommon for volunteers to be on call nearly 24 hours a day. Today, however, increased time demands, the rise in families' needs for dual incomes, and vying interests create an environment in which volunteers may donate one specific weeknight or a few hours on a weekend. As a result, rural EMS agencies in particular are currently faced with volunteer staffing shortages, particularly during weekday work hours.

Many systems are a combination of volunteer- and career-based because of the challenges of maintaining an entirely volunteer system. Such combined systems represent an attempt to achieve cost savings while ensuring adequate services to the public. However, the sustainability of each type of system—career, volunteer, and combination—is unclear as a result of the resource demands on career systems and the lack of personnel for volunteer systems.

Air Ambulance Systems

Air medical operations have grown substantially since their inception in the 1970s. Today there are an estimated 650–700 medical helicopters operating in the United States (Gearhart et al., 1997; Helicopter Association International, 2005; Meier, 2005; Baker et al., 2006), up from approximately 230 in 1990 (Blumen and UCAN Safety Committee, 2002; Helicopter Association International, 2005). These helicopter operations are owned and managed by a variety of entities, including for-profit providers, nonprofit organizations such as local hospitals, government agencies such as the state police, and military air medical service providers. Many air medical providers were originally employed as hospital contractors but now work on an independent basis. Typically, the base helipads for these providers are located in airports, independent hangars and helipads, and designated areas of a hospital (Branas et al., 2005).

Air ambulance operations have served thousands of critically ill or injured persons over the past several decades (Blumen and UCAN Safety Committee, 2002). However, there has been growing concern about the safety of these operations. Approximately 200 people have lost their lives as a result of air medical crashes since 1972, and these deaths have been increasing as the industry continues to expand (Blumen and UCAN Safety Committee, 2002; Bledsoe, 2003; Baker et al., 2006). Crashes are often attributable to pilots flying in poor weather or at night. Li and colleagues (2001) found a four-fold risk of a fatal crash in flights that encountered reduced visibility. Baker and colleagues (2006) found that crashes in darkness represented 48 percent of all crashes and 68 percent of all fatal crashes. In addition, some companies are flying older, single-engine helicopters that lack the instruments needed to help pilots navigate safely (Meier, 2005). In 2004 and 2005 a total of 12 fatal air ambulance crashes occurred—the highest number of fatal crashes in two consecutive years experienced in the industry's history (Isakov, 2006). Recent increases in Medicare payments have led to greater competition in the industry, which has added to concerns regarding safety (Meier, 2005).

Air medical services are believed to improve patient outcomes because of two primary factors: reduced transport time to definitive care and a higher skill mix applied during transport. However, presumed gains in transport time do not necessarily occur, given the time it takes the helicopter crew to launch, find a suitable landing position, and provide care at the scene. This is especially true when the distance to the scene is short. Questions have also been raised regarding the appropriateness of air ambulance deployments in specific patient care situations (Schiller et al., 1988; Moront et al., 1996; Cunningham et al., 1997; Arfken et al., 1998; Dula et al., 2000). A 2002 study found that helicopters were used excessively for patients who were not severely injured and that they often did not deliver patients to the hospital more rapidly than ground ambulances (Levin and Davis, 2005).

On the other hand, a number of other studies suggest benefits of air ambulance service relative to ground transport. Davis and colleagues (2005) found that patients with moderate to severe traumatic brain injury who received care through air ambulance had improved outcomes. In addition, the study found that out-of-hospital intubation among air-transported patients resulted in better outcomes than ED intubation among ground-transported patients. Patients with more severe injuries appeared to derive the greatest benefit from air medical transport. And Gearhart and colleagues (1997) reviewed the literature and reported 1–12 additional survivors per 100 patients flown.

EMS in Rural Areas

According to the 2000 U.S. Census, 21 percent of the nation's population lives in rural and frontier areas. Residents of these areas experience significant health disparities relative to their urban counterparts (Pollock, 2001). A large portion of these disparities results from the distinctive cultural, social, economic, and geographic characteristics that define rural America, but the situation also reflects the difficulty of applying medical systems designed for urban environments to rural and frontier communities.

Rural EMS Challenges

Rural EMS systems face a multitude of challenges. A particularly daunting challenge is providing adequate access to care given the distances involved and the limited assets available. Ensuring the delivery of quality EMS to rural populations is also complicated by the makeup and skill level of prehospital EMS personnel and associated issues of management, funding, and medical direction for rural EMS systems. In 1989, the Office of Technology Assessment estimated that three-quarters of rural prehospital EMS personnel were volunteers (U.S. Congress, Office of Technology Assessment, 1989). A more recent national assessment found that 77 percent of EMS personnel in rural areas were volunteers, compared with 33 percent in urban areas (Minnesota Department of Health, Office of Rural Health Primary Care, 2003).

State health directors list access to quality EMS care as a major rural health concern (O'Grady et al., 2002). In a 2003 survey of national and state rural health experts, 73 percent identified access to health care as a priority issue, and EMS access was cited as a primary concern (Gamm et al., 2003; Rawlinson and Crewes, 2003). In its 2004 report *Quality Through*

Collaboration: The Future of Rural Health, the Institute of Medicine cited EMS as one of four essential health care services for rural residents, along with primary, dental, and mental health care (IOM, 2004).

As noted in Chapter 1, EMS response times from the instigating event to arrival at the hospital are significantly longer in rural than in urban areas. These prolonged response times occur at each step in EMS activation and response, including time to EMS notification, time from EMS notification to arrival at the scene, and time from arrival at the scene to arrival at the hospital. A 2002 survey found that 30 percent of rural patients fatally injured in a crash (compared with 8.3 percent in urban areas) arrived at the hospital more than 60 minutes after the crash, after the "golden hour" had expired (NHTSA, 2005). These prolonged response times are attributable to the increased distances involved, but also to other factors, such as the limits of 9-1-1 availability in sparsely populated areas. While the availability of 9-1-1 extends to the vast majority of the U.S. population, 4 percent of the nation's counties still do not have access to basic 9-1-1 (see Chapter 5). Moreover, enhanced 9-1-1, which provides geographic data to the dispatch center so the location of an incident can be pinpointed, is difficult to implement when a large portion of the rural population uses rural routes and post office boxes to designate addresses (Gausche and Seidel, 1999). In addition, the small number of ambulances available in some rural regions and the inability to priority dispatch these ambulances if there is only one unit available remain a challenge (Key, 2002).

One of the first obstacles to timely EMS activation in rural areas is the delay that commonly occurs in the discovery of crash scenes. On infrequently traveled rural roads, a long time may elapse before victims are discovered. This delay may be the single largest contributor to prolonged times until transport to a hospital (Esposito et al., 1995). In a study of rural Missouri, only 39 percent of calls alerting EMS came within 5 minutes of the collision, compared with 90 percent in urban study areas (Brodsky, 1992). Automated collision notification systems offer the potential for significant improvement in this area (see Chapter 5). In a rural demonstration project conducted by NHTSA during 1995–2000, this technology was demonstrated not only to work, but also to reduce response times (NHTSA, 2001).

When prehospital EMS is activated, there is significant local variation in the type and quality of services provided. Rural EMTs working in an isolated environment while treating a critically ill or injured patient will spend more time with the patient and use fewer resources than urban EMTs or paramedics. Certain clinical scenarios may actually require a greater skill level and more multitasking on the part of rural EMTs as compared with their urban counterparts. As noted, however, EMS systems in rural areas are staffed largely by volunteers with highly variable levels of expertise, training, and experience. A rural EMT may encounter highly critical cases very infrequently as a result of the small size of the local population and the number of volunteers required to cover a schedule. For the limited number of EMS personnel in a largely volunteer system, formal training and critical care experience are often lacking, and even when such training is attained, the low volume of calls contributes to the degradation of critical care skills. Moreover, access to continuing education may be scarce in rural areas (Key, 2002). Additionally, volunteer organizations experience a higher level of provider turnover, which may reduce the number of experienced volunteers. Taken together, these factors mean that rural EMS providers may be less proficient than urban providers.

A high percentage of rural EMS personnel may be trained only in BLS, and indeed, many rural programs offer only BLS services (Minnesota Department of Health, Office of Rural Health Primary Care, 2003). Even when rural EMTs are trained to perform critical tasks, such as endotracheal intubation, their success rate is poor (Sayre et al., 1998), in part because of the infrequent need to exercise such skills noted above. In one study, despite training, rural EMS personnel were able to intubate only 49 percent of their patients successfully. Cited as possible explanations for this low success rate were training deficiencies, infrequent intubation opportunities, and inconsistent supervision (Bradley et al., 1998). Likewise, Spaite (1998) pointed out that rural EMS personnel with defibrillator training may defibrillate a patient only two or three times in a decade, emphasizing a pivotal role for the use of automated external defibrillators. In addition, even when ALS is available in rural areas, the services have repeatedly been demonstrated to be provided at much lower levels of quality than in urban settings (Gausche et al., 1989; Svenson et al., 1996; Seidel et al., 1999).

The availability and qualifications of EMS medical directors are also an issue. Many of these individuals have little or no experience in EMS medical direction. A survey of state EMS directors indicated that recruitment of medical directors is frequently very difficult and that providers serving in that role are often primary care physicians with little or no emergency medicine training. While on-line continuing medical education is becoming more available, it has been slow to take hold; moreover, such training can impart cognitive information, but typically does not teach technical and procedural skills. Nevertheless, the use of telemedicine and distance learning allows previously inaccessible training to penetrate remote areas, while new, more realistic and dynamic patient simulators enable case-based honing of critical skills and decision-making abilities. These tools may be able to offset some of the problems with skill deterioration due to the limited experience attained in rural areas (McGinnis, 2004).

Addressing Rural EMS Challenges

A number of strategies for optimizing EMS resources have been proposed to deal with the paucity of funding, response units, and other resources in rural areas. One such proposal is the dynamic load-responsive deployment of ambulance units. With this approach, ambulances are positioned strategically throughout an area and are dispatched centrally in an effort to reduce response times. Determination of where to position individual units is based on the demand in each area combined with the distance to be traveled, using an established average response time. In one study, load-responsive deployment in a rural area resulted in a 32 percent increase in the number of calls responded to within the established time allowance of 8 minutes (Peleg and Pliskin, 2004). While promising, however, this approach is not possible in very isolated rural communities where EMS units are staffed by volunteers who respond from home.

Another method found to increase the efficiency of EMS systems in rural areas is the establishment of regionally based systems. Such systems may be organized in countywide or larger areas, with ambulances being prepositioned in strategic locations and dispatched centrally (Key, 2002). Basic EMS providers and fire departments scattered throughout the area can act as first responders, with fully equipped units responding after dispatch. Such a system has been used successfully on San Juan Island, a rural island off the coast of Washington State. Killien and colleagues (1996) demonstrated a survival to discharge rate for out-of-hospital cardiac arrest of 22 percent employing this type of system, whereas most studies in rural areas have found survival rates of less than 10 percent (Killien et al., 1996). One of the largest rural regional EMS systems in the United States is that of the East Texas Medical Center. This system serves nearly 17,000 square miles over 17 counties, with 85 ambulance units and two helicopters. Units are dispatched through a central 9-1-1 dispatcher using a modern global positioning system for geographic information (East Texas Medical Center Regional Healthcare System, 2004). In this way, a large rural area encompassing many counties can be served by an EMS system with up-to-date equipment and resources that could not be sustained financially by any one county alone.

Another issue pertinent to rural settings is the involvement of citizens or lay first responders who can provide first aid, start CPR, and take other measures while awaiting the arrival of EMS. The 2005 World Health Organization report *Prehospital Trauma Care Systems* strongly recommends such citizen engagement, particularly in resource-poor communities that cannot afford costly or sophisticated EMS systems (Sasser et al., 2005). Training dispatchers to give prearrival instructions can help reinforce citizen involvement, with or without prior CPR and first-aid training. Although the current standard for CPR training is a 4-hour class taught by a paid instructor, research has shown that citizens can teach themselves CPR with a video and inexpensive manikin in 30 minutes (see Chapter 4). Numerous benefits can result, including more consistent provision of first aid, rapid access to bystander CPR, enhanced community response to disasters and mass-casualty events, and possibly more rational use of EDs and EMS assets.

Role of EMS in Rural Public Health

Individuals in rural communities have less access to the full range of essential public health services than their urban counterparts (U.S. Congress, Office of Technology Assessment, 1989). Many such areas have no local county or city public health agency, and those public health departments that do serve rural areas have few if any staff with formal public health training (Pollock, 2001). As a result, the rural EMS system often assumes a broader role in the community than the typical urban system with regard to both the medical needs of individuals and the public health and safety of the community overall. Because of the lack of physicians and nurses and other medical facilities, it is not unusual in rural communities for EMS to provide informal evaluation, advice, and care that are never reflected in an EMS patient's record and do not involve transportation (McGinnis, 2004). The lack of public health departments may require rural EMS personnel to assume leadership roles in tasks performed traditionally by public health departments, such as immunizations (Pollock, 2001). Finally, the lack of capacity of rural public health departments and a limited rural public safety infrastructure result in greater reliance on rural EMS personnel to participate in disaster preparedness relative to their urban counterparts (Spaite et al., 2001).

REFERENCES

AAA (American Ambulance Association). 2004. *Community Guide to Ensure High-Performance Emergency Ambulance Service*. McLean, VA: AAA.

AAA. 2006. *Ambulance Facts*. [Online]. Available: http://www.the-aaa.org/media/Ambulance-Facts.htm [accessed January 5, 2006].

AEMS (Advocates for Emergency Medical Services). 2005a. *FICEMS Bill*. [Online]. Available: http://www.advocatesforems.org/default.cfm/PID=1.9.24/ [accessed October 1, 2005].

AEMS. 2005b. *EMS Related Fiscal Year 2006 Federal Funding*. [Online]. Available: http://www.advocatesforems.org/Library/upload/EMS_funding_summary_chart3.pdf [accessed October 1, 2005].

Arfken CL, Shapiro MJ, Bessey PQ, Littenberg B. 1998. Effectiveness of helicopter versus ground ambulance services for interfacility transport. *Journal of Trauma-Injury Infection & Critical Care* 45(4):785–790.

Baker SP, Grabowski JG, Dodd RS, Shanahan DF, Lamb MW, Li GH. 2006. EMS helicopter crashes: What influences fatal outcome? *Annals of Emergency Medicine* 47(4):351–356.

Bledsoe BE. 2003. Air medical helicopter accidents in the United States: A five-year review. *Prehospital Emergency Care* 7(1):94–98.

Blumen IJ, UCAN Safety Committee. 2002. *A Safety Review and Risk Assessment in Air Medical Transport.* Salt Lake City, UT: Air Medical Physician Association.

Bradley JS, Billows GL, Olinger ML, Boha SP, Cordell WH, Nelson DR. 1998. Prehospital oral endotracheal intubation by rural basic emergency medical technicians. *Annals of Emergency Medicine* 32(1):26–32.

Branas CC, MacKenzie EJ, Williams JC, Schwab CW, Teter HM, Flanigan MC, Blatt AJ, ReVelle CS. 2005. Access to trauma centers in the United States. *Journal of the American Medical Association* 293(21):2626–2633.

Brodsky H. 1992. Delay in ambulance dispatch to road accidents. *American Journal of Public Health* 82(6):873–875.

Brown WE Jr, Dawson DE, Levine R. 2003. Compensation, benefits, and satisfaction: The Longitudinal Emergency Medical Technical Demographic Study (LEADS) project. *Prehospital Emergency Care* 7(3).

Burt CW, McCaig LF, Valverde RH. 2006. *Analysis of Ambulance Transports and Diversions Among U.S. Emergency Departments.* Hyattsville, MD: National Center for Health Statistics.

Center for Catastrophe Preparedness and Response NYU. 2005. *Emergency Medical Services: The Forgotten First Responder—A Report on the Critical Gaps in Organization and Deficits in Resources for America's Medical First Responders.* New York: Center for Catastrophe Preparedness and Response, New York University.

City and County of San Francisco, Office of the Budget Analyst. 2002. *Management Audit of the San Francisco Fire Department: Introduction.* [Online]. Available: http://www.sfgov.org/site/budanalyst_page.asp?id=4844 [accessed April 20, 2006].

Cunningham P, Rutledge R, Baker CC, Clancy TV. 1997. A comparison of the association of helicopter and ground ambulance transport with the outcome of injury in trauma patients transported from the scene. *Journal of Trauma-Injury Infection & Critical Care* 43(6):940–946.

Davis DP, Hoyt DB, Ochs M, Fortlage D, Holbrook T, Marshall LK, Rosen P. 2003. The effect of paramedic rapid sequence intubation on outcome in patients with severe traumatic brain injury. *Journal of Trauma-Injury Infection & Critical Care* 54(3):444–453.

Davis DP, Peay J, Serrano JA, Buono C, Vilke GM, Sise MJ, Kennedy F, Eastman AB, Velky T, Hoyt DB. 2005. The impact of aeromedical response to patients with moderate to severe traumatic brain injury. *Annals of Emergency Medicine* 46(2):115–122.

Davis R. 2003a, July. Many lives are lost across USA because emergency services fail. *USA Today.* P. 1A.

Davis R. 2003b. The Method: Measure How Many Victims Leave the Hospital Alive. [Online]. Available: http://www.usatoday.com/news/nation/ems-day1-method.htm [accessed January 27, 2007].

Davis R. 2004, August 26. D.C. EMS chief's firing illustrates conflicts over lifesaving reform: Turf wars hamper efforts across USA. *USA Today.* P. B14.

Delbridge TR, Bailey B, Chew JL Jr, Conn AK, Krakeel JJ, Manz D, Miller DR, O'Malley PJ, Ryan SD, Spaite DW, Stewart RD, Suter RE, Wilson EM. 1998. EMS agenda for the future: Where we are . . . where we want to be. *Prehospital Emergency Care* 2(1):1–12.

DHHS (Department of Health and Human Services). 2003. *Emergency Medical Treatment and Labor Act (EMTALA) Interim Guidance. Center for Medicare and Medicaid Services' Center for Medicaid and State Operations, Survey and Certification Group.* Baltimore, MD: DHHS.

Dula DJ, Palys K, Leicht M, Madtes K. 2000. Helicopter versus ambulance transport of patients with penetrating trauma. *Air Medical Journal* 36(4):S76.

East Texas Medical Center Regional Healthcare System. 2004. *ETMC EMS.* [Online]. Available: http://emsservices.etmc.org [accessed September 2004].

Elting K, Toddy M. 2003. *New Rules Clarify EMTALA Obligations.* [Online]. Available: http://www.jonesday.com/pubs/pubs_detail.aspx?pubID=S1820 [accessed May 24, 2006].

EMS Insider. 2005. *EMS Employers Struggle with Paramedic Shortages.* [Online]. Available: http://www.jems.com/insider/4_04.html [accessed April 4, 2005].

Esposito TJ, Sanddal ND, Hansen JD, Reynolds S. 1995. Analysis of preventable trauma deaths and inappropriate trauma care in a rural state. *The Journal of Trauma* 39(5):955–962.

Franks PE, Kocher N, Chapman S. 2004. *Emergency Medical Technicians and Paramedics in California.* San Francisco, CA: University of California, San Francisco Center for the Health Professions.

Gamm L, Hutchison L, Dabney BJ, Dorsey A, eds. 2003. *Rural Healthy People 2010: A Companion Document to Healthy People 2010* (Volume 1). College Station, TX: Southwest Rural Health Research Center.

GAO (U.S. Government Accountability Office). 2001a. *Emergency Care. EMTALA Implementation and Enforcement Issues.* Washington, DC: Government Printing Office.

GAO. 2001b. *Emergency Medical Services: Reported Needs Are Wide-Ranging, with a Growing Focus on Lack of Data* (GAO-2-28). Washington, DC: Government Printing Office.

GAO. 2003. *Hospital Emergency Departments: Crowded Conditions Vary among Hospitals and Communities.* Washington, DC: Government Printing Office.

Gausche M, Seidel JS. 1999. Out-of-hospital care of pediatric patients. *Pediatric Clinics of North America* 46(6):1305–1327.

Gausche M, Seidel JS, Henderson DP, Ness B, Ward PM, Wayland BW, Almeida B. 1989. Pediatric deaths and emergency medical services (EMS) in urban and rural areas. *Pediatric Emergency Care* 5(3):158–162.

Gausche M, Lewis RJ, Stratton SJ, Haynes BE, Gunter CS, Goodrich SM, Poore PD, McCollough MD, Henderson DP, Pratt FD, Seidel JS. 2000. Effect of out-of-hospital pediatric endotracheal intubation on survival and neurologic outcome: A controlled clinical trial. *Journal of the American Medical Association* 283(6):783–790.

Gearhart PA, Wuerz R, Localio AR. 1997. Cost-effectiveness analysis of helicopter EMS for trauma patients. *Annals of Emergency Medicine* 30(4):500–506.

Hauert SA. 1990. *The MPDS and Medical-Legal Danger Zones.* [Online]. Available: http://www.emergencydispatch.org/articles/medicallegal1.htm [accessed February 24, 2006].

Helicopter Association International. 2005. *White Paper: Improving Safety in Helicopter Emergency Medical Services (HEMS) Operations.* Alexandria, VA: Helicopter Association International.

IOM (Institute of Medicine). 1985. *Injury in America.* Washington, DC: National Academy Press.

IOM. 1993. *Emergency Medical Services for Children.* Washington, DC: National Academy Press.

IOM. 2000. *To Err Is Human: Building a Safer Health System.* Washington, DC: National Academy Press.

IOM. 2004. *Quality through Collaboration: The Future of Rural Health.* Washington, DC: The National Academies Press.

Isakov AP. 2006. Souls on board: Helicopter emergency medical services and safety. *Annals of Emergency Medicine* 47(4):357–360.

JCAHO (Joint Commission for the Accreditation of Healthcare Organizations). 2002. Delays in treatment. *Sentinel Event Alert* (26):1–3.

Kaiser Commission on Medicaid and the Uninsured. 2003. *Medicaid Benefits.* [Online]. Available: http://www.kff.org/medicaid/benefits/index.cfm [accessed August 20, 2004].

Keim SM, Spaite DW, Maio RF, Garrison HG, Desmond JS, Gregor MA, O'Malley PJ, Stiell IG, Cayten CG, Chew JL Jr, Mackenzie EJ, Miller DR. 2004. Risk adjustment and outcome measures for out-of-hospital respiratory distress. *Academic Emergency Medicine* 11(10):1074–1081.

Key CB. 2002. Operational issues in EMS. *Emergency Medicine Clinics of North America* 20(4):913–927.

Killien SY, Geyman JP, Gossom JB, Gimlett D. 1996. Out-of-hospital cardiac arrest in a rural area: A 16–year experience with lessons learned and national comparisons. *Annals of Emergency Medicine* 28(3):294–300.

Levin A, Davis R. 2005, July 18. Surge in crashes scars air ambulance industry. *USA Today*. P. 1A.

Lewis RJ, Berry DA, Cryer H III, Fost N, Krome R, Washington GR, Houghton J, Blue JW, Bechhofer R, Cook T, Fisher M. 2001. Monitoring a clinical trial conducted under the food and drug administration regulations allowing a waiver of prospective informed consent: The diaspirin cross-linked hemoglobin traumatic hemorrhagic shock efficacy trial. *Annals of Emergency Medicine* 38(4):397–404.

Li G, Baker SP, Grabowski JG, Rebok GW. 2001. Factors associated with pilot error in aviation crashes. *Aviation, Space, and Environmental Medicine* 72(1):52–58.

Margolis G, Studnek J. 2006. How many volunteers are there really? *Journal of Emergency Medical Services* 31(3).

Martinez R. 1998. New vision for the role of emergency medical services. *Annals of Emergency Medicine* 32(5):594–599.

McGinnis K. 2004. *Rural and Frontier Emergency Medical Services Agenda for the Future.* Kansas City, MO: National Rural Health Association.

Mears G. 2004. *2003 Survey and Analysis of EMS Scope of Practice and Practice Settings Impacting EMS Services in Rural America: Executive Brief and Recommendations.* Chapel Hill, NC: University of North Carolina at Chapel Hill Department of Emergency Medicine.

MedPAC (Medicare Payment Advisory Committee). 2003. *Appendix A: How Medicare Pays for Services: An Overview.* Washington, DC: MedPAC.

Meier B. 2005, February 28. Fatal crashes provoke debate on safety of sky ambulances. *The New York Times.* P. A1.

Minnesota Department of Health, Office of Rural Health Primary Care. 2003. *Profile of Rural Ambulance Services in Minnesota.* [Online]. Available: http://www.health.state.mn.us/divs/chs/rhpc/Worddocs/RHProfile-EMS.doc [accessed December 18, 2005].

Monosky KA. 2004. The JEMS 2003 200 city survey. *Journal of Emergency Medical Services* 29(2):38–53.

Moront ML, Gotschall CS, Eichelberger MR. 1996. Helicopter transport of injured children: System effectiveness and triage criteria. *Journal of Pediatric Surgery* 31(8):1183–1186; discussion 1187–1188.

Murray JA, Demetriades D, Berne TV, Stratton SJ, Cryer HG, Bongard F, Fleming A. 2000. Prehospital intubation in patients with severe head injury. *The Journal of Trauma* 49(6):1065–1070.

NAS, NRC (National Academy of Sciences, National Research Council). 1966. *Accidental Death and Disability: The Neglected Disease of Modern Society.* Washington, DC: NAS.

NAS, NRC. 1972. *Roles and Resources of Federal Agencies in Support of Comprehensive Emergency Medical Services.* Washington, DC: NAS.

NAS, NRC. 1978. *Emergency Medical Services at Midpassage.* Washington, DC: NAS.

NASEMSD (National Association of State EMS Directors). 2005. *Special Report: Implementation Status of the EMS Agenda for the Future.* Falls Church, VA: NASEMSD.

National Commission on Terrorist Attacks upon the United States. 2004. *The 9/11 Commission Report.* Washington, DC: National Commission on Terrorist Attacks upon the United States.

National Emergency Number Association. 2004. *The Development of 9-1-1.* [Online]. Available: http://www.nena.org/PR_Pubs/Devel_of_911.htm [accessed September 28, 2004].

National Fire Protection Association. 2005. *Fire Department Calls.* Quincy, MA: National Fire Protection Association.

National Registry of Emergency Medical Technicians. 2003. *Longitudinal Emergency Medical Technician Attributes and Demographics Survey (LEADS) Data.* [Online]. Available: http://www.nremt.org/about/lead_survey.asp [accessed November 28, 2005].

NHTSA (National Highway Traffic Safety Administration). 1996. *Emergency Medical Services Agenda for the Future.* Washington, DC: U.S. Department of Transportation. [Online]. Available: http://www.nhtsa.dot.gov/people/injury/ems/agenda/emsman.html [accessed May 25, 2006].

NHTSA. 2001. Automatic collision notification field test summary. *Annals of Emergency Medicine* 38(4):453–454.

NHTSA. 2005. *Fatality Analysis Reporting System (FARS) Web-Based Encyclopedia.* [Online]. Available: http://www-fars.nhtsa.dot.gov [accessed January 1, 2006].

NHTSA Technical Assistance Program. 2000. *Statewide EMS Reassessments: Program Guide.* Washington, DC: NHTSA.

O'Grady MJ, Mueller C, Wilensky GR. 2002. *Essential Research Issues in Rural Health: The State Rural Health Director's Perspective* (Policy Analysis Brief, Series W.5). Bethesda, MD: Project Hope, Walsh Center for Rural Analysis.

Overton J. 2002. *Reimbursement Trends.* Kuehl AE, ed. Dubuque, IA: Kendall/Hunt Publishing Company.

Peleg K, Pliskin JS. 2004. A geographic information system simulation model of EMS: Reducing ambulance response time. *American Journal of Emergency Medicine* 22(3):164–170.

Pollock DA. 2001. Barriers to health care access: What counts and who's counting? *Academic Emergency Medicine* 8(11):1016–1018.

Pozner CN, Zane R, Nelson S, Levine M. 2004. International EMS systems: The United States: Past, present, and future. *Resuscitation* 60:239–244.

Rawlinson C, Crewes P. 2003. Access to quality health services in rural areas: Emergency medical services. In: *Rural Healthy People 2010: A Companion Document to Healthy People 2010.* College Station, TX: The Texas A&M University System Health Science Center, School of Rural Public Health, Southwest Rural Health Research Center.

Sasser S, Varghese M, Kellermann A, Lormand JD. 2005. *Prehospital Trauma Care Systems.* Geneva, Switzerland: World Health Organization.

Sayre MR, Sakles JC, Mistler AF, Evans JL, Kramer AT, Pancioli AM. 1998. Field trial of endotracheal intubation by basic EMTs. *Annals of Emergency Medicine* 31(2):228–233.

Schiller WR, Knox R, Zinnecker H, Jeevanandam M, Sayre M, Burke J, Young DH. 1988. Effect of helicopter transport of trauma victims on survival in an urban trauma center. *Journal of Trauma-Injury Infection & Critical Care* 28(8):1127–1134.

Schmitt K, Shimberg B. 1996. *Demystifying Occupational and Professional Regulation: Answers to Questions You Have Been Afraid to Ask.* Lexington, KY: Council on Licensure, Enforcement and Regulation.

Seidel J, Henderson D, Tittle S, Jaffe D, Spaite D, Dean J, Gausche M, Lewis R, Cooper A, Zaritsky A, Espisito T, Maederis D. 1999. Priorities for research in emergency medical services for children: Results of a consensus conference. *Annals of Emergency Medicine* 33(2):206–210.

Shimberg B, Roederer D. 1994. *Questions a Legislator Should Ask.* Lexington, KY: Council on Licensure, Enforcement and Regulation.

Spaite D. 1998. Intubation by basic EMTs: Lifesaving advance or catastrophic complication? *Annals of Emergency Medicine* 31(2):276–277.

Spaite DW, Maio R, Garrison HG, Desmond JS, Gregor MA, Stiell IG, Cayten CG, Chew JL Jr, Mackenzie EJ, Miller DR, O'Malley PJ. 2001. Emergency medical services outcomes project (EMSOP) II: Developing the foundation and conceptual models for out-of-hospital outcomes research. *Annals of Emergency Medicine* 37(6):657–663.

Svenson JE, Spurlock C, Nypaver M. 1996. Factors associated with the higher traumatic death rate among rural children. *Annals of Emergency Medicine* 27(5):625–632.

U.S. Congress, Office of Technology Assessment. 1989. *Rural Emergency Medical Services—Special Report*. Washington, DC: U.S. Government Printing Office.

U.S. Fire Administration. 2005. *Federal Interagency Committee on Emergency Medical Services (FICEMS)*. [Online]. Available: http://www.usfa.fema.gov/subjects/ems/ficems.shtm [accessed January 5, 2006].

Wanerman R. 2002. The emtala paradox. Emergency medical treatment and labor act. *Annals of Emergency Medicine* 40(5):464–469.

Wang HE, Peitzman AB, Cassidy LD, Adelson PD, Yealy DM. 2004. Out-of-hospital endotracheal intubation and outcome after traumatic brain injury. *Annals of Emergency Medicine* 44(5):439–450.

Williams D. 2005. 2004 JEMS 200-city survey. *Journal of Emergency Medical Services* 30(2):42–60.

3

Building a 21st-Century Emergency and Trauma Care System

While today's emergency and trauma care system offers significantly more medical capability than was available in years past, it continues to suffer from severe fragmentation, an absence of systemwide coordination, and a lack of accountability. These shortcomings diminish the care provided to emergency patients and often result in worsened medical outcomes (Davis, 2003). To address these challenges and chart a new direction for emergency and trauma care, the committee envisions a system in which all communities will be served by well-planned and highly coordinated emergency and trauma care systems that are accountable for performance and serve the needs of patients of all ages within the system.

In this new system, 9-1-1 dispatchers, emergency medical services (EMS) personnel, medical providers, public safety officers, and public health officials will be fully interconnected and united in an effort to ensure that each patient receives the most appropriate care, at the optimal location, with the minimum delay. From the patient's point of view, delivery of services for every type of emergency will be seamless. All service delivery will also be evidence-based, and innovations will be rapidly adopted and adapted to each community's needs. Hospital emergency department (ED) closures and ambulance diversions will never occur, except in the most extreme situations, such as a hospital fire or a communitywide mass casualty event. Standby capacity appropriate to each community based on its disaster risks will be embedded in the system. The performance of the system will be transparent, and the public will be actively engaged in its operation through prevention, bystander training, and monitoring of system performance.

While these objectives will require substantial, systemwide change, they are achievable. Early progress toward the goal of more integrated, coordinated, and regionalized emergency and trauma care systems became derailed over the last two decades (see Chapter 2). Efforts stalled because of deeply entrenched interests and cultural attitudes, as well as funding cutbacks and practical impediments to change. These obstacles remain today and represent the primary challenges to achieving the committee's vision. However, the problems are becoming more apparent, and this provides a catalyst for change. The committee calls for concerted, cooperative efforts at multiple levels of government and the private sector to finally break through and achieve these goals.

This chapter describes the committee's vision for a 21st-century emergency and trauma care system. This vision rests on the broad goals of improved coordination, expanded regionalization, and increased transparency and accountability, each of which is discussed in turn. The chapter then profiles current approaches of states and local regions that exhibit these features. Finally, the chapter details the committee's recommendation for a federal demonstration program to support additional state and local efforts aimed at attaining the vision of a more coordinated and effective emergency and trauma care system.

IMPROVING COORDINATION

Today's emergency and trauma care system suffers from fragmentation along a number of different dimensions. As described in Chapter 2, EMS occupies a space that overlaps three major silos: health care, public health, and public safety. In most cases, these three systems are not aligned, and their means of communicating or coordinating with one another are highly limited. Within health care, there is considerable fragmentation along a number of dimensions relating to EMS. For example, coordination among 9-1-1 dispatch, prehospital EMS, air medical providers, and hospital and trauma centers is often lacking (NHTSA, 1996). EMS personnel arriving at the scene of an incident often do not know what to expect regarding the number of injured or their condition (McGinnis, 2005). They also are frequently unaware of which hospitals are on diversion status and which are ready to receive the type of patient they are transporting. Lack of coordination between EMS and hospitals can result in delays that compromise care. In addition, deployment of air medical services is often not well coordinated. While air medical providers are not permitted to self-dispatch, a lack of coordination at the ground EMS and dispatch level sometimes results in multiple air ambulances arriving at the scene of a crash even when all are not needed. Similarly, police, fire, and EMS personnel and equipment often overcrowd a crash scene because of insufficient coordination regarding the appropriate response.

In addition, in many communities there is little interaction between emergency care services and community safety net providers, even though the two share a common base of patients, and their actions may affect one another substantially. The absence of coordination represents missed opportunities for enhanced access, improved diagnosis, patient follow-up and compliance, and enhanced quality of care and patient satisfaction.

Coordination between EMS and public health agencies could also be improved. Through their regular activities, EMS providers have information that could serve as a barometer for both illness and injury trends within the community, potentially assisting state and local public health departments. However, communication links between these agencies are often not well established. Moreover, although prevention activities are generally limited in the emergency care setting, utilization of emergency services represents an important opportunity for imparting information on injury prevention to patients. Emergency care providers could benefit from the resources and experiences of public health agencies and experts in establishing injury prevention activities.

Finally, perhaps now more than ever, with the threat of bioterrorism and outbreaks of diseases such as avian influenza, it is essential that EMS, EDs, trauma centers, and state and local public health agencies partner to conduct surveillance for disease prevalence and outbreaks and other health risks. Emergency responders can recognize the diagnostic clues that may indicate an unusual infectious disease outbreak so that public health authorities can respond quickly (GAO, 2003c). However, a partnership that allows for improved communication of information between emergency care providers and public health officials must first be in place.

Movement Toward Greater Coordination

The value of integrating and coordinating emergency and trauma care has long been recognized. For example, the 1966 National Academy of Sciences/National Research Council (NAS/NRC) report *Accidental Death and Disability: The Neglected Disease of Modern Society* called for better coordination of emergency and trauma care through community councils on emergency medical services, which would bring together physicians, medical facilities, EMS, public health agencies, and others to procure equipment, construct facilities, and ensure optimal emergency care on a day-to-day basis, as well as in a disaster or national emergency (NAS and NRC, 1966).

Although the drive toward system development waned when federal funding of EMS was folded into state block grants in 1981, the goal of system planning and coordination has remained paramount within the emergency and trauma care community. In 1996, the National Highway Traffic

Safety Administration's (NHTSA) *Emergency Medical Services Agenda for the Future* also emphasized the goal of system integration:

> EMS of the future will be community-based health management that is fully integrated with the overall health care system. It will have the ability to identify and modify illness and injury risks, provide acute illness and injury care and follow-up, and contribute to treatment of chronic conditions and community health monitoring. . . . [P]atients are assured that their care is considered part of a complete health care program, connected to sources for continuous and/or follow-up care, and linked to potentially beneficial health resources. . . . EMS maintains liaisons, including systems for communication with other community resources, such as other public safety agencies, departments of public health, social service agencies and organizations, health care provider networks, community health educators, and others. . . . EMS is a community resource, able to initiate important follow-up care for patients, whether or not they are transported to a health care facility. (NHTSA, 1996, pp. 7, 10)

While the concept of a highly integrated emergency and trauma care system as articulated by NHTSA was not new, progress toward its realization has been slow. Nevertheless, there have been important successes in the coordination of emergency and trauma care services that point the way toward solutions to the problem of fragmentation. The most important example of such successes is the trauma system, which has developed a comprehensive and coordinated approach to the care of injured patients. Children's hospitals have been successful in effecting regional coordination to ensure transport and appropriate care for children with specialized needs. The pediatric intensive care system is a leading example of regional coordination among hospitals, community physicians, and EMS providers (Gausche-Hill and Wiebe, 2001). These examples demonstrate the possibilities for enhanced coordination across the system as a whole.

Importance of Communication

Communication is critical to establishing systemwide coordination. An effective communications system is the glue that can hold together effective, integrated emergency and trauma care services. It provides the key link between 9-1-1 dispatch and EMS responders and is necessary to ensure that on-line medical direction is available when needed. It enables dispatchers to offer prearrival instructions to callers requesting an ambulance. An effective communications system also enables ambulance dispatchers to assist EMS personnel in directing patients to the most appropriate facilities based on the nature of their injuries and the facilities' fluctuating capacity. Good communication is necessary to link EMS personnel with other public safety providers, such as police, fire and emergency management, and public health, and can facilitate coordination and incident command in disaster situations. Effective communication also facilitates medical and operational oversight and quality control within the system. In Chapter 5, the committee stresses the importance of fully integrated communications systems to link EMS with hospital, public safety, public health, and emergency management personnel.

SUPPORTING REGIONALIZATION

The objective of regionalization is to improve patient outcomes by directing patients to facilities with experience in and optimal capabilities for any given type of illness or injury. Substantial evidence demonstrates that doing so improves outcomes and reduces costs across a range of high-risk conditions and procedures, including cardiac arrest and stroke (Grumbach et al., 1995; Imperato et al., 1996; Nallamothu et al., 2001; Chang and Klitzner, 2002; Bardach et al., 2004). The literature also supports the benefits of regionalization of treatment for severely injured trauma patients in improving patient outcomes of care, reducing mortality from traumatic injury, and lowering costs (Jurkovich and Mock, 1999; MacKenzie, 1999; Mann et al., 1999; Mullins, 1999; Mullins and Mann, 1999; Nathens et al., 2000; Chiara and Cimbanassi, 2003; Bravata et al., 2004; MacKenzie et al., 2006), although the evidence here is not uniformly positive (Glance et al., 2004). Formal protocols within a region for prehospital and hospital care contribute to improved patient outcomes as well (Bravata et al., 2004). In addition, organized trauma systems have been shown to add value in facilitating performance measurement and promoting research.

While regionalization of trauma services to high-volume centers is optimal when feasible, Nathens and Maier (2001) argued for an inclusive trauma system in which smaller facilities have been verified and designated as lower-level trauma centers. They suggested that the quality of care may be substantially better in such facilities than in those outside the system, and comparable to national norms. Inclusive trauma systems are designed to cover the entire continuum of care of the injured patient, from the site of injury through acute care and, when appropriate, rehabilitation. Such a system requires the committed involvement of all qualified medical facilities in the region. An efficient triage system, coupled with established transfer agreements, is required to ensure that patients receive the right care in the right place at the right time. In addition, all facilities caring for injured patients must be evaluated for standards of care and must contribute at least a minimal dataset to support systemwide quality/performance improvement programs.

Regionalization may also be a cost-effective strategy for developing and training teams of response personnel. Regionalization benefits triage, medical care, outbreak investigations, security management, and emergency management. Indeed, both the Health Resources and Services Administration (HRSA) and the Centers for Disease Control and Prevention (CDC) have made regional planning a condition for preparedness funding (GAO, 2003a).

Concerns About Regionalization

The case for regionalization of emergency services is strong, but not absolute. Regionalization can adversely impact the overall availability of clinical services in a community if directing a large number of patients to a regional program leads to elimination of needed services at other facilities. For example, the loss of a profitable set of patients, such as those with suspected acute myocardial infarction (AMI), could result in the closure of a smaller hospital's cardiac unit or even the entire hospital. The survival of small rural facilities may require the identification and treatment of patients who do not require the capacities and capabilities of larger facilities, as well as repatriation to a local facility for long-term care and follow-up after stabilization at a tertiary center. It is important to take a systems approach that considers the full effects of regionalization on a community.

Determining the appropriate metrics for this type of analysis and defining the process for applying those metrics within each region raise significant research and practical issues. Nonetheless, in the absence of rigorous evidence to guide the process, planning authorities should take the above factors into account in developing regionalized systems of emergency and trauma care. Also, the committee is wary of regionalization that results in directing patients to specialty hospitals that do not provide comprehensive emergency services, as these facilities can drain financial resources from those hospitals that do provide such care (GAO, 2003b; Dummit, 2005).

Configuration of Services

The design of the emergency and trauma care system envisioned by the committee bears similarities to the inclusive trauma system originally conceived and first proposed and developed by CDC, and adapted and disseminated by the American College of Surgeons (ACS). Under this approach, every hospital in a community can play a role in the trauma system by undergoing state verification and designation as a level I to level IV/V trauma center based on its capabilities. Trauma care is optimized in the region through protocols and transfer agreements that are designed to direct trauma patients to the most appropriate level of care available given the type of injury and relative travel times to each center.

In addition to trauma center verification, ACS, along with the American

College of Emergency Physicians (ACEP), state EMS directors, NHTSA, HRSA, trauma nurses, and others, has developed the nascent Trauma Systems Consultation program. Under this program, on-site consultation is provided when requested by the lead agency of a region. The consultation is performed by a multidisciplinary team, which evaluates all components of the system and offers specific recommendations for raising the system to the next level, regardless of how embryonic or mature the system may be. An important feature of these consultations is that they cover the entire continuum of care. A number of regions have sought and received such a consultation.

The committee's vision expands the concept of an inclusive trauma system to encompass all illnesses and injuries, as well as the entire continuum of emergency care—including 9-1-1 dispatch, prehospital EMS, and clinics and urgent care providers that may take part in emergency care. All providers can play a role in supplying emergency care in their community according to their capabilities. Under the committee's vision, providers would undergo a process by which their capabilities would be identified and categorized in a manner not unlike trauma verification and designation; the result would be a complete inventory of emergency and trauma care providers within a community. Initially, this categorization might simply be based on the existence of a service—for example, the availability of a cardiac catheterization laboratory or coverage by a neurosurgeon. Eventually, the categorization process might evolve to include more detailed information—for example, the availability of specific emergency procedures and on-call specialty care and indicators of quality, including both service-specific outcomes and general indicators, such as time to treatment, frequency of diversion, and ED boarding. Prehospital EMS could be similarly categorized according to ambulance capacity, availability, credentials of EMS personnel, advanced life support (ALS) and pediatric ALS, treat and release and search and rescue capabilities, disaster readiness (e.g., personal protective equipment), and outcomes (e.g., survival rate from witnessed cardiac arrest due to ventricular fibrillation).

A standard national approach to the categorization of emergency and trauma care providers is needed. Categories should reflect meaningful differences in the types of emergency and trauma care available, yet be simple enough to be understood easily by the provider community and the public. The use of national definitions would ensure that the categories would be understood by providers and by the public across states or regions of the country and would promote benchmarking of performance. Therefore, the committee recommends that the **Department of Health and Human Services and the National Highway Traffic Safety Administration, in partnership with professional organizations, convene a panel of individuals with multidisciplinary expertise to develop evidence-based categorization systems for** emergency medical services, emergency departments, and trauma centers based on adult and pediatric service capabilities (3.1). The results of this process would be a complete inventory of emergency and trauma care assets for each community, which should be updated regularly to reflect the rapid changes in delivery systems nationwide. The development of the initial categorization system should be completed within 18 months of the release of this report.

Treatment, Triage, and Transport

Once understood, the basic classification system proposed above could be used to determine the optimal destination for patients based on their condition and location. However, more research and discussion are needed to determine the circumstances under which patients should be brought to the closest hospital for stabilization and transfer as opposed to being transported directly to the facility offering the highest level of care, even if that facility is farther away. Debate continues over whether EMS personnel should perform ALS procedures in the field, or rapid transport to definitive care is best (Wright and Klein, 2001). The answer to this question likely depends, at least in part, on the type of emergency condition. It is evident, for example, that whether a patient will survive out-of-hospital cardiac arrest depends almost entirely on actions taken at the scene, including rapid defibrillation, provision of cardiopulmonary resuscitation (CPR), and perhaps other ALS interventions. Delaying these actions until the unit reaches a hospital results in dismal rates of survival and poor neurological outcomes. Conversely, there is little that prehospital personnel can do to stop internal bleeding from major trauma. In this instance, rapid transport to definitive care in an operating room offers the victim the best odds of survival.

EMS responders who provide stabilization before the patient arrives at a critical care unit are sometimes subject to criticism because of a strongly held belief among many physicians that out-of-hospital stabilization only delays definitive treatment without adding value; however, there is little evidence that the prevailing "scoop and run" paradigm of EMS is always optimal (Orr et al., 2006). In cases of out-of-hospital cardiac arrest, properly trained and equipped EMS personnel can provide all needed interventions at the scene. In fact, research has shown that failure to reestablish a pulse on the scene virtually ensures that the patient will not survive, regardless of what is done at the hospital (Kellermann et al., 1993). On the other hand, the scoop and run approach makes sense when a critical intervention needed by the patient can be provided only at the hospital.

Decisions regarding the appropriate steps to take should be resolved using the best available evidence. Therefore, the committee recommends that **the National Highway Traffic Safety Administration, in partnership** with professional organizations, convene a panel of individuals with multidisciplinary expertise to develop evidence-based model prehospital care protocols for the treatment, triage, and transport of patients (3.2). The transport protocols should also reflect the state of readiness of given facilities within a region at a particular point in time. Real-time, concurrent information on the availability of hospital resources and specialists should be furnished to EMS personnel to support transport decisions. Development of an initial set of model protocols should be completed within 18 months of the release of this report. These protocols would facilitate much more uniform treatment of injuries and illnesses nationwide so that all patients would receive the current standard of care at the most appropriate location. The protocols might require modification to reflect local resources, capabilities, and transport times; however, they would acknowledge the fact that the basic pathophysiology of human illness is the same in all areas of the country. Once in place, the national protocols could be tailored to local assets and needs. The process for updating the protocols will also be important because it will dictate how rapidly patients will receive the current standard of care.

The 1966 NAS/NRC report *Accidental Death and Disability* anticipated the need to categorize care facilities and improve transport decisions:

> The patient must be transported to the emergency department best prepared for his particular problem. . . . Hospital emergency departments should be surveyed . . . to determine the numbers and types of emergency facilities necessary to provide optimal emergency treatment for the occupants of each region. . . . Once the required numbers and types of treatment facilities have been determined, it may be necessary to lessen the requirements at some institutions, increase them in others, and even redistribute resources to support space, equipment, and personnel in the major emergency facilities. Until patient, ambulance driver, and hospital staff are in accord as to what the patient might reasonably expect and what the staff of an emergency facility can logically be expected to administer, and until effective transportation and adequate communication are provided to deliver casualties to proper facilities, our present levels of knowledge cannot be applied to optimal care and little reduction in mortality and/or lasting disability can be expected. (NAS and NRC, 1966, p. 20)

These views were echoed in the 1993 Institute of Medicine (IOM) report *Emergency Medical Services for Children*, which stated that "categorization and regionalization are essential for full and effective operation of systems" (IOM, 1993, p. 171).

Once the decision has been made to transport a patient, the responding ambulance unit should be instructed—either by written protocol or by on-line medical direction—which hospital should receive the patient (see Figure 3-1). This instruction should be based on developed transport

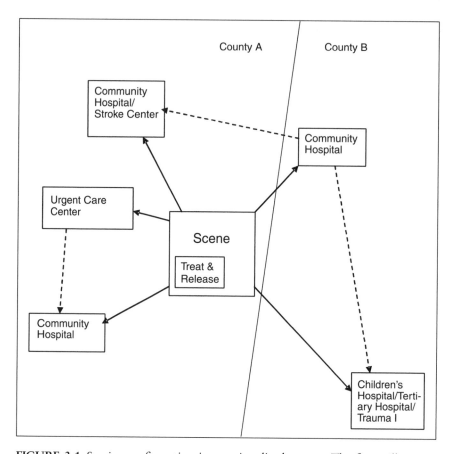

FIGURE 3-1 Service configuration in a regionalized system. The figure illustrates some potential transport options within a regionalized system. The basic structure of current EMS systems is not altered, but protocols are refined to ensure that patients go to the optimal facility given their type of illness or injury, the travel time involved, and facility status (e.g., availability of ED and intensive care unit [ICU] beds). For example, instead of taking a stroke victim to the closest general community hospital or to a tertiary medical center that is farther away, there may be a third option—transport to a community hospital with a stroke center. Over time, based on evidence on the effectiveness of alternative delivery models, some patients may be transported to a nearby urgent care center for stabilization or treated on the street and released. Whichever pathway the patient follows, communications are enhanced, data collected, and the performance of the system evaluated and reported so that future improvements can be made.

protocols to ensure that the patient is taken to the optimal facility given the severity and nature of the illness or injury, the status of the various care facilities, and the travel times involved. Ideally, this decision should take into account a number of complex and fluctuating factors, such as hospital ED closures and diversions and traffic congestion that hinders transport times for the EMS unit (The SAFECOM Project, 2004).

In addition to using ambulance units and the EMS system to direct patients to the optimum location for emergency and trauma care, hospital emergency and trauma care designations should be posted prominently to improve patients' self-triage decisions. Such postings can educate the public about the types of emergency services available in their community and enable patients who are not using EMS to direct themselves to the optimal facility.

FOSTERING ACCOUNTABILITY

Fostering accountability is perhaps the most important of the committee's three goals because it is necessary to achieve the other two. Lack of accountability has contributed to the failure of the emergency and trauma care system to adopt needed changes in the past. Without accountability, participants in the system need not accept responsibility for their failures and can avoid making changes necessary to avoid them in the future.

Accountability has failed to take hold in EMS systems because responsibility is dispersed across many different components of the system; thus it is difficult for policy makers to determine when a system breakdown occurs, much less where it is located or how it can be adequately addressed. EMS diversion is a good example. When a city recognizes it has an unacceptably high frequency of diversions, the locus of responsibility for the problem remains unclear. EMS can blame the ED for crowded conditions and excessively long off-loading times; EDs can blame their hospital for not transporting admitted patients to inpatient units promptly; hospitals can blame on-call specialists or the discharging physician, as well as long-term care facilities that are unwilling to take additional referrals; and all players in the system can blame the state public health department for inadequate funding of community-based alternatives or community physicians for failing to manage their patients adequately so as to keep them out of the ED.

The unpredictable and infrequent nature of emergency and trauma care contributes to the lack of accountability. Most people have limited exposure to the emergency and trauma care system and consider it unlikely that they will ever require an ambulance transport. Consequently, public awareness of specific problem areas in the system is limited. In fact, however, Americans visit EDs more than 114 million times a year, and more than 16 million of these visits involve transport by ambulance (Burt et al., 2006).

Public awareness is also hindered by the lack of nationally defined indicators of system performance. Few localities can answer basic questions about their emergency and trauma care services, such as "What is the overall performance of the emergency care system?"; "How well do 9-1-1, dispatch, prehospital EMS, hospital emergency and trauma care, and other components of the system perform?"; "What is the system's success rate for resuscitating victims of out-of-hospital cardiac arrest compared with other cities of similar size?"; and "How does the system's performance compare with that in other regions and the rest of the nation?" By and large, the public assumes that the system functions better than it actually does (Harris Interactive, 2004), and awareness of the problems plaguing the system is very limited.

The committee believes several steps are required to bring accountability into the emergency and trauma care system. These include the development of national performance indicators, the measurement of system performance, and public dissemination of performance information.

Development of National Performance Indicators

There is currently no shortage of performance measurement and standards-setting projects. For example, ED performance measures have been developed by Qualis Health and Lindsay (Lindsay et al., 2002). In addition, the Data Elements for Emergency Department Systems (DEEDS) project and Health Level Seven (HL7) are working to develop uniform specifications for ED performance data (Pollock et al., 1998; CDC and NCICP, 2001; HL7, 2005).

The EMS Performance Measures Project is coordinated by the National Association of State EMS Officials in partnership with the National Association of EMS Physicians, and is supported by NHTSA and HRSA. The project is working to develop consensus measures of EMS system performance that will assist in demonstrating the system's value and defining an adequate level of EMS capacity and preparedness for a given community (measureEMS.org, 2005). The consensus process of the project has sought to unify disparate efforts to measure performance previously undertaken nationwide that have lacked consistency in definitions, indicators, and data sources. Work undertaken under the project in 2004 resulted in the development of 138 indicators of EMS performance. This list was pared down to 25 indicators in 2005. The list included system measures, such as "What are the time intervals in a call?" and "What percentage of transports is conducted with red lights and sirens?", and clinical measures, such as "How well was my pain relieved?" The questions were defined using data elements from the National EMS Information System (NEMSIS) dataset so that results could be compared with validity across EMS systems (see Chapter 5).

In addition, statewide trauma and EMS systems are evaluated by ACS, NHTSA's Office of EMS, and (in the past) HRSA's Division of Trauma and EMS. There are also various components of the system with independent accrediting bodies. Hospitals, for example, are accredited by the Joint Commission on Accreditation of Healthcare Organizations (JCAHO); ambulance services are accredited by the Commission on Accreditation of Ambulance Services (CAAS); and air medical services are voluntarily accredited by the Commission on Accreditation of Medical Transport Systems (CAMTS). Each of these organizations collects performance information.

What is missing is a standard set of measures that can be used to assess the performance of the full emergency and trauma care system within each community, as well as the ability to benchmark that performance against statewide and national performance metrics. A credible entity to develop such measures would not be strongly tied to any one component of the emergency care continuum.

One approach would be to form a collaborative entity that would include representation from all of the system components, including hospitals, trauma centers, EMS agencies, physicians, nurses, and others. Another approach would be to work with an existing organization, such as the National Quality Forum (NQF), to develop a set of emergency care–specific measures. NQF grew out of the President's Advisory Commission on Consumer Protection and Quality in the Health Care Industry in 1998. It operates as a not-for-profit membership organization made up of national, state, regional, and local groups representing consumers, public and private purchasers, employers, health care professionals, provider organizations, health plans, accrediting bodies, labor unions, supporting industries, and organizations involved in health care research or quality improvement. NQF has reviewed and endorsed measure sets applicable to several health care settings and clinical areas and services, including hospital care, home health care, nursing-sensitive care, nursing home care, cardiac surgery, and diabetes care (NQF, 2002, 2003, 2004a,b, 2005).

The committee recommends that **the Department of Health and Human Services convene a panel of individuals with emergency and trauma care expertise to develop evidence-based indicators of emergency and trauma care system performance (3.3).** Because of the need for an independent, national process that involves the broad participation of every component of emergency and trauma care, the federal government should play a lead role in promoting and funding the process. The development of the initial set of performance indicators should be completed within 18 months of the release of this report.

The measures developed should include structure and process measures, but evolve toward outcome measures over time. They should be nationally standardized so that statewide and national comparisons can be made.

Measures should evaluate the performance of individual providers within the system, as well as that of the system as a whole. Measures should also be sensitive to the interdependence among the components of the system; for example, EMS response times may be adversely affected by ED diversions.

Furthermore, because an episode of emergency and trauma care can span multiple settings, each of which can have a significant impact on the final outcome, it is important that patient-level data from each setting be captured and combined. Currently it is difficult to piece together an episode of emergency and trauma care. To address this need, states should develop guidelines for the sharing of patient-level data from dispatch through post–hospital release. The federal government should support such efforts by sponsoring the development of model procedures that can be adopted by states to minimize their administrative costs and liability exposure as a result of sharing these data.

Measurement of Performance

Performance data should be collected on a regular basis from all of the emergency and trauma care providers in a community. Over time, emerging technologies may support more simplified and streamlined data collection methods, such as wireless transmission of clinical data and direct links to patient electronic health records. However, these types of technical upgrades would likely require federal financial support, and EMS personnel would have to be persuaded to transition from paper-based run records, which are less amenable to efficient performance measurement. The collected data should be tabulated in ways that can be used to measure, report on, and benchmark system performance, generating information useful for ongoing feedback and process improvement. Using their regulatory authority over health care services, states should play a lead role in collecting and analyzing these performance data.

While a full-blown data collection and performance measurement and reporting system is the desired ultimate outcome, the committee believes a handful of key indicators of regional system performance should be collected and promulgated as soon as possible. These could include, for example, indicators of 9-1-1 call processing times, EMS response times for critical calls, and ambulance diversions. In addition, consensus measurement of EMS outcomes could be applied to two to three sentinel conditions. For example, emergency and trauma care systems across the country might be tasked with providing data on such conditions as cardiac arrest (see Box 3-1), pediatric respiratory arrest, and major blunt trauma with shock. Data from the different system components would allow researchers to measure how well the system performs at each level of care (9-1-1, first response, EMS, and ED).

BOX 3-1
Cardiac Arrest Registry to Enhance Survival

A new 18-month initiative funded by the Centers for Disease Control and Prevention (CDC) is under way in Fulton County, Georgia. Cardiac Arrest Registry to Enhance Survival (CARES) is intended to develop a prototype national registry to help local EMS administrators and medical directors identify when and where cardiac arrest occurs, which elements of their EMS system are functioning properly in dealing with these cases, and what changes can be made to improve outcomes. The initiative is engaging Atlanta-area 9-1-1, EMS and first-responder services, and EDs in systematically collecting minimum data essential to improving survival in cases of cardiac arrest and submitting these data to the registry. Area hospitals log on to a simple, Health Insurance Portability and Accountability Act (HIPAA)–compliant website to report each patient's outcome. Data compilation and analysis are conducted by researchers at Emory University. Using information gathered from the CARES registry, a community consortium organized by the American Heart Association (AHA) will orchestrate various community interventions to reduce disparities and improve outcomes among victims of cardiac arrest. CARES is designed to enable cities across the country to collect similar data quickly and easily, and use these data to improve cardiac arrest treatment and outcomes.

Sudden cardiac arrest results from an abrupt loss of heart function and is the leading cause of death among adults in the United States. Its onset is unexpected, and death occurs minutes after symptoms develop (AHA, 2005). Survival rates in the event of sudden cardiac arrest are low, but vary as much as 10-fold across communities. Victims' chances of survival increase with early activation of 9-1-1 and prompt handling of the call, early provision of bystander cardiopulmonary resuscitation (CPR), rapid defibrillation, and early access to definitive care. CARES is designed to allow communities to measure each link in their "chain of survival" quickly and easily and use this information to save more lives.

Public Dissemination of Information on System Performance

Public dissemination of performance data is crucial to drive the needed changes in the delivery of emergency and trauma care services. Dissemination can take various forms, including public report cards, annual reports, and state public health reports, which can be viewed either in hard copy format or online. A key to success is ensuring that important information regarding the performance of the community's emergency and trauma care system can be retrieved by the public with a minimum of effort in a format that is highly organized and visually compelling.

Public dissemination of health care information is still in a state of development, despite the proliferation of such initiatives over the past two decades. Problems include the costs associated with data collection, the sensitivity of individual provider information, concerns about interpretation of data by the public, and lack of public interest. There are many examples from which to learn—the Health Plan Employer Data and Information Set (HEDIS), which reports on managed care plans to purchasers and consumers; the Centers for Medicare and Medicaid Services' (CMS) reports on home health and nursing home care—the *Home Health Compare* and *Nursing Home Compare* websites, respectively (CMS, 2005a); and *Hospital Compare* from the Hospital Quality Alliance, which reports comparative quality data on hospitals (CMS, 2005b). A number of states and regional business coalitions have also developed report cards on managed care plans and hospitals (State of California Office of the Patient Advocate, 2005). Because of the unique status of the emergency and trauma care system as an essential public service and the public's limited awareness of the significant problems facing the system, the public is likely to take an active interest in this information. The committee believes dissemination of these data will have an important impact on public awareness and the development of integrated regional systems.

Public reporting can be at a detailed or aggregate level. Because of the potential sensitivity of performance data, they should initially be reported in the aggregate at the national, state, and regional levels, rather than at the level of the individual provider organization. Prematurely reporting organizational performance data may inhibit participation and divert providers' resources to public relations rather than corrective efforts. At the same time, however, individual provider organizations should have full access to their own data so they can understand and improve their individual performance, as well as their contribution to the overall system. Over time, information on individual provider organizations should become an important part of the public information on the system. Eventually, the data may be used to drive performance-based payment for emergency and trauma care.

Aligning Payments with Incentives

In addition to public data reporting, financial incentives can play a major role in improving health care service and performance (Bailit Health Purchasing, 2001). The way emergency and trauma care services are currently reimbursed reinforces certain modes of delivery that are inefficient and stand in the way of achieving the committee's vision. Historically, payment for EMS has been based on transport of a sick or injured person to the hospital. This approach has created a financial incentive to transport patients to the hospital even when doing so may not be required or when out-of-hospital "treat and release" may be more appropriate.

It has been estimated that anywhere from 11 to 61 percent of ambulance transports to EDs are not medically necessary (Gratton et al., 2003). Current financial incentives are suspected of adding unnecessary costs to the health care system and burdening already overburdened hospital-based providers. Under the current system, a patient with a sprained ankle may be transported by ambulance and treated at the ED, incurring substantial costs from both providers, when a simple splint by an EMT and a car or taxi ride to a primary care provider would achieve essentially the same outcome at a much lower cost. On the opposite end of the spectrum, allowing paramedics to terminate an unsuccessful cardiac resuscitation in the field could reduce costs by preventing futile care in the hospital and might also reduce the danger to EMS personnel and the public by limiting the number of high-speed transports. However, current financial incentives discourage EMS agencies from making determinations regarding the need for transport to a hospital.

To determine whether incentives are properly aligned, CMS should investigate whether Medicare and Medicaid payment methodologies ought to be revised to support payment for emergency care services in the most appropriate setting (including treat and release), perhaps encompassing payments for medical directors who assume responsibility for release decisions. The committee believes CMS should consider using demonstration projects to test various options, to ensure that the models are safe, and to assess whether downstream savings may result.

Another example of misaligned incentives is that many hospitals do not have a strong economic motivation to address the problems of ED crowding, boarding, and ambulance diversion. In fact, hospitals may benefit financially from these practices. Several payment approaches could eliminate this perverse incentive. One would be to eliminate or compensate for the differential in payment between scheduled and ED admissions. Another would be to assess direct financial rewards or penalties for hospitals based on their management of patient throughput. Through its purchaser and regulatory power, CMS has the ability to drive hospitals to address and manage patient flow and ensure timely access to quality care for its clients. All payers, including Medicare, Medicaid, and private insurers, should also develop contracts that reward hospitals for timely and efficient emergency care and penalize those in which chronic delays in treatment, crowding, and EMS diversions occur. CMS should lead the way in the development of innovative payment approaches that can accomplish these objectives; all payers should be encouraged to do the same.

MODEL SYSTEMS CURRENTLY IN OPERATION

A number of current efforts to establish emergency and trauma care systems achieve some or all of the committee's goals of coordination, regionalization, and accountability. Some are purely voluntary, while others have the force of state regulation. Some are local and regional in scope, while others are statewide or national. This section highlights several such efforts that provide insights for future initiatives.

The Maryland EMS and Trauma System

Maryland has a unique statewide system that coordinates emergency care, including prehospital care, EDs, and trauma and specialty centers. The Maryland Institute for EMS Systems (MIEMSS) is the administrative lead agency for the system. MIEMSS is an independent state agency governed by an 11-member multidisciplinary board that is appointed by the governor. The system is funded through a surcharge on vehicle registrations that provides support for a broad range of statewide services, including the Maryland State Police medevac program, training and licensure of EMS personnel, medical oversight, prehospital care and triage protocols, trauma and specialty center designation, data management, quality improvement, and an EMS communications system.

Coordination

A key component of the effective operational coordination of the emergency care system in Maryland is the statewide EMS communications system. This system includes a communications center in Baltimore that dispatches the Maryland State Police medevac helicopters and provides communications and coordination among all components of the state EMS system, including EMS, hospitals, trauma and specialty centers, and 9-1-1 dispatch facilities. For example, a paramedic in western Maryland can talk directly with a local ED physician or obtain on-line consultation with a specialty center in Baltimore. While local 9-1-1 centers initiate dispatch, they typically are too busy to follow patients through the continuum of care and to coordinate health care facilities and major incidents. The EMS communications system provides these critical linkages that enable medical direction, coordination of patient distribution, and continuity of care on a day-to-day basis. The communications center also has direct links to incident command to facilitate the coordination of EMS and health care resources during major incidents. Over the past decade, the state has enhanced the communications system through the development of a digital microwave network, which now connects EMS with other public safety (police, fire, emergency management) and public health entities throughout the state.

In addition, the state has developed a County Hospital Alert Tracking System (CHATS) that monitors the status of hospitals so that ambulances can be directed to less crowded facilities. The system can also be used for individual services—for example, patients with acute coronary syndrome can be directed to facilities according to the current availability of reperfusion suites. The Facility Resource Emergency Database (FRED) system was designed to gather electronically detailed information from hospitals on bed availability, staffing, medications, and other critical capacity issues during disasters, but is also used to communicate information to and from hospitals on a day-to-day basis.

The state ensures coordination and compliance with protocols through a system of EMS operational programs that are required to undertake credentialing, medical oversight, and quality improvement activities.

Regionalization

While EMS and 9-1-1 are operated locally, EMS providers use statewide treatment and triage protocols that promote regionalization of care at state-designated facilities. In addition to trauma centers, these facilities currently include neurotrauma, hyperbaric, burn, eye, perinatal, and hand centers. Regulations have recently been promulgated to designate stroke centers, and the relatively new prehospital stroke protocol will triage acute stroke patients to these designated stroke centers. The state is divided into five regions, each with an advisory council that includes representatives from EMS, hospitals, and trauma and specialty centers. Each region has a representative on the 29-member State EMS Advisory Council.

Accountability

The Maryland system monitors the performance of providers, as well as that of the system itself. Providers are monitored through their affiliated EMS operational programs, and when necessary, quality assurance issues are referred to the state-level Provider Review Panel. EMS operational programs are required to submit performance data, and as a state agency, MIEMSS reports on system performance. The CHATS system enables EMS programs, participating hospitals, and the public to view the status of hospitals, including availability of ICU beds, ED beds, and trauma beds, at all times through its website. CHATS also collects and reports historical information on trends in hospital diversion, which are reviewed on a regular basis. A statewide web-based EMS patient care report is replacing paper ambulance run sheets so that data can be collected and analyzed more quickly and accurately, thereby facilitating real-time performance improvement.

Conclusion

While Maryland is relatively advanced in achieving the goals of coordination, regionalization, and accountability, it is not clear how easily its system could be replicated in other states. Over the years, the system has benefited from stable leadership, strong support of government leaders and the public, a steady and reliable source of funding, a high concentration of career and volunteer EMS personnel and health care resources, and limited geography—features that many states do not currently enjoy.

Austin/Travis County, Texas

Austin/Travis County and four surrounding counties in Texas agreed to form a single EMS and trauma system to provide seamless care to emergency and trauma patients throughout the region. The initiative, which required a decade of planning, started with a fragmented delivery system consisting of the Austin EMS system, 13 separate fire departments, and a 9-1-1 service run through the sheriff's office that lacked unified protocols. These different entities agreed to come together to form a unified system that would coordinate all emergency care within the region. The system operates through a Combined Clinical Council that includes representatives of the different agencies and providers within the geographic area, including fire departments, 9-1-1, EMS, air medical services, and corporate employers. This is a "third service" system—it is separate from fire and other public safety entities. The system is supported financially by the individual entities.

Coordination

Coordination of care is achieved through several means. A unified set of clinical guidelines was developed and is maintained by the system in accordance with current clinical evidence. These guidelines provide a common framework for the care and transport of patients throughout the system. Any changes to the guidelines must be evaluated and approved by the Combined Clinical Council.

All providers in the region have a common set of credentials and are given badges that identify them as certified providers within the system, substantially reducing the multijurisdictional fragmentation that is common across metropolitan areas. In addition, there is no distinction within the system between volunteer and career providers. The integrated structure facilitates both incident command and disaster planning.

Regionalization

The unified system supports the regional emergency and trauma system through clinical operating guidelines that determine the care and transport of all emergency and trauma patients. But the system is focused more on coordination and medical direction of EMS than on regionalization of care.

Accountability

A Healthcare Quality Committee is charged with reviewing the performance of the system and recommending specific actions to improve quality.

Palm Beach County, Florida

An initiative currently under way in Palm Beach County, Florida, is more limited in scope than the Maryland and Austin systems. The goal of the initiative is to find regional solutions to the limited availability of physician specialists who provide on-call emergency care services. In spring 2004, physician leaders, hospital executives, and public health officials formed the Emergency Department Management Group to address this problem. The initiative is in the early stages of development, and approaches are evolving. One approach is to attack the rising cost of malpractice insurance for emergency care providers, which discourages specialists from serving on on-call panels. The organization is developing a group captive insurance company to offer liability coverage for physicians providing care in county EDs.

Coordination

The Emergency Department Management Group is developing a web-based, electronic ED call schedule so the EMS system can track which specialists are available at all hospitals throughout the county. This will enable the system to direct transport to the most appropriate facility based on a patient's type of injury or illness.

Regionalization

The Emergency Department Management Group is exploring the regionalization of certain high-demand specialties, such as hand surgery and neurosurgery, so that the high costs of maintaining full on-call coverage can be concentrated in a few high-volume hospitals, where the volume of cases makes it feasible to maintain such coverage. Hospitals throughout the county would pay a "subscription fee" to support the cost of on-call coverage at designated hospitals. The fee would be set at a level below what it would cost to have hospitals manage their on-call coverage problems individually.

Accountability

The initiative includes the development of a countywide quality assurance program under which all hospitals would submit certain data elements for assessment. It is unclear at this time how far this system would go toward public disclosure of system performance.

San Diego County, California

San Diego County has a regionalized trauma system that is characterized by a strong public–private partnership between the county and its five adult and one children's trauma centers. Public health, assessment, policy development, and quality assurance are core components of the system, which operates under the auspices of the state EMS Authority.

Coordination

A countywide electronic system (QA Net) provides the real-time status of every trauma center and ED in the county, including the reason for diversion status, ICU bed availability, and trauma resuscitation capacity. The system has been in place for over 10 years and is a critical part of the coordination of emergency and trauma care in the county.

A regional communications system serves as the backbone of the emergency and trauma care system for both day-to-day operations and disasters. It includes an enhanced 9-1-1 system and a countywide network that allows all ambulance providers and hospitals to communicate. The network is used to coordinate decisions on EMS destinations and bypass information, and allows each hospital and EMS provider to know the status of every other hospital and provider on a real-time basis. Because the system's authority comes from the state to the local level, all prehospital and emergency hospital services are coordinated through one lead agency. This arrangement provides continuity of services, standardized triage, treatment and transport protocols, and an opportunity to improve the system as issues are identified.

Regionalization

The county is divided into five service areas, each of which has at least a level II trauma center. Adult trauma patients are triaged and transported to the appropriate trauma center, while the children's hospital provides trauma care to all seriously injured children below the age of 14. Serious burn cases are taken to the University of California-San Diego Burn Center. The county is considering regionalization for other conditions, such as stroke and heart attack, based on the trauma model. The system includes the designation of regional trauma centers, designation of base hospitals to provide medical direction to EMS personnel, establishment of regional medical policies and procedures, and licensure of EMS.

Accountability

Accountability is driven by a quality improvement program in which a medical audit committee meets monthly to review systemwide patient deaths and complications. The committee includes trauma directors; trauma nurse managers; the county medical examiner; the chief of EMS; and representatives of key specialty organizations, including orthopedic surgeons and neurosurgeons, as well as a representative for nondesignated facilities. A separate prehospital audit committee that includes ED physicians and prehospital providers also meets monthly and discusses any relevant prehospital issues.

DEMONSTRATING FUTURE MODELS

States and regions face a variety of situations, and no one approach to building emergency and trauma care systems will achieve the goals discussed in this chapter. There is, for example, substantial variation across states and regions in the level of development of trauma systems; the effectiveness of state EMS offices and regional EMS councils; and the degree of coordination and integration among fire departments, EMS, hospitals, trauma centers, and emergency management. The baseline conditions and needs also vary. For example, rural areas face very different problems from those of urban areas, and an approach that works for one may be counterproductive for the other.

In addition to these varying needs and conditions, the problems involved are too complex for the committee to prescribe an a priori solution. A number of different avenues should be explored and evaluated to determine what does and does not work. Over time and over a number of controlled initiatives, such a process should yield important insights about what works and under what conditions. These insights can provide best-practice models that can be widely adopted to advance the nation toward the committee's vision.

The process described here is one that can be supported effectively through federal demonstration projects. Such an approach can provide funding critical to project success; guidance for design and implementation; waivers from federal laws that might otherwise impede the process; and standardized, independent evaluations of projects and overall national assessment of the program. At the same time, the demonstration approach allows for significant variations according to state and regional needs and conditions within a set of clearly defined parameters. The IOM report *Fostering Rapid Advances in Health Care: Learning from System Demonstrations* articulated the benefits of the demonstration approach: "There is no accepted blueprint for redesigning the health care sector, although there is widespread recognition that fundamental changes are needed. . . . For many important issues, we have little experience with alternatives to the status quo. . . . [T]he committee sees the launching of a carefully crafted set of demonstrations as a way to initiate a 'building block' approach" (IOM, 2002).

The committee therefore recommends that **Congress establish a demonstration program, administered by the Health Resources and Services Administration, to promote coordinated, regionalized, and accountable emergency and trauma care systems throughout the country, and appropriate $88 million over 5 years to this program (3.4).** The essential features of the program are described below.

Recipients

Grants would be targeted at states, which could develop projects at the state, regional, or local level; cross-state collaborative proposals would be encouraged. Grantees would be selected through a competitive process based on the quality of proposals and an assessment of the likelihood of success in achieving the stated goal(s). Grantees could propose approaches that would address one, two, or all three of the goals of coordination, regionalization, and accountability.

Purpose of the Grants

Each proposal would be required to describe the proposed approach in detail, explain how it would achieve the stated goal(s), identify who would carry out the responsibilities associated with the initiative, identify the costs associated with its implementation, and describe how success would be measured. Proposals should describe the state's current stage of development and sophistication with regard to the stated goal(s) and explain how the grant would be used to enhance system performance in that regard.

Grants could be used in a number of different ways. Grant funds could be used to enhance communications so as to improve coordination of services; of particular interest would be the development of centralized communications centers at the regional or state level. Grants could be used to establish convening and planning functions, such as the creation of a regional or state advisory group of stakeholders for the purposes of building collaboration and designing and executing plans to improve coordination. Grant funds could be used to hire consultants and staff to manage the planning and coordination functions, as well as to pay for data collection, analysis, and public reporting. In very limited circumstances, the funds could also be used to implement information systems for the purpose of improving coordination of services. Grant funds should not, however, be used for routine functions that would be performed in the absence of the demonstration project, such as the hiring or training of pediatric specialists or the purchase of pediatric equipment.

The central objective of the grants would be to promote the coordination of emergency and trauma care assets within selected regional areas and to drive improvements in performance. This objective might be achieved in any number of ways, and one basis for awarding the grants would be the level of innovation shown by the applicants. In many urban and suburban areas of the country, for example, emergency care resources are often allocated inefficiently. Multiple EMS agencies of different types (including ground and air ambulances) may all be called to a scene, duplicating care capacity and creating unnecessary confusion. An applicant might devise a method of dispatch that would improve the allocation of resources, avoid redundancy, and improve care. An applicant might propose investing in technology that would promote better positioning of ambulances to reflect the most frequent "hot spots." Or an applicant might propose establishing a creative means of tracking the performance of the EMS system, such as a direct feedback loop in which EMS personnel could ascertain (e.g., through a web-based program) the outcomes of the patients they treated. A region might elect to keep this information confidential to support voluntary improvements or supply it to medical directors to support improvements in specific performance measures. Such a system might seek to improve data flow through each point along the care continuum, including 9-1-1 dispatch, EMS, hospital EDs and trauma centers, and subsequent care, allowing for a better understanding of systemwide performance. These data might also be used to assess the cost-effectiveness of prehospital care.

In addition, regional emergency and trauma care systems might examine patient outcomes to inform EMS treatment and transport decisions and to make local modifications to the national protocols proposed in this report. The system might also track workforce safety issues, such as injuries, exposures, and stress-related conditions of paramedics and emergency medical technicians (EMTs).

The above are just a few of the many uses for the proposed grants that might be devised by states and regions.

Funding Levels

The committee proposes a two-phase program. In phase I, the program would fund up to 10 projects at up to $6 million each over 3 years. The committee recommends support for this number of projects for two reasons. First, the committee hopes that the recommendations presented in this report will stimulate a desire among states and communities to undertake efforts aimed at achieving the committee's vision. Resources should be available to encourage and support these efforts. Second, there is likely to be considerable variation in the types of projects proposed. A certain number of projects will be needed to generate appropriate lessons learned.

Based on successful results that appeared to be replicable and sustainable in other states, the program would launch phase II, in which smaller, 2-year demonstration grants—up to $2 million each—would be made available to up to 10 additional states. This phase of the program would also include a technical assistance program designed to disseminate results and practical guidance to all states. Program administration would encompass evaluation of the program throughout its 5 years, including reports and public comments at 2.5 and 5 years after project initiation. The committee estimates funding for the program as follows:

- Phase I grants: $60 million (over 3 years)
- Phase II grants: $20 million (over 2 years)
- Phase II technical assistance: $4 million (over 2 years)
- Overall program administration: $4 million (over 5 years)
- Total program funding: $88 million (over 5 years)

Granting Agency

No single agency has responsibility for the multiple components of the nation's emergency and trauma care system. As noted earlier, this responsibility is currently shared among multiple agencies—principally NHTSA, HRSA, CDC, and the Department of Homeland Security (DHS). If, as recommended below, a lead federal agency is established to consolidate funding and provide leadership for these multiple activities, it would be the appropriate agency to lead this proposed effort. Until that consolidation occurs, however, the committee believes this demonstration program should be placed within HRSA. HRSA has directed a successful related demonstration program—Emergency Medical Services for Children (EMS-C)—and sponsors the Trauma-EMS Systems Program, both of which share many of the broad goals of the proposed demonstration program (although both have been targeted for elimination in recent federal budgets). HRSA has already demonstrated a willingness and ability to collaborate effectively with other relevant federal agencies, including NHTSA, CDC, and, increasingly, DHS, and should be encouraged to consider them as partners in this enterprise.

NEED FOR SYSTEM INTEGRATION
AND A FEDERAL LEAD AGENCY

The committee's vision of a coordinated, regionalized, and accountable emergency and trauma care system is impeded by the structure of federal programs that currently support emergency and trauma care. To function effectively, the components of the emergency and trauma care system must be highly integrated. Operationally, this means that all of the key players in a given region—hospital emergency and trauma departments, 9-1-1 dispatchers, state public health officials, trauma surgeons, EMS agencies, ED nurses, hospital administrators, firefighters, police, community safety net providers, and others—must work together to make decisions, deploy resources, and monitor and adjust system operations based on performance feedback.

As documented throughout this report, however, fragmentation, silos, and entrenched interests prevail throughout emergency and trauma care. The organization of federal government programs that support and regulate emergency and trauma care services reflects to a large degree the fragmentation of those services at the local level. Responsibility for emergency and trauma care is widely dispersed among multiple federal agencies within the Department of Health and Human Services (DHHS), the U.S. Department of Transportation (DOT), and DHS. This situation reflects the history and inherent nature of emergency and trauma care—essential public services that operate at the intersection of medical care, public health, and public safety (police and fire departments and emergency management agencies). In the 1960s, the mounting toll of highway deaths led NHTSA to become the first government home for EMS, and it has remained the informal lead agency for EMS ever since. Thus although EMS is first and foremost a medical discipline, federal responsibility for EMS rests with DOT. This responsibility was recently reinforced by the elevation of NHTSA's EMS program to the status of the Office of EMS within the agency. Today, NHTSA actively supports a number of workforce and research initiatives, the development of NEMSIS, and a major nationwide initiative to promote the development of next-generation 9-1-1 service.

DHHS has played an important supporting role in the development of EMS and has taken the lead role with respect to hospital-based emergency and trauma care. It has housed the Division of Emergency Medical Services and the Division of Trauma and EMS for many years and, most recently, the Trauma/EMS Systems Program. All of these programs have since been eliminated; the latter was zeroed out in the fiscal year 2006 federal budget. DHHS continues to support CDC's National Center for Injury Prevention and Control, the EMS-C program, and the National Bioterrorism Hospital Preparedness Program. These programs have made important contributions to emergency and trauma care despite inconsistent funding and the frequent threat of elimination. The Agency for Healthcare Research and Quality (AHRQ), another DHHS agency, has historically been the principal federal agency funding research in emergency care delivery, including much of the early research on management of out-of-hospital cardiac arrest. Recently, AHRQ has funded important studies of ED crowding, operations management, and patient safety issues. It is active as well in funding research on preparedness, bioterrorism planning, and response.

DHS also plays an important role in emergency and trauma care. The Federal Emergency Management Agency (FEMA), once an independent cabinet-level agency now housed in DHS, provides limited amounts of grant funding to local EMS agencies through the U.S. Fire Administration. DHS also houses the Metropolitan Medical Response System (MMRS), a grant program designed to enhance emergency and trauma preparedness in major population centers. This program moved from DHHS to DHS in 2003. In addition, DHS houses the Disaster Medical Assistance Team (DMAT) program, through which health professionals volunteer and train as locally organized units so they can be deployed rapidly, under federal direction, in response to disasters nationwide.

Efforts have been made to improve interagency collaboration at the federal level, especially in recent years. Over the last decade, federal agencies have worked collaboratively to provide leadership to the emergency and trauma care field, to minimize gaps and overlaps across programs, and to pool resources to jointly fund promising research and demonstration programs. For example, NHTSA and HRSA jointly supported the development of the *Emergency Medical Services Agenda for the Future*, as well as a number of other important EMS reports. This degree of collaboration has not been universal among federal agencies, however. Moreover, collaborative efforts are limited by the constraints of agency authorization and funding. At some point, agencies must pursue their own programmatic goals at the expense of joint initiatives. Furthermore, to the degree that successful collaboration has occurred, it has generally depended on the good will of key individuals in positions of leadership, which may limit the sustainability of these efforts when personnel changes occur.

In an effort to enhance the sustainability of collaborative initiatives, a number of agencies have participated in informal planning groups. For example, the Interagency Committee on EMSC Research (ICER), which is sponsored by HRSA, brings together representatives from a number of federal programs for the purposes of sharing information and improving research in emergency and trauma care for children.

A broader initiative is the Federal Interagency Committee on EMS

(FICEMS), a planning group designed to coordinate the efforts of the various federal agencies involved in emergency and trauma care (see Box 3-2). FICEMS was originally established in the late 1970s. The organization had no statutory authority until 2005, when it was given formal status by the Safe, Accountable, Flexible, Efficient Transportation Equity Act: A Legacy for Users (SAFETEA-LU), DOT's reauthorization legislation (P.L. 109-59). While the focus of FICEMS is EMS, the group has in practice reached beyond the strict boundaries of prehospital care to facilitate coordination and collaboration with agencies involved in other aspects of hospital-based emergency and trauma care. NHTSA is charged with providing administrative support for FICEMS, which must submit a report to Congress annually. The central aims of the group are as follows:

• To ensure coordination among the federal agencies involved with state, local, or regional EMS and 9-1-1 systems.
• To identify state, local, or regional needs in EMS and 9-1-1 services.

BOX 3-2
FICEMS Membership

The 2005 Safe, Accountable, Flexible, Efficient Transportation Equity Act: A Legacy for Users designated the following agencies as members of FICEMS. Each year, members elect a representative from one of these member organizations as the FICEMS chairperson:

• National Highway Traffic Safety Administration (DOT)
• Preparedness Division, Directorate of Emergency Preparedness and Response (DHS)
• Health Resources and Services Administration (DHHS)
• Centers for Disease Control and Prevention (DHHS)
• U.S. Fire Administration, Directorate of Emergency Preparedness and Response (DHS)
• Centers for Medicare and Medicaid Services (DHHS)
• Under Secretary of Defense for Personnel and Readiness (Department of Defense [DOD])
• Indian Health Service (DHHS)
• Wireless Telecommunications Bureau, Federal Communications Commission
• Another relevant federal agency (appointed by DOT or DHS in consultation with DHHS)
• A state EMS director

- To recommend new or expanded programs, including grant programs, for improving state, local, or regional EMS and implementing improved EMS communications technologies, including wireless 9-1-1.
- To identify ways of streamlining the process through which federal agencies support state, local, or regional EMS.
- To assist state, local, or regional EMS in setting priorities based on identified needs.
- To advise, consult, and make recommendations on matters relating to the implementation of coordinated state EMS programs.

Problems with the Current Structure

Despite recent efforts at improved federal collaboration, there is widespread agreement that the various components of emergency and trauma care (EMS for adults and children, trauma care, hospital-based care) have not received sufficient attention, stature, and funding within the federal government. The scattered nature of federal responsibility for emergency and trauma care limits the visibility necessary to secure and maintain funding within the federal government. The result has been marked fluctuations in budgetary support and the constant risk that key programs will be dramatically downsized or eliminated. The lack of a clear point of contact for the public and for stakeholders makes it difficult to build a unified constituent base that can advocate effectively for funding and provide feedback to the government on system performance. The lack of a unified budget has created overlaps, gaps, and idiosyncratic funding of various programs (for example, separate hospital surge capacity initiatives are currently taking place in AHRQ, CDC, HRSA, and DHS). Finally, lack of unified accountability disperses responsibility for system failures and perpetuates divisions between public safety and medical-based emergency and trauma care professionals. The degree to which the scattered responsibility for emergency and trauma care at the federal level has contributed to this disappointing performance is unclear. Regardless, the committee believes a new approach is warranted.

Alternative Approaches

Strong federal leadership for emergency and trauma care is at the heart of the committee's vision for the future, and continued fragmentation of responsibility at the federal level is not consistent with these goals. Consequently, the committee considered two options for remedying the situation: (1) maintain the status quo, giving the FICEMS approach time to strengthen and mature, or (2) designate or create a new lead agency within the federal government for emergency and trauma care. Some of the key differences between these two approaches are summarized in Table 3-1.

TABLE 3-1 Comparison of the Current FICEMS Approach and the Committee's Lead Agency Proposal

	Maintain the Status Quo, Allowing FICEMS to Gain Strength	Designate or Create a New Lead Agency
Description	• Current agencies retain autonomy, but the FICEMS process fosters collaboration in planning.	• Combines emergency care functions from several agencies into a new lead agency.
Authority	• FICEMS has the authority to convene meetings, but no authority to enforce planning, evaluation, and coordination of programs and funding.	• Lead agency would have planning and budgetary authority over the majority of emergency care activities at the federal level.
Funding	• No guarantee of coordinated program funding. • Distributed responsibility for federal functions means that if programs are cut, others remain, reducing the risk of losing all federal support for emergency and trauma care.	• Consolidates visibility and political representation of emergency care, enhancing federal funding opportunities. • Emergency care funding is fully coordinated. • Risk of losing significant funding for emergency care in a hostile budget environment.
Collaboration	• Brings together the key emergency and trauma care agencies. • FICEMS cannot enforce coordination or collaboration.	• Unified agency would drive collaboration among all components of emergency and trauma care to achieve systemwide performance goals.
Public Identity	• Still lacks a unified point of authority from the public's perspective. • FICEMS, especially through its advisory council, facilitates response to the public.	• Provides for a unified federal emergency and trauma care presence for interaction with the public and stakeholder groups.
Professional Identity	• Fragmented federal representation makes it difficult to break down silos in the field.	• Provides a home for emergency and trauma care, which can project and enhance the professional identity of emergency and trauma care providers over time. • Lead agency could consolidate constituencies and engender stronger political representation.

continued

TABLE 3-1 Continued

	Maintain the Status Quo, Allowing FICEMS to Gain Strength	Designate or Create a New Lead Agency
Efficiency	• May reduce redundancy through enhanced collaboration. • Very low administrative overhead costs.	• Eliminates redundant administrative structure, reducing administrative overhead costs. • Consolidated funding would allow for better allocation of federal dollars across the various emergency care needs (e.g., would eliminate overlapping programs).
Transition	• FICEMS is established in law, and implementation is under way. • Given FICEMS' limited powers, risks to individual programs and constituencies are minimal.	• Substantial startup costs associated with the transition to a single agency. • Potential for changes in program and funding emphasis during the transition, which could create winners and losers. • Potential dissension among emergency care agencies and constituencies could impact the organization's effectiveness.

Option 1: Maintain the Status Quo and Allow FICEMS to Strengthen

The committee considered the ramifications of maintaining the status quo. The problems associated with fragmented federal leadership of emergency care, documented above, include variable funding, periodic program cuts, programmatic duplications and critical program gaps. With the recent enactment of a statutory framework for FICEMS, however, the committee considered the possibility that the need for a lead federal agency has diminished. The committee carefully examined the rationale for delaying the move toward a lead federal agency and allowing FICEMS time to gain strength. The central argument in support of this strategy is that there have been a number of recent improvements in the level of collaboration at the federal level, and these efforts should be given a chance to work before an unproven and politically risky approach is pursued. A number of recent developments support this view: the enactment of a statutory framework for FICEMS; the increasing level of collaboration among some federal agencies; the substantial new NHTSA funding for a next-generation 9-1-1 initiative; and the elevation of the NHTSA EMS program to the Office of EMS, which has the potential to improve visibility and funding for EMS, and perhaps other aspects of emergency and trauma care, within the federal government.

While the committee applauds these positive developments, setbacks have occurred as well. As noted above, DHHS's Division of Emergency Medical Services, its Division of Trauma and EMS, and most recently its Trauma/EMS Systems Program have been zeroed out of the federal budget. Federal funding for AHRQ, nonbioterrorism programs at CDC, and other federal programs related to emergency and trauma care at the federal level have been cut. These developments suggest that a fragmented organizational structure at the federal level would significantly hinder the creation of a coordinated, regionalized, accountable emergency and trauma care system. FICEMS can be a valuable body, but it is a poor substitute for formal agency consolidation. FICEMS is expressly focused on EMS, and ultimately has limited power even within this sphere. It is not a federal agency and therefore cannot regulate, spend, or withhold funding. It cannot even hold its own member agencies accountable for their actions—or lack of action.

Option 2: Designate or Create a New Federal Lead Agency

The possibility of a lead agency for emergency and trauma care has been discussed for years and was highlighted in the 1996 report *Emergency Medical Services Agenda for the Future*. While the concept of a lead agency promoted in that report was focused on prehospital EMS, the committee believes a lead agency should encompass all components involved in the provision of emergency and trauma care. This federal lead agency would unify federal policy development related to emergency and trauma care, provide a central point of contact for the various constituencies in the field, serve as a federal advocate for emergency and trauma care within the government, and coordinate grants so that federal dollars would be allocated efficiently and effectively.

A lead federal agency could better move the emergency and trauma care system toward improved integration; unify funding and other decisions; and represent all emergency and trauma care patients, providers, and settings, including prehospital EMS (both ground and air), hospital-based emergency and trauma care, pediatric emergency and trauma care, rural emergency and trauma care, and medical disaster preparedness. Specifically, a federal lead agency could:

- Create unified accountability for the performance of the emergency and trauma care system.
- Rationalize funding across the various aspects of emergency and trauma care to optimize the allocation of resources in achieving system outcomes.

• Coordinate programs to eliminate overlaps and gaps in current and future funding.

• Provide consistent federal leadership on policy issues that cut across agency boundaries.

• Create a large combined federal presence, increasing the visibility of emergency and trauma care within the government and among the public.

• Provide a recognizable entity that would serve as a single point of contact for stakeholders and the public, resulting in consolidated and efficient data collection and dissemination and coordinated program information.

• Enhance the professional identity and stature of emergency and trauma care practitioners.

• Bring together multiple professional groups and cultures, creating cross-cultural and interdisciplinary interaction and collaboration that would model and reinforce the integration of services envisioned by the committee.

Although creating a lead agency could yield many benefits, such a move would also involve significant challenges. Numerous questions must be addressed regarding the location of such an agency in the federal government, its structure and functions, and the possible risk of weakening or losing current programs. HRSA's rural EMS and EMS/Trauma System programs have already been defunded, and the EMS-C program is under the constant threat of elimination. There is real concern that proposing an expensive and uncertain agency consolidation could jeopardize programs already at risk, such as EMS-C, as well as cripple new programs just getting started, such as NHTSA's enhanced 9-1-1 program. This is particularly likely if there is resistance to the consolidation from within the current agency homes for these programs.

A related concern is that the priority currently given to certain programs could shift, resulting in less support for existing programs. EMS advocates have expressed concern that hospital-based emergency and trauma care issues would dominate the agenda of a new unified agency. The pediatric community is worried about getting lost in a new agency and has fought hard to establish and maintain strong categorical programs supported by historically steady funding streams. There is concern that under the proposed new structure, the EMS-C program could become diminished or simply lose visibility amid the multitude of programs addressed by the new agency.

There is also the potential for administrative and funding disruptions. Combining similar agencies, particularly those that reside within the same department, may be straightforward. But combining agencies with different missions across departments with different cultures may prove highly difficult. The problems experienced during the consolidation of programs in DHS increase anxiety about this proposal.

Another concern is that removing medical-related functions from DHS and DOT could exacerbate rather than reduce fragmentation. Operationally, nearly half of EMS operations are fire department–based. Thus, there is concern that separating EMS and fire responsibilities at the federal level could splinter rather than strengthen relationships.

The Committee's Recommendation

Despite the concerns outlined above, the committee believes the potential benefits of consolidation outweigh the potential risks. A lead federal agency is required to fully realize the committee's vision of a coordinated, regionalized, and accountable emergency and trauma care system. The committee recognizes that a number of challenges are associated with the establishment of a new lead agency, though it believes these concerns can be mitigated through appropriate planning. The committee therefore recommends that **Congress establish a lead agency for emergency and trauma care within 2 years of the release of this report. This lead agency should be housed in the Department of Health and Human Services, and should have primary programmatic responsibility for the full continuum of emergency medical services and emergency and trauma care for adults and children, including medical 9-1-1 and emergency medical dispatch, prehospital emergency medical services (both ground and air), hospital-based emergency and trauma care, and medical-related disaster preparedness. Congress should establish a working group to make recommendations regarding the structure, funding, and responsibilities of the new agency, and design and monitor the transition to its assumption of the responsibilities outlined above. The working group should include representatives from federal and state agencies and professional disciplines involved in emergency care (3.5).**

Objectives of the Lead Agency

The lead agency's mission would be to enhance the performance of the emergency and trauma care system as a whole, as well as to improve the performance of the various components of the system, such as prehospital EMS, hospital-based emergency care, trauma systems, pediatric emergency and trauma care, prevention, rural emergency and trauma care, and disaster preparedness. The lead agency would set the overall direction for emergency and trauma care planning and funding; would be the primary collector and repository of data in the field; and would be the key source of information about emergency and trauma care for the public, the federal government, and practitioners themselves. It would be responsible for allocating federal resources across all of emergency and trauma care to achieve systemwide goals, and should be held accountable for the performance of the system and its components.

Location of the Lead Agency

The lead agency would be housed within DHHS. The committee considered many factors in selecting DHHS over DOT and DHS. The factor that drove this decision above all others was the need to unify emergency and trauma care within a medical care/public health framework. Emergency and trauma care is by its very nature involved in multiple arenas—medical care, public safety, public health, and emergency management. The multiple identities that result from this multifaceted involvement reinforce the fragmentation that is endemic to the emergency and trauma care system. For too long, the gulf between EMS and hospital care has hindered efforts at communication, continuity of care, patient safety and quality of care, data collection and sharing, collaborative research, performance measurement, and accountability. It will be difficult for emergency and trauma care to achieve seamless and high-quality performance across the system until the entire system is organized within a medical care/public health framework, while also retaining its operational linkages with public safety and emergency management.

Only DHHS, as the department responsible for medical care and public health in the United States, can encompass all of these functions effectively. Although DOT has played an important role in both EMS and acute trauma care and has collaborated effectively with other agencies, its EMS and highway safety focus is too narrow to represent all of emergency and trauma care. DHS houses the Fire Service, which is closely allied with EMS, particularly at the field operations level. But the focus of DHS on disaster preparedness and bioterrorism is also too narrow to encompass the broad scope of emergency and trauma care.

Because emergency and trauma care functions would be consolidated in a department oriented toward medical care and public health, there is a risk that public safety and emergency management components could receive less attention, stature, or funding. Therefore, the committee considers it important that the mission of the new agency be understood and clearly established by statute so that the public safety and emergency management aspects of emergency and trauma care will not be neglected.

Programs Included Under the Lead Agency

The committee envisions that the lead agency would have primary programmatic responsibility for the full continuum of EMS; emergency and trauma care for adults and children, including medical 9-1-1 and emergency medical dispatch; prehospital EMS (both ground and air); hospital-based emergency and trauma care; and medical-related disaster preparedness. The agency's focus would be on program development and strategic funding to improve the delivery of emergency and trauma care nationwide. It would not be primarily a research funding agency, with the exception of existing grant programs mentioned above. Funding for basic, clinical, and health services research in emergency and trauma care would remain the primary responsibility of existing research agencies, including the National Institutes of Health (NIH), AHRQ, and CDC. Because of the limited research focus of the lead agency, it would be important for existing research agencies, NIH in particular, to work closely with the new agency and strengthen their commitment to emergency and trauma care research. On the other hand, it may be appropriate to keep certain clinical and health services research initiatives with the programs in which they are housed, and therefore bring them into the new agency. For example, the Pediatric Emergency Care Applied Research Network could be moved into the new agency along with the rest of the EMS-C program.

In addition to existing functions, the lead agency would become the home for future programs related to emergency and trauma care, including new programs that would be dedicated to the development of inclusive systems of emergency and trauma care.

Working Group

While the committee envisions consolidation of most of the emergency care–related functions currently residing in other agencies and departments, it recognizes that many complex issues are involved in determining which programs should be combined and which left in their current agency homes. A deliberate process should be established to determine the exact composition of the new agency and to coordinate an effective transition. For these reasons, the committee is recommending the establishment of an independent working group to make recommendations regarding the structure, funding, and responsibilities of the new agency and to coordinate and monitor the transition process. The working group would include representatives from federal and state agencies and professional disciplines involved in emergency care. The committee considered whether FICEMS would be an appropriate entity to assume this advisory and oversight role and concluded that, as currently constituted, it lacks the scope and independence to carry out this role effectively.

Role of FICEMS

FICEMS is a highly promising entity that is complementary to the proposed new lead agency. FICEMS would play a vital role during the proposed interim 2-year period by continuing to enhance coordination and collaboration among agencies and providing a forum for public input. In addition, it could play an important advisory role to the independent working group. Once the lead agency had been established, FICEMS would continue to coordinate work between the lead agency and other agencies, such as NIH, CMS, and the Department of Defense (DoD), that would remain closely involved in various emergency and trauma care issues.

Structure of the Lead Agency

While the principle of integration across the multiple components of emergency and trauma care should drive the structure, operation, and funding of the new lead agency, the committee envisions distinct program offices to provide focused attention and programmatic funding for key areas, such as the following:

- Prehospital EMS, including 9-1-1, dispatch, and both ground and air medical services
  - Hospital-based emergency and trauma care
  - Trauma systems
  - Pediatric emergency and trauma care
  - Rural emergency and trauma care
  - Disaster preparedness

To ensure that current programs would not lose visibility and stature within the new agency, each program office should have equal status and reporting relationships within the agency's organizational structure. The committee envisions a national dialogue over the coming year—coordinated by the proposed independent working group, aided by input from FICEMS, and with the involvement of the Office of Management and Budget and the congressional committees with jurisdiction—to specify the organizational structure in further detail and implement the committee's recommendation.

Funding for the Lead Agency

Existing programs transferring to the new agency would bring with them their full current and projected funding, although this may not be possible for some funds, such as the Highway Trust Funds, which contribute to the operational funding for the Office of EMS. Congress should also establish additional funding to cover the costs associated with the transition to and the new administrative overhead associated with the lead agency. In addition, Congress should add new funding for the offices of hospital-based emergency and trauma care, rural emergency and trauma care, and trauma systems. In light of the pressing challenges confronting emergency care providers and the American public, this would be money well spent. While the committee is unable to estimate the costs associated with establishing a unified lead agency, it recognizes that these costs would be substantial. At the same time, however, the committee believes that countervailing cost savings would result from reduced duplication and lower overhead. Consequently, new funding that flowed into the agency would result in new programming, rather than an increase in existing overhead.

Mitigation of Concerns Regarding the Establishment of a Lead Federal Agency

The committee recognizes that transitioning to a single lead agency would be a difficult challenge under any circumstances, but would be especially difficult for an emergency and trauma care system that is already under duress from funding cutbacks, elimination of programs, growing public demand on the system, and pressure to enhance disaster preparedness. During this critical period, it is important that support for emergency and trauma care programs already in place in the various federal agencies be sustained. In particular, the Office of EMS within NHTSA has ongoing programs that are critical to the EMS system. Similarly, existing emergency care–related federal programs, such as those in HRSA's EMS-C program and Office of Rural Health Policy and at CDC, should be supported during the transition period. If the committee's proposal is to be successful, the constituencies associated with established programs must not perceive that they are being politically weakened during the transition period.

The committee believes the proposed consolidation of agencies would enhance support for emergency and trauma care across the board, benefiting all current programs. But it also believes avoiding disruptions that could adversely affect established programs is critically important. Therefore, the committee believes legislation creating the new agency should protect current levels of funding and visibility for existing programs. The new agency should balance its funding priorities by adding to existing funding levels, not by diverting funds away from existing programs.

The committee acknowledges the concern that removing medical-related emergency and trauma functions from DHS and DOT would create additional fragmentation. The committee believes the public safety aspects of emergency and trauma care must continue to be addressed as a core element of the emergency and trauma care system. But the primary focus of the system should be medical care and public health if the recognition, stature, and outcomes that are critical to the system's success are to be achieved.

Adapting the Legal and Regulatory Framework

The way hospitals and EMS agencies deliver emergency care is shaped largely by federal and state laws—in particular, the Emergency Medical Treatment and Active Labor Act (EMTALA) of 1986, the Health Insurance Portability and Accountability Act (HIPAA), and medical malpractice laws. The application of these laws to the actual provision of care is guided by sometimes baffling regulatory rules and advisories, enforcement decisions, and court decisions, as well as by providers' understanding of the laws. EMTALA and HIPAA are discussed below.

Emergency Medical Treatment and Active Labor Act of 1986

EMTALA was enacted to prevent hospitals from refusing to serve uninsured patients and "dumping" them on other hospitals. The act established a mandate for hospitals and physicians who provide emergency and trauma care to provide a medical screening exam to all patients and appropriately stabilize patients or transfer them to an appropriate facility if an emergency medical condition exists (GAO, 2001).

EMTALA has implications for the regional coordination of care. The act was written to provide individual patient protections—it focuses on the obligations of an individual hospital to an individual patient (Rosenbaum and Kamoie, 2003). While it serves an important purpose, the statute is not clearly adaptable to a highly integrated regional emergency care system in which the optimal care of patients may diverge from conventional patterns of emergency treatment and transport.

Until recently, EMTALA appeared to hinder the regional coordination of services in several specific ways—for example, requiring a hospital-owned ambulance to transport a patient to the parent hospital even if it is not the optimal destination for that patient, requiring a hospital to interrupt the transfer to administer a medical screening exam for a patient being transferred from ground transport to helicopter using the hospital's helipad, and limiting the ability of hospitals to direct nonemergent patients who enter the ED to an appropriate and readily available ambulatory care setting or clinic. Interim guidance published by CMS in 2003 appeared to mitigate these problems (DHHS, 2003). This guidance established, for example, that a patient visiting an off-campus hospital site that does not normally provide emergency care does not create an EMTALA obligation, that a hospital-owned ambulance need not return the patient to the parent hospital if it is operating under the authority of a communitywide EMS protocol, and that hospitals are not obligated to provide treatment for clearly nonemergency situations as determined by qualified medical personnel. Further, hospitals involved in disasters need not adhere strictly to EMTALA if operating under a community disaster plan. Despite these changes, however, uncertainty surrounding the interpretation and enforcement of EMTALA remains a damper on the development of coordinated, integrated emergency care systems.

In 2005, CMS convened a technical advisory group to study EMTALA and address additional needed changes (CMS, 2005a,b,c). To date, the advisory group has focused on incremental modifications to the act.

While the recent CMS guidance and deliberations of the EMTALA advisory group are positive steps, the committee envisions a more fundamental rethinking of EMTALA that would support and facilitate the development of regionalized emergency systems, rather than simply addressing each obstacle on a piecemeal basis. The new EMTALA would continue to protect patients from discrimination in treatment while enabling and encouraging communities to test innovations in the design of emergency care systems, such as direct transport of patients to non–acute care facilities—dialysis centers and ambulatory care clinics, for example—when appropriate.

Health Insurance Portability and Accountability Act

HIPAA was enacted to facilitate electronic transmission of data between providers and payers while protecting the privacy of patient health information. In protecting patient confidentiality, HIPAA can present certain challenges for providers, such as making it more complicated for a physician to send information about a patient to another physician for a consultation. Regional coordination is based on the seamless delivery of care across multiple provider settings. Patient-specific information must flow freely between these settings—from dispatch to emergency response to hospital care—to ensure that appropriate information will be available for clinical decision making and coordination of services in emergency situations. In addition, retrospective patient-level data are needed to measure the performance of the system and to develop protocols based on outcomes of care across providers. Current interpretations of HIPAA would make it difficult to achieve the required degree of information fluidity.

Recommendation

Both EMTALA and HIPAA protect patients from potential abuses and serve invaluable purposes. As written and frequently interpreted, however, they can impede the exchange of lifesaving information and hinder the development of regional systems. The committee believes appropriate modifications can be made to both acts that would preserve their original purpose while reducing their adverse impact on the development of regional systems. The committee recommends that **the Department of Health and Human Services adopt regulatory changes to the Emergency Medical Treatment and Active Labor Act and the Health Insurance Portability and Accountability**

Act so that the original goals of the laws will be preserved, but integrated systems can be further developed (3.6).

Financing System Costs

In addition to the above and other regulatory issues that should be addressed by the federal government, there are outstanding issues related to the financing of the emergency care system. While the establishment of the proposed federal lead agency would help rationalize the federal grant payments allocated to EMS and the emergency care system more broadly, these grants represent a small share of total payments to EMS providers. Payments for EMS are made primarily through public and private insurance reimbursements and local subsidies. A large percentage of EMS transports are for elderly patients, making the federal Medicare program a particularly important payer.

EMS costs include the direct costs of each emergency response, as well as the readiness costs associated with maintaining the capability to respond quickly, 24 hours a day, 7 days a week—costs that are not adequately reimbursed by Medicare. In addition, by paying only when a patient is transported, Medicare limits the flexibility of EMS in providing the most appropriate care for each patient. Therefore, the committee recommends that **the Centers for Medicare and Medicaid Services convene an ad hoc working group with expertise in emergency care, trauma, and emergency medical services systems to evaluate the reimbursement of emergency medical services and make recommendations with regard to including readiness costs and permitting payment without transport (3.7).** A key objective of this working group would be to develop a strategy and a mechanism to ensure that federal, state, and local governments each would pay a fair share toward maintaining EMS readiness capacity. The working group would examine the role played by the Medicare and Medicaid programs in establishing a basic level of EMS readiness across the country and assess the extent to which local self-determination should be the basis for deciding whether to extend service beyond this level. In addition, the working group would consider whether pay-for-performance principles should be applied to EMS. Finally, the group would examine the costs and burden sharing required for local EMS systems to make needed upgrades in communications and information technology.

SUMMARY OF RECOMMENDATIONS

3.1: The Department of Health and Human Services and the National Highway Traffic Safety Administration, in partnership with professional organizations, should convene a panel of indi-

viduals with multidisciplinary expertise to develop evidence-based categorization systems for emergency medical services, emergency departments, and trauma centers based on adult and pediatric service capabilities.

3.2: The National Highway Traffic Safety Administration, in partnership with professional organizations, should convene a panel of individuals with multidisciplinary expertise to develop evidence-based model prehospital care protocols for the treatment, triage, and transport of patients.

3.3: The Department of Health and Human Services should convene a panel of individuals with emergency and trauma care expertise to develop evidence-based indicators of emergency and trauma care system performance.

3.4: Congress should establish a demonstration program, administered by the Health Resources and Services Administration, to promote coordinated, regionalized, and accountable emergency and trauma care systems throughout the country, and appropriate $88 million over 5 years to this program.

3.5: Congress should establish a lead agency for emergency and trauma care within 2 years of the release of this report. This lead agency should be housed in the Department of Health and Human Services, and should have primary programmatic responsibility for the full continuum of emergency medical services and emergency and trauma care for adults and children, including medical 9-1-1 and emergency medical dispatch, prehospital emergency medical services (both ground and air), hospital-based emergency and trauma care, and medical-related disaster preparedness. Congress should establish a working group to make recommendations regarding the structure, funding, and responsibilities of the new agency, and design and monitor the transition to its assumption of the responsibilities outlined above. The working group should include representatives from federal and state agencies and professional disciplines involved in emergency and trauma care.

3.6: The Department of Health and Human Services should adopt regulatory changes to the Emergency Medical Treatment and Active Labor Act and the Health Insurance Portability and Accountability Act so that the original goals of the laws will be preserved, but integrated systems can be further developed.

3.7: The Centers for Medicare and Medicaid Services should convene an ad hoc working group with expertise in emergency care, trauma, and emergency medical services systems to evaluate the reimbursement of emergency medical services and make recommendations with regard to including readiness costs and permitting payment without transport.

REFERENCES

AHA (American Heart Association). 2005. *Sudden Cardiac Death: AHA Scientific Position.* [Online]. Available: http://www.americanheart.org/presenter.jhtml?identifier=4741 [accessed February 15, 2006].

Bailit Health Purchasing. 2001. *The Growing Case for Using Physician Incentives to Improve Health Care Quality.* Washington, DC: National Health Care Purchasing Institute, Academy for Health Services Research and Health Policy.

Bardach NS, Olson SJ, Elkins JS, Smith WS, Lawton MT, Johnston SC. 2004. Regionalization of treatment for subarachnoid hemorrhage: A cost-utility analysis. *Circulation* 109(18):2207–2212.

Bravata D, McKonald K, Owens D, Wilhelm ER, Brandeau ML, Zaric, GS, Holty, JC, Sundaram V. 2004. Regionalization of bioterrorism preparedness and response. Rockville, MD: Agency for Healthcare Research and Quality.

Burt CW, McCaig LF, Valverde RH. 2006. *Analysis of Ambulance Transports and Diversions among U.S. Emergency Departments.* Hyattsville, MD: National Center for Health Statistics.

CDC, NCICP (Centers for Disease Control and Prevention, National Center for Injury Control and Prevention). 2001. *Web-based Injury Statistics Query and Reporting System (WISQARS).* [Online]. Available: http://www.cdc.gov/ncipc/wisqars/ [accessed September 2004].

Chang RK, Klitzner TS. 2002. Can regionalization decrease the number of deaths for children who undergo cardiac surgery? A theoretical analysis. *Pediatrics* 109(2):173–181.

Chiara O, Cimbanassi S. 2003. Organized trauma care: Does volume matter and do trauma centers save lives? *Current Opinion in Critical Care* 9(6):510–514.

CMS (Centers for Medicare and Medicaid Services). 2005a. *Report Number One to the Secretary, U.S. Department of Health and Human Services, From the Inaugural Meeting of the Emergency Medical Treatment and Labor Act Technical Advisory Group.* Washington, DC: CMS.

CMS. 2005b. *Report Number Two to the Secretary, U.S. Department of Health and Human Services, From the Emergency Medical Treatment and Labor Act Technical Advisory Group.* Washington, DC: CMS.

CMS. 2005c. *Report Number Three to the Secretary, U.S. Department of Health and Human Services, From the Emergency Medical Treatment and Labor Act Technical Advisory Group.* Washington, DC: CMS.

Davis R. 2003, July. The Method: Measure How Many Victims Leave the Hospital Alive. *USA Today.* [Online]. Available: http://www.usatoday.com/news/nation/ems-day1-method.htm [accessed January 27, 2007].

DHHS (Department of Health and Human Services). 2003. *Emergency Medical Treatment and Labor Act (EMTALA) Interim Guidance. Center for Medicare and Medicaid Services' Center for Medicaid and State Operations, Survey and Certification Group.* Baltimore, MD: DHHS.

Dummit LA. 2005. Specialty hospitals: Can general hospitals compete? *National Health Policy Forum Issue Brief* (804):1–12.

GAO (U.S. Government Accountability Office). 2001. *Emergency Care. EMTALA Implementation and Enforcement Issues*. Washington, DC: U.S. Government Printing Office.

GAO. 2003a. *Hospital Preparedness: Most Urban Hospitals Have Emergency Plans but Lack Certain Capacities for Bioterrorism Response*. Washington, DC: U.S. Government Printing Office.

GAO. 2003b. *Specialty Hospitals: Geographic Location, Services Provided, and Financial Performance*. Washington, DC: U.S. Government Printing Office.

GAO. 2003c. *Infectious Diseases: Gaps Remain in Surveillance Capabilities of State and Local Agencies*. Washington, DC: GAO.

Gausche-Hill M, Wiebe R. 2001. Guidelines for preparedness of emergency departments that care for children: A call to action. *Pediatrics* 107(4):773–774.

Glance LG, Osler TM, Dick A, Mukamel D. 2004. The relation between trauma center outcome and volume in the national trauma databank. *Journal of Trauma-Injury Infection & Critical Care* 56(3):682–690.

Gratton MC, Ellison SR, Hunt J, Ma OJ. 2003. Prospective determination of medical necessity for ambulance transport by paramedics. *Prehospital Emergency Care* 7(4):466–469.

Grumbach K, Anderson GM, Luft HS, Roos LL, Brook R. 1995. Regionalization of cardiac surgery in the United States and Canada: Geographic access, choice, and outcomes. *Journal of the American Medical Association* 274(16):1282–1288.

Harris Interactive. 2004. *Trauma Care: Public's Knowledge and Perception of Importance*. Rochester, NY: The Coalition for American Trauma Care.

HL7 (Health Level Seven). 2005. *Health Level Seven*. [Online]. Available: http://www.hl7.org [accessed December 1, 2005].

Imperato PJ, Nenner RP, Starr HA, Will TO, Rosenberg CR, Dearie MB. 1996. The effects of regionalization on clinical outcomes for a high risk surgical procedure: A study of the Whipple procedure in New York state. *American Journal of Medical Quality* 11(4):193–197.

IOM (Institute of Medicine). 1993. *Emergency Medical Services for Children*. Washington, DC: National Academy Press.

IOM. 2002. *Fostering Rapid Advances in Health Care: Learning from System Demonstrations*. Corrigan JM, Greiner A, Erickson SM, eds. Washington, DC: The National Academies Press.

Jurkovich GJ, Mock C. 1999. Systematic review of trauma system effectiveness based on registry comparisons. *Journal of Trauma-Injury Infection & Critical Care* 47(Suppl. 3): S46–S55.

Kellermann AL, Hackman BB, Somes G, Kreth TK, Nail L, Dobyns P. 1993. Impact of first-responder defibrillation in an urban emergency medical services system. *Journal of the American Medical Association* 270(14):1708–1713.

Lindsay P, Schull M, Bronskill S, Anderson G. 2002. The development of indicators to measure the quality of clinical care in emergency departments following a modified-delphi approach. *Academic Emergency Medicine* 9(11):1131–1139.

MacKenzie EJ. 1999. Review of evidence regarding trauma system effectiveness resulting from panel studies. *Journal of Trauma-Injury Infection & Critical Care* 47(Suppl. 3): S34–S41.

MacKenzie EJ, Rivara FP, Jurkovich GJ, Nathens AB, Frey KP, Egleston BL, Salkever DS, Scharfstein DO. 2006. A national evaluation of the effect of trauma-center care on mortality. *New England Journal of Medicine* 354(4):366–378.

Mann NC, Mullins RJ, MacKenzie EJ, Jurkovich GJ, Mock CN. 1999. Systematic review of published evidence regarding trauma system effectiveness. *Journal of Trauma-Injury Infection & Critical Care* 47(Suppl. 3):S25–S33.

McGinnis KK. 2005. *EMS Communications Needs of the Future.* Presentation at the meeting of the ITS America 2005: 16th Annual Meeting & Exposition, Philadelphia, PA.

measureEMS.org. 2005. *Performance Measures in EMS.* [Online]. Available: http://www. measureems.org/performancemeasures2.htm [accessed January 5, 2006].

Mullins RJ. 1999. A historical perspective of trauma system development in the United States. *Journal of Trauma-Injury Infection & Critical Care* 47(Suppl. 3):S8–S14.

Mullins RJ, Mann NC. 1999. Population-based research assessing the effectiveness of trauma systems. *Journal of Trauma-Injury Infection & Critical Care* 47(Suppl. 3):S59–S66.

Nallamothu BK, Saint S, Kolias TJ, Eagle KA. 2001. Clinical problem-solving of nicks and time. *New England Journal of Medicine* 345(5):359–363.

Nathens AB, Maier RV. 2001. The relationship between trauma center volume and outcome. *Advances in Surgery* 35:61–75.

Nathens AB, Jurkovich GJ, Rivara FP, Maier RV. 2000. Effectiveness of state trauma systems in reducing injury-related mortality: A national evaluation. *The Journal of Trauma* 48(1):25–30; discussion 30–31.

NAS, NRC (National Academy of Sciences, National Research Council). 1966. *Accidental Death and Disability: The Neglected Disease of Modern Society.* Washington, DC: National Academy Press.

NHTSA (National Highway and Traffic Safety Administration). 1996. *Emergency Medical Services Agenda for the Future.* Washington, DC: U.S. Government Printing Office.

NQF (National Quality Forum). 2002. *National Voluntary Consensus Standards for Adult Diabetes Care.* [Online]. Available: http://www.qualityforum.org/txdiabetes-public.pdf [accessed November 23, 2005].

NQF. 2003. *Safe Practices for Better Health Care.* Washington, DC: NQF.

NQF. 2004a. *National Voluntary Consensus Standards for Nursing Home Care.* [Online]. Available: http://www.qualityforum.org/txNursingHomesReportFINALPUBLIC.pdf [accessed November 23, 2005].

NQF. 2004b. *National Voluntary Consensus Standards for Nursing-Sensitive Care: An Initial Performance Measure Set.* [Online]. Available: http://www.qualityforum.org/txNCFI-NALpublic.pdf [accessed November 23, 2005].

NQF. 2005. *National Voluntary Consensus Standards for Home Health Care.* [Online]. Available: http://www.qualityforum.org/webHHpublic09–23–05.pdf_ [accessed November 23, 2005].

Orr RA, Han YY, Roth K. 2006. Pediatric transport: Shifting the paradigm to improve patient outcome. In: Fuhrman B, Zimmerman J, eds. *Pediatric Critical Care* (3rd edition). Mosby, Elsevier Science Health. Pp. 141–150.

Pollock DA, Adams DL, Bernardo LM, Bradley V, Brandt MD, Davis TE, Garrison HG, Iseke RM, Johnson S, Kaufmann CR, Kidd P, Leon-Chisen N, MacLean S, Manton A, McClain PW, Michelson EA, Pickett D, Rosen RA, Schwartz RJ, Smith M, Snyder JA, Wright JL. 1998. Data elements for emergency department systems, release 1.0: A summary report. Deeds Writing Committee. *Journal of Emergency Nursing* 24(1):35–44.

Rosenbaum S, Kamoie B. 2003. Finding a way through the hospital door: The role of EMTALA in public health emergencies. *Journal of Law, Medicine & Ethics* 31(4):590–601.

The SAFECOM Project. 2004. *Statement of Requirements for Public Safety Wireless Communications & Interoperability.* Washington, DC: Department of Homeland Security.

State of California Office of the Patient Advocate. 2005. *2005 HMO Report Card.* [Online]. Available: http://www.opa.ca.gov/report_card/ [accessed January 12, 2006].

Wright JL, Klein BL. 2001. Regionalized pediatric trauma systems. *Clinical Pediatric Emergency Medicine* 2:3–12.

4

Supporting a High-Quality EMS Workforce

Emergency medical services (EMS) is provided by dedicated professionals, both career and volunteer, who administer essential care to patients in need across the country. These services form a continuum of care that includes the dispatcher in the 9-1-1 emergency call center, fire and/or EMS personnel arriving on scene, and providers at the hospital emergency department (ED) or trauma center. How efficiently and effectively this care is delivered can mean the difference between life and death.

Qualifications for becoming an EMS provider vary widely nationwide. Education and training requirements and scope of practice designations are substantially different from one state to another, and limited reciprocity for providers seeking to move from one area of the country to another can pose a substantial burden. National efforts to promote greater uniformity have been progressing in recent years, but significant variation still remains.

EMS personnel face a difficult, often hazardous work environment, and they are not well paid. As a result, recruitment and retention are perennial challenges for EMS systems. However, surveys of EMS personnel indicate that many find their work to be highly rewarding. As the baby boomers reach retirement age and demand for EMS is expected to increase, it will be important to ensure that the available workforce is sufficient to meet that demand.

The first section of this chapter presents the committee's findings and recommendations with regard to restructuring the requirements for EMS personnel. This is followed by an overview of the EMS workforce—its roles and responsibilities, demographics, and size. Next is a discussion of issues associated with recruitment and retention. The final two sections address two key groups of ancillary EMS personnel: emergency medical dispatchers (EMDs) and EMS medical directors

RESTRUCTURING OF WORKFORCE REQUIREMENTS

EMS personnel have become part of the health care workforce only within the past 40 years. Over the past 10–15 years, concerted efforts have been made to change professional education and training standards for EMS personnel, as well as their scope of practice requirements. In 1993, a national, multidisciplinary consensus process culminated in the publication of the *National EMS Education and Practice Blueprint* (NREMT, 1993). This report sought to establish recognized levels of EMS personnel, nationally recognized scopes of practice, and frameworks for curriculum development and workforce reciprocity (NHTSA, 2000). The report established standard knowledge and practice expectations for four levels of EMS personnel: first responder, emergency medical technician (EMT)-B (Basic), EMT-I (Intermediate), and EMT-P (Paramedic). At the time, more than 40 different levels of EMT certification existed (NHTSA, 1996).

The 1996 report of the National Highway Traffic Safety Administration (NHTSA) *Emergency Medical Services Agenda for the Future* included education systems as one of its 14 priority areas for improvement. The report emphasized the need to develop national core content for curricula for providers at various levels and asserted that all EMS education must be conducted with the benefit of qualified medical direction (NHTSA, 1996). Goals included in the report are detailed in Box 4-1.

The *Emergency Medical Services Agenda for the Future: Implementation Guide*, released in 1998, expanded upon these goals, providing specific objectives and timeframes for accomplishing the goals (NHTSA, 1998). The report emphasized the need to update and adopt the *National EMS Education and Practice Blueprint* to promote consistency in the levels of EMS practice, and asserted that core content for EMS curricula should comply with the guidelines of the *Blueprint*. In addition, the *Implementation Guide* advocated the creation of a system for reciprocity of EMS provider credentials, with the goal of eliminating legal barriers to intra- and interstate reciprocity (NHTSA, 1998).

One of the outgrowths of the *Emergency Medical Services Agenda for the Future* was the development of the *Emergency Medical Services Education Agenda for the Future: A Systems Approach*, published in 2000 (NHTSA, 2000). The purpose of the *Education Agenda* was to create a more logical and uniform approach to EMS education and to maximize student competence. The report called for an education system with five integrated primary components: National EMS Core Content, National EMS Scope of Practice Model, National EMS Education Standards, National EMS

BOX 4-1
Education System Goals Set Forth in
Emergency Medical Services Agenda for the Future

- Ensure the adequacy of EMS education programs.
- Update the objectives of care curricula frequently enough so they reflect the health care needs of EMS patients.
- Incorporate research, quality improvement, and management learning objectives in higher-level EMS education.
- Commission the development of national core curriculum content to replace existing EMS program curricula.
- Conduct EMS education with medical direction.
- Seek accreditation of EMS education programs.
- Establish innovative and collaborative relationships between EMS education programs and academic institutions.
- Recognize EMS education as an academic achievement.
- Develop bridging and transition programs.
- Include EMS-related objectives in the education of all health professionals.

SOURCE: NHTSA, 1996.

Education Program Accreditation, and National EMS Certification (see Figure 4-1).

Under this model, the Core Content forms the foundation for the Scope of Practice Model, and the Scope of Practice Model forms the foundation for the Education Standards (NHTSA and HRSA, 2005). Education Program Accreditation impacts the process for educating EMS personnel, and National Certification specifies the end product.

This vision for the future of EMS education has been partially developed since its initial release 6 years ago. Work on the National EMS Core Content and the Scope of Practice Model has been completed; the remaining components of the model are still in the development stage.

National EMS Core Content

The National EMS Core Content encompasses the entire domain of out-of-hospital medicine. It provides a list of knowledge, skills, and tasks required to provide care in out-of-hospital settings, detailing what EMS personnel must know and how they must practice (NHTSA and HRSA, 2005). The Core Content is broad enough so that state-of-the-art changes

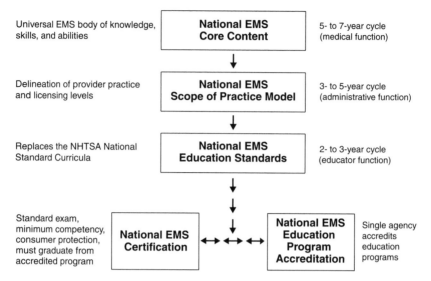

FIGURE 4-1 The five primary integrated components of the EMS education system.
SOURCES: Adapted from NHTSA and HRSA, 2005.

and regional practice patterns can be incorporated within its framework (NHTSA, 2000).

While the *Emergency Medical Services Agenda for the Future: Implementation Guide* sought to update and adopt the *National EMS Education and Practice Blueprint*, the *Education Agenda* suggested that the validity and utility of the *Blueprint* could be enhanced by separating the development of the core content and the scope of practice for the various provider levels. This approach allowed leadership for each of these elements to be assumed by the most appropriate group (see Figure 4-2) (NHTSA, 2000). The medical community is responsible for leading the development of the Core Content, with input from regulators and educators.

National EMS Scope of Practice Model

Based on the direction provided by the *Education Agenda*, the *Blueprint* was revised and renamed the National EMS Scope of Practice Model. This model defines, by name and by function, the levels of out-of-hospital EMS personnel based on the National EMS Core Content (NHTSA, 2000). Regulators are responsible for making these designations, with input from educators and physicians.

The National EMS Scope of Practice Model Task Force has created

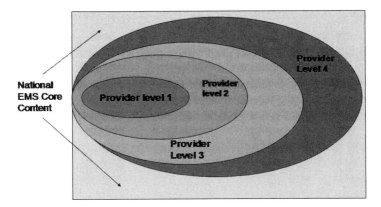

FIGURE 4-2 Core content and scope of practice for various provider levels.
NOTE: The figure is illustrative only. It does not include the numbers and names of EMS provider levels determined by the process for the National EMS Scope of Practice Model.
SOURCES: NHTSA and HRSA, 2005.

a national model to aid states in developing and refining their scopes of practice and licensure requirements for EMS personnel. The purpose of the effort is not to impose national scope of practice standards, but to encourage greater consistency across the states. The committee supports this effort, but further recommends that **state governments adopt a common scope of practice for emergency medical services personnel, with state licensing reciprocity (4.1).** Doing so would promote greater uniformity in provider services across states and would alleviate current limitations relating to workforce mobility (see below).

The task force released its final report in 2005. The report describes scope of practice models for emergency medical responders (EMRs), EMTs, and paramedics. It also creates scope of practice standards for a new category of personnel termed advanced emergency medical technicians (AEMTs). Plans for a proposed advanced practice paramedic level have been deferred (NHTSA, 2005).

National EMS Education Standards

Curricula developed on behalf of the U.S. Department of Transportation (DOT) have provided the basis for the education of first responders, EMT-Bs, EMT-Is, and EMT-Ps. These National Standard Curricula (NSC) have undergone revision over time to reflect changes in accepted practice patterns and the evidence base for specific procedures. The curriculum for first responders was updated most recently in 1995, that for EMT-Bs in 1994, that for EMT-Is in 1999, and that for EMT-Ps in 1998 (NHTSA, 2006). Because the revision of these NSC documents is the only setting in which national discussions regarding EMS scopes of practice occur, the revision process is time-consuming and expensive (NHTSA, 2000).

Education standards are needed to guide program managers and instructors in making appropriate decisions about what material to cover in classroom instruction. Currently, the content of most EMS education programs is based on the NSC. But while use of the NSC has contributed to the standardization of EMS education, the quality and length of programs still vary nationally, as do state licensure requirements for each position.

The NSC for basic life support (BLS) includes a minimum of 110 hours of didactic training, but states vary in their requirements from under 110 to more than 400 hours. For advanced life support (ALS) at the EMT-P level, applicants must receive 1,000 to 1,200 hours of didactic training beyond the EMT-B level, with additional practicum time (DOT, 1998); however states vary in their requirements from 270 to 2,000 hours (Mears, 2004). Based on the NSC, the EMT-I level requires 300 to 400 total training hours beyond the EMT-B level (DOT, 1998), but the number of hours varies across states from 50 to 492 (Mears, 2004).

The overwhelming majority of states and territories require both a written and a practical exam for initial credentialing (Mears, 2004). For all EMT levels and in all 50 states, a written exam is required, although the level of difficulty of these exams varies widely (NHTSA, 2000). All states require that licensure be renewed, typically every 2–3 years. Renewal usually entails completion of continuing education courses, verification of skills by a medical director, and current affiliation with an EMS provider (the latter requirement is common for ALS but less so for BLS). Standards for EMTs developed by the National Registry of Emergency Medical Technicians (NREMT) require initial training and recertification every 2 years.

Although state variation in educational requirements is substantial, the *Education Agenda* asserted that reliance on the highly prescriptive NSC has resulted in a significant loss of flexibility. The report concluded that a strict focus on the NSC could result in the development of narrow technical and conceptual skills without consideration for the broad range of professional competencies now expected of entry-level EMS personnel. The report advocated greater flexibility in meeting preestablished education standards, as well as more creativity in delivery methods, including problem-based learning and computer-aided instruction. However, the *Education Agenda* noted that accreditation of education programs and national certification need to be in place before the transition from the NSC to the National EMS Education Standards can take place (NHTSA, 2000).

EMS Education and Training Programs

The majority of EMTs and paramedics receive their education and training in programs offered by EMS agencies, community colleges, universities, hospitals and medical centers, fire departments, or private training programs. Increasing numbers of colleges offer bachelor's degrees in EMS (Delbridge et al., 1998). However, medical education for EMS careers varies widely across the country, and it is frequently inadequate. Adherence to the NSC does not in itself ensure quality (NHTSA, 2000), and as noted, considerable state-level variation continues to exist.

This situation mirrors the challenges faced by the broader medical education system in the early 20th century. At the time, there were no standards for medical education programs and no adequate system to ensure quality. A report issued by Abraham Flexner in 1910 called for the establishment of more rigorous standards for medical education programs (Beck, 2004). Flexner visited 168 graduate and postgraduate medical schools in the United States and Canada and evaluated them on the basis of several criteria, including entrance requirements, faculty training, and financing to support the institution. The report was highly critical of the majority of schools visited. In the years following the report's release, a large percentage of those schools closed, while others merged (Hiatt and Stockton, 2003). Consequently, the report is credited with triggering reforms in the standards, organization, and curriculum of medical schools across North America. In many respects, today's EMS education system calls for a similar response.

The *Education Agenda* proposed national EMS education program accreditation as a way to address this problem. Currently, most states have some process for approving EMS education programs; however, these requirements vary widely. Some states require only that proper paperwork be filed (NHTSA, 2000). State education program approvals typically focus only on the paramedic level, and national accreditation is usually optional. The only nationally recognized accreditation available for EMS education is through the Committee on Accreditation of Emergency Medical Services Professions (CoAEMSP) under the auspices of the Commission on Accreditation of Allied Health Education Programs (CAAHEP). The *Education Agenda* advocated that a single national accreditation agency be identified and accepted by state regulatory offices.

The committee maintains that greater standardization and higher quality standards are needed to improve EMS education nationally and at the state level. Therefore, **the committee recommends that states require national accreditation of paramedic education programs (4.2)**. However, the committee recognizes that this requirement would increase the cost of and thus likely reduce access to paramedic education in many states. Access to EMS education programs is a critical issue in many areas of the country but especially in rural states, where reasonable access is necessary for communities to train and maintain sufficient numbers of EMS providers. There are many paramedic training programs in rural areas that do not fit typical "higher education" models and therefore would have a difficult time meeting accreditation standards. Cost is also an issue in that many municipal and volunteer services are already struggling to fund training. The committee recognizes that not all states are prepared to move to national accreditation requirements and proposes that the federal government provide technical assistance and possibly financial support to state governments to help with the transition.

National EMS Certification

Certification is designed to verify competency at a predetermined level of proficiency. The *Education Agenda* anticipated that national EMS certification would be accepted by all state EMS offices as verification of entry-level competency. It envisioned that all EMS graduates would complete an accredited program of instruction and would obtain national certification to qualify for state licensure. Certifying exams would be based on practice analysis and the National EMS Scope of Practice Model (NHTSA, 2000).

NREMT currently offers certification examinations for the first responder, EMT-B, EMT-I, and EMT-P levels, which are accepted by many states as evidence of competency (NHTSA, 1996). Two-thirds of the states use NREMT for initial credentialing of EMTs, and 84 percent of states use it for EMT-Ps (Mears, 2004).

The *Education Agenda* identified several barriers to the universal use of national exams, including the cost of implementation and administration, political issues, the use of a mandated practical exam, lack of local support, and perceived failure rates. Accordingly, it recommended a graduated phase-in plan whereby states would identify a timeline for adoption (NHTSA, 2000).

The committee supports the goals of the *Education Agenda* and recommends that **states accept national certification as a prerequisite for state licensure and local credentialing of emergency medical services providers (4.3).** This measure would support professionalism and consistency among and between the states. However, the committee is cognizant of the fact that requiring national certification would increase the cost of licensure—a significant issue for the volunteer workforce and also for EMS personnel generally, given their low wages. This, along with the difficulty of the national exams, could result in a reduction in the provider pool. While fewer, better-trained personnel may represent an improvement in the long run, this benefit must be weighed against the potential decline in the workforce available to respond to patients in many areas across the country.

For these and other reasons, the National Association of State EMS Officials (NASEMSO) has endorsed the *Education Agenda*, but on the condition that no definite timetable be set for implementation. Within states there is still significant resistance to a national certification requirement, and some state legislatures have moved to reduce or remove these requirements. NHTSA and NASEMSO are currently ramping up an initiative to support states in their efforts to implement these components of the *Education Agenda*; however, state EMS directors remain concerned about reducing the overall number of EMS providers by changing current state requirements. The committee supports efforts to facilitate an eventual transition to national certification.

EMERGENCY MEDICAL SERVICES PERSONNEL

EMTs and paramedics are the backbone of prehospital emergency care in the United States. They provide essential care for patients in emergency situations and are frequently able to reduce patient morbidity and mortality. As noted earlier, although the work they do can be extremely arduous and is not well paid, surveys indicate that many EMS professionals find the job to be highly rewarding (Patterson et al., 2005).

Roles and Responsibilities of EMS Personnel

As described above, EMS personnel have different levels of training and qualifications. The scope of practice of first responders, EMT-Bs, EMT-Is, and EMT-Ps varies by state, but the tasks most commonly performed by each are detailed here (see Boxes 4-2, 4-3, 4-4, and 4-5). First responders provide basic care to patients. Many firefighters, police officers, and other emergency workers have this most basic level of training. They are typically the first to arrive on scene and are therefore able to provide vital care. For example, fire department first responders have been demonstrated to take significantly less time than ambulance attendants to provide defibrillation to victims (Shuster and Keller, 1993). Likewise, police first responders have been shown to perform well in using automated external defibrillators on victims of sudden cardiac arrest (Davis and Mosesso, 1998).

EMT-Bs are generally trained to provide basic, noninvasive prehospital care (although some states may allow them to perform selected invasive procedures). These personnel provide care to patients at the scene of a medical emergency and during transport to the hospital.

EMT-Is perform all the tasks of an EMT-B but may also perform some of the tasks of an EMT-P. The scope of practice for EMT-Is varies widely by state, but is always broader than the scope of practice for an EMT-B in the same state and narrower than the scope of practice for an EMT-P. Nationwide, there are over 40 identifiable versions of licensure between EMT-B and EMT-P.

BOX 4-2
Tasks Performed by the Majority of First Responders

- Obtain vital signs
- Obtain a medical history
- Deliver supplemental oxygen
- Perform an assessment to determine the need for spinal immobilization
- Perform spinal immobilization
- Perform a rapid trauma assessment
- Control severe external bleeding with direct pressure, a pressure dressing, and/or pressure points
- Splint an extremity
- Auscultate breath sounds
- Use a bag valve mask
- Perform manual cardiopulmonary resuscitation
- Perform a physical examination
- Use an automated or semiautomated external defibrillator
- Perform manual airway maneuvers
- Perform eye irrigation
- Manually remove a foreign body airway obstruction
- Use a pulse oximeter

SOURCE: NREMT, 2005.

BOX 4-3
Tasks Performed by the Majority of EMT-Basics

All tasks performed by first responders, plus:

- Insert an oropharyngeal or nasopharyngeal airway
- Perform upper airway suctioning
- Perform manual airway maneuvers
- Determine the Glasgow Coma Score (GCS)
- Administer oral glucose
- Assist patients in taking their own prescribed medications
- Use a glucometer to determine blood glucose level

SOURCE: NREMT, 2005.

BOX 4-4
Tasks Performed by the Majority of EMT-Intermediates

All tasks performed by EMT-Basics, plus:

- Use a stroke scale
- Administer aspirin
- Deliver a medication orally
- Deliver medications using a nebulizer
- Use a sharps protection intravenous (IV) catheter
- Establish a peripheral IV, and monitor during transport

SOURCE: NREMT, 2005.

BOX 4-5
Selected Tasks Performed by the Majority
of EMT-Paramedics

All tasks performed by EMT-Basics and EMT-Intermediates, plus:

- Administer drugs (e.g., epinephrine, sedatives, seizure medications, opioid and nonopioid analgesics, aspirin, oral glucose, nebulizers, metered dose inhalers)
- Administer intravenous fluids
- Obtain and interpret a 12-lead electrocardiograph (ECG)
- Use manual and automated external defibrillators to administer lifesaving shocks to a stopped or erratically beating heart
- Use advanced airway techniques and equipment to assist those patients experiencing a respiratory emergency
- Perform endotracheal and nasotracheal intubations
- Perform needle chest decompression

SOURCE: NREMT, 2005.

EMT-Ps are the most highly skilled emergency medical workers, and they provide the most extensive care. They are trained in all phases of emergency prehospital care, including ALS treatment.

In addition to providing prehospital care, some EMTs now work as technicians in hospital EDs (Franks et al., 2004). These EMT-trained technicians are able to perform basic emergency care in the ED setting, allowing

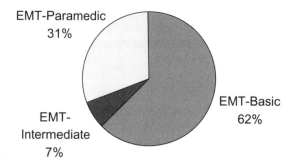

EMT-Paramedic
31%

EMT-Intermediate
7%

EMT-Basic
62%

FIGURE 4-3 NREMT registration status of EMTs, United States, 2003.
SOURCE: NREMT, 2003.

nurses and physicians more time to treat complex cases and perform more intensive procedures. The scope of practice for such personnel is limited, but has increased in some EDs to include intravenous infusions, splinting, and phlebotomy.

The largest group of EMS personnel by far is EMT-Bs, who constituted 62.2 percent of all EMS personnel in 2003 (see Figure 4-3). EMT-Ps constituted another 31.3 percent, while only 6.5 percent were registered as EMT-Is. (Note that these data, and much of the data that follow, are based on the NREMT, which certifies a significant minority of EMS personnel in the United States. As described below, most states use the NREMT for initial licensure of EMT-Bs and EMT-Ps, but very few states require that registration be maintained. This likely results in a bias in the survey results that follow because the pool of respondents is probably younger and different in other ways from those who remain registered. However, broader data reflecting a more representative pool of EMS personnel are not available.)

Demographics of the EMS Workforce

The majority of EMS personnel in the United States are young, white males, although in some rural jurisdictions, females outnumber males in the volunteer workforce. Fully 65 percent of EMS personnel nationwide were men in 2003, compared with 35 percent women. EMS personnel were also substantially younger than the U.S. civilian labor force as a whole (see Figure 4-4). In addition, EMT-Bs were younger than EMT-Ps (20.7 and 8.2 percent, respectively, were under age 25).

Finally, in 2003 the vast majority of EMS personnel were non-Hispanic white—86.1 percent, compared with 67.9 percent of the total U.S. population. African Americans, Hispanics, and Asians/Pacific Islanders were sub-

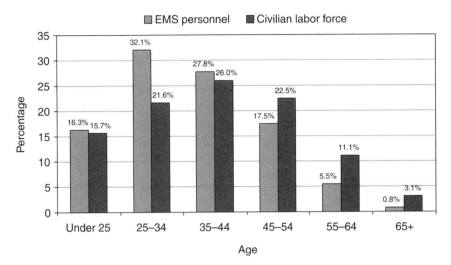

FIGURE 4-4 Age distribution of EMS personnel (2003) and the civilian labor force (2002), United States.
SOURCES: NREMT, 2003; BLS, 2004a.

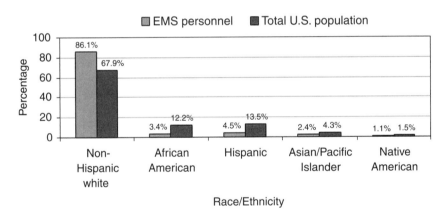

FIGURE 4-5 Race/ethnicity of EMS personnel and the total U.S. population, 2003.
SOURCES: NREMT, 2003; U.S. Bureau of the Census, 2004.

stantially underrepresented relative to their percentage of the population (see Figure 4-5). Racial/ethnic distribution varied between urban and rural areas: while only 2.1 percent of EMS personnel in rural areas were African American and only 1.2 percent Hispanic, the numbers in large cities were 7.8 and 12.4 percent, respectively.

EMT is an occupation primarily of rural areas and small towns. In 2003, 32.5 percent of EMS personnel reported that they were employed in a small town, 21.6 percent that they were employed in a rural community, and 16.4 percent that they were employed in a medium-sized town. Only 9.9 percent of EMS personnel reported employment in a large city (see Figure 4-6).

Reflecting this preponderance of employment in rural areas, the majority of EMS personnel (57.4 percent) responded to fewer than 10 calls per week in 2003 (see Figure 4-7). Among EMS personnel in rural communities, only 9.1 percent responded to 10 or more calls per week, versus 80.7 percent in large cities.

In urban areas, there has been an increasing trend for emergency medical/ambulance services to be assumed by municipal fire departments. In 2003, EMS personnel were most likely to be employed by fire department–based services (37.6 percent), followed by county- or municipal-based services (24.3 percent) and volunteer rescue services (21.7 percent). A smaller number of EMS personnel worked for hospital-based services (15.5 percent), including private ambulance companies (see Figure 4-8).

Size of the EMS Workforce

It is difficult to know how many EMS personnel are currently employed in the United States because registration requirements vary across states and because so many EMS personnel are volunteers (see Table 4-1). There were

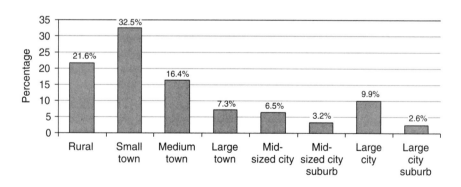

FIGURE 4-6 Type of community in which EMS personnel employed, United States, 2003.
SOURCE: NREMT, 2003.

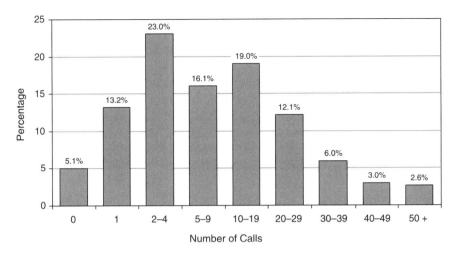

FIGURE 4-7 Number of calls responded to by EMS personnel per week, United States, 2003.
SOURCE: NREMT, 2003.

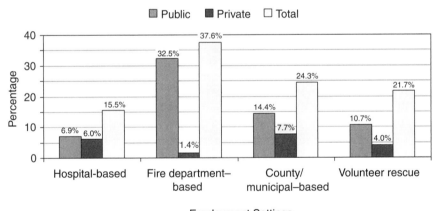

FIGURE 4-8 Public versus private employment settings of EMS personnel, United States, 2003.
SOURCE: NREMT, 2003.

192,182 EMTs in NREMT in 2004; as noted earlier, however, while many states require initial national registration for their EMS personnel, not all require that active EMTs maintain their national registration. As a result, the NREMT figure is in all likelihood an undercount. Bureau of Labor Statistics (BLS) data show 192,000 EMTs employed nationwide in 2004. However,

TABLE 4-1 Estimates of the EMS Workforce in the United States

Type	Description	Number	Source
State-Licensed EMTs	Individuals who, regardless of their employment status, are state-licensed as EMTs	775,000	State licensure lists, 2005
Employer-Classified EMT Jobs	Paid jobs classified by employers, regardless of training or licensure requirements, as "EMT"	192,000	BLS, 2004
Nationally Registered EMTs	Individuals who, regardless of their employment status, are nationally registered as EMTs	192,182	NREMT, 2004
Self-Reported EMTs as Primary Paid Job	Individuals who, regardless of training or licensure, self-report EMT as their primary paid employment	132,000	2000 Census Public Use Microdata Sample

SOURCES: NREMT, 2004; BLS, 2004b; Lindstrom, 2006.

these data are employer-reported and do not include volunteer EMS person-nel. The 2000 Census Public Use Microdata Sample shows 132,398 EMTs employed as their primary job, but again, many EMT positions are only part-time or on a volunteer basis. Approximately 775,000 EMTs held state licenses in 2005, but this figure includes individuals who are no longer active EMTs and is likely an overcount.

BLS projects that EMS positions will increase by 59,000 between 2002 and 2012, an estimated growth rate of 33 percent. Total job openings for the period, including replacement positions, are estimated at 80,000 (BLS, 2004a).

Population growth and increasing urbanization are fueling this pro-jected increase. The aging of the population will further stimulate demand for EMS, as older Americans will be more likely to have medical emergen-cies. Demand for EMS personnel will also continue to be strong in rural and smaller metropolitan areas (BLS, 2006). This is especially true given that it takes more EMS personnel to run a volunteer service now than was the case a decade ago (see below).

Even before factoring in this added demand, there is currently a per-ceived shortage of EMS personnel in the United States. This perception has been driven in part by reported shortages of paramedics in major cities such as Washington, D.C. In 2005, the District announced that 57 of its 166 para-medic positions were unfilled. As a result, 12 of its 14 ALS ambulances were being staffed by tiered units, including a paramedic and an EMT, rather than

TABLE 4-2 NREMT Exams per Year (Timeframe July 1–June 30)

	2000	2001	2002	2003	2004
First Responder	4,086	6,090	5,209	7,108	7,363
EMT-Basic	46,346	63,067	65,398	75,594	83,692
EMT-Intermediate 85	5,243	5,900	5,284	5,169	5,413
EMT-Intermediate 95		332	439	681	1,327
Paramedic	8,749	11,284	13,738	12,806	14,803
Total	64,424	86,673	90,068	101,358	112,598

SOURCE: NREMT, 2004.

two paramedics (Wilber, 2005). The decision as to the appropriate staffing of ambulance units is one factor determining whether a paramedic shortage is perceived to exist in any given jurisdiction. In addition, numerous issues relating to recruitment and retention of personnel play significant roles.

The number of personnel available for recruitment varies according to the number of individuals in the EMT education pipeline. For the most part, graduations from EMT education programs increased steadily from the 1995–1996 through the 2001–2002 academic years (National Center for Education Statistics, 2000). In addition, the number of individuals who were tested by NREMT increased markedly from 2000 to 2004 (see Table 4-2) (NREMT, 2004). However, the number of paramedics tested remained relatively flat during 2002–2004, perhaps contributing to the perceived shortage in many parts of the country.

NHTSA and the Health Resources and Services Administration (HRSA) are currently funding an EMS Workforce for the 21st Century project that will provide a systematic assessment of the nation's EMS workforce. The project will examine the future of the EMS workforce in the United States and establish a National EMS Workforce Policy Agenda. The project is managed by the Center for the Health Professions at the University of California-San Francisco.

RECRUITMENT AND RETENTION

EMS personnel have indicated in surveys that their work provides them with a sense of accomplishment and belonging in the community. However, overall job satisfaction is often very low because of concerns regarding personal safety, stressful working conditions, irregular hours, limited potential for career advancement, excessive training requirements, and modest pay and benefits (Cydulka et al., 1997; Brown et al., 2003; Patterson et al., 2005).

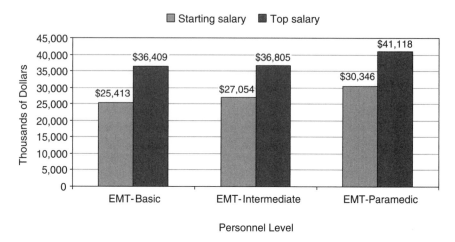

FIGURE 4-9 Average annual starting and top salaries for EMS personnel, United States, 2002.
SOURCE: Monosky, 2002.

Nationwide, salaries for EMS personnel in 2002 averaged between $25,413 (starting) and $36,409 (top) for EMT-Bs, between $27,054 and $36,805 for EMT-Is, and between $30,346 and $41,118 for EMT-Ps (see Figure 4-9). Salaries for EMS personnel have been increasing, but they are still lower than those for other health care professionals. For example, BLS data indicate that the mean average salary for registered nurses was $52,410 in 2004 (BLS, 2004b).

In addition, there is no well-defined career ladder for EMS personnel (Patterson et al., 2005). EMS personnel in fire department–based services sometimes must transition out of EMS work to assume other duties in order to advance within their organization. Others work as EMS personnel as a step toward becoming a physician assistant or a registered nurse.

Safety

Working conditions for EMS personnel are physically demanding and often dangerous. Injury rates for EMS workers are high; back injuries are especially common, as are other "sprains, strains, tears" (Maguire et al., 2005). The most dangerous times for EMS personnel are when they are inside an ambulance while it is moving or when they are working at a crash scene near other moving vehicles (Garrison, 2002). In addition, EMS personnel are frequently exposed to the threat of violence and other unpredictable and uncontrolled situations (Franks et al., 2004). Moreover, EMS personnel can be exposed to potentially infectious bodily fluids and airborne pathogens.

As a result of the emotional and psychological stresses of their job, EMS personnel may experience burnout and even post-traumatic stress disorder. Moreover, Maguire and colleagues (2002) found that EMS workers' occupational fatality rates were comparable to those of police and fire department personnel. The researchers estimated a rate of 12.7 fatalities per 100,000 EMS workers annually, compared with 14.2 for police, 16.5 for firefighters, and an overall national average of 5.0. These health and safety hazards for EMS personnel can contribute to high rates of job-related illnesses, low job satisfaction, and high turnover.

Workforce Mobility

Another key challenge is that EMS personnel who are licensed in one state but want to practice in another are often restricted in their ability to do so. As noted earlier, the legal scope of practice for EMS personnel is not consistent across states, and many states have extensive paperwork and testing requirements that can be burdensome for EMS personnel. For other professionals, such as physicians and nurses, transfer from one state to another is often much easier.

The *Emergency Medical Services Agenda for the Future: Implementation Guide* described the need to eliminate legal barriers to intra- and interstate reciprocity for EMS provider credentials. The committee supports this position, and maintains that reciprocity for licensing across states should be improved and requirements standardized. For example, paperwork requirements (e.g., diploma, current unencumbered license, continuing education credits) and testing requirements should be largely similar across states. While deciding which of the many different state requirements to standardize is challenging, improving reciprocity is an important objective that states should actively pursue. In addition, the movement toward national certification will help institute greater uniformity and will allow for improved reciprocity.

The Volunteer Workforce

EMS is different from all other health care occupations in that a substantial number of its workers serve in a volunteer capacity. According to data gathered by NREMT, 36.5 percent of registered EMS personnel were volunteers in 2003. In some states, the number of EMS personnel who were volunteers was well above 50 percent. The vast majority of volunteer EMS personnel were EMT-Bs (89.5 percent). Figures 4-10a and 4-10b, respectively, show the percentages of EMS personnel at the EMT-B, EMT-I, and EMT-P levels who are volunteers and paid employees.

In 2003, 75 percent of EMS personnel in rural areas were volunteers, compared with 7.5 percent in large cities (see Figure 4-11). Nearly 86 percent of rural EMTs were EMT-Bs, compared with 48.1 percent in large cities, where almost half of EMTs (47.7 percent) were EMT-Ps. As a result, rural Americans frequently do not have access to the same level of prehospital care as urban Americans.

Volunteer personnel have traditionally been the lifeblood of rural EMS agencies (see also Chapter 3). Since the development of EMS systems began in the 1960s, countless millions of hours have been contributed by rural EMS personnel to the care of neighbors, friends, and complete strangers. For a variety of reasons, however, volunteer staffing has become increasingly difficult.

The demographic characteristics of rural communities are changing rapidly. In many rural areas, the population is aging as younger residents move away. During the 1990s, more than 300 rural counties in the United States experienced a 15 percent or greater increase in their elderly population as a result of migration (IOM, 2004). This demographic shift can impact EMS systems in two ways; first, as noted earlier, increased demand on EMS systems is associated with a more fragile elderly population; second, the pool of potential volunteers is reduced. Moreover, those who migrate to rural areas from city environments often have unrealistic expectations of rural EMS systems and place considerable demands on the volunteer workforce.

In addition, the face of volunteerism is changing overall (Putnam, 2000). As discussed in Chapter 3, during the early stages of EMS, it was not uncommon for volunteers to be on call virtually 24 hours a day. Today there are more demands on volunteers' time as a result of the need for two-income families, as well as competing interests, and volunteers are more likely to donate one specific weeknight or a few hours on a weekend. As a result, rural EMS agencies are faced with volunteer staffing shortages, particularly during the weekday work hours.

Demands on remaining volunteers have been exacerbated by the closure or restructuring of many rural hospital facilities. While these changes have increased the efficiency and viability of the remaining rural hospitals, they have increased the demands placed on rural EMS agencies because of the need for long-distance and time-consuming interfacility transfers. It is not uncommon for such transfers to keep volunteers away from their jobs or families for 3 to 6 hours or more.

New staffing models are needed for rural EMS systems. These might include consolidation and regionalization of transporting EMS programs, augmented locally by nontransporting quick-response units that provide immediate care and stabilization. Additionally, paid staffing, either alone or

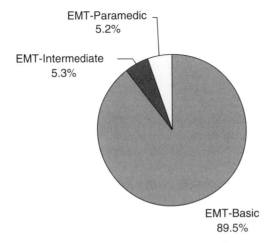

FIGURE 4-10a Volunteer NREMT registrants, United States, 2003.
SOURCE: NREMT, 2003.

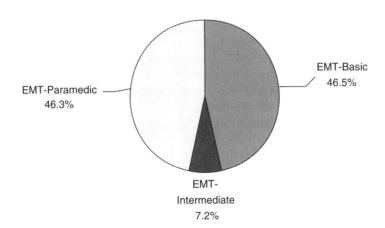

FIGURE 4-10b Paid NREMT registrants, United States, 2003.
SOURCE: NREMT, 2003.

to augment the volunteer force, must be considered. Finally, opportunities for rural prehospital personnel to expand their responsibilities within the health care or public health arena should be explored. Such opportunities would enable these personnel to receive competitive compensation while maintaining a variety of skills and contributing to the overall well-being of the community (McGinnis, 2004). Long undervalued, EMS must become an essential health care service that is publicly supported.

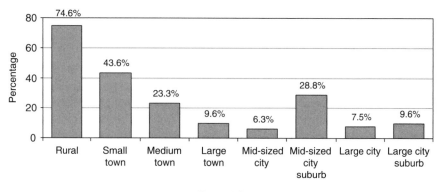

FIGURE 4-11 Percentage of volunteer EMS personnel by type of community, United States, 2003.
SOURCE: NREMT, 2003.

Bystander Care

Although not a part of the EMS workforce, bystanders are often first on the scene in emergency medical situations. Because time is such a crucial factor, they may be in the best position to render immediate care while EMS personnel are in transit. EMDs typically have protocols for delivering prearrival instructions to bystanders so they can administer such treatments as cardiopulmonary resuscitation (CPR) for heart attack victims and the Heimlich maneuver for choking victims. Provision of instructions for CPR by telephone, for example, is associated with a 50 percent improvement in the odds of survival compared with cases in which no CPR is administered before the arrival of EMS (Rea et al., 2001; Idris and Roppolo, 2003).

As a result, efforts are under way to increase rates of bystander care, for example, through public service announcements (Becker et al., 1999). Such efforts are particularly important for minority populations, who are less likely to receive CPR training than whites (Brookoff et al., 1994). In addition, bystander training in CPR is shifting from lengthy programs offered in large classes to video self-instruction (Todd et al., 1999; Brennan and Braslow, 2000). Web-based formats for such training have also been developed.

Placement of automated external defibrillators (AEDs) in public areas such as airports provides bystanders with additional capabilities to provide needed care. Bystanders can thereby act as an extension of the emergency care workforce and dramatically improve outcomes for out-of-hospital emergency patients. The Public Access Defibrillation trial, the largest EMS clinical trial completed in the United States to date, found that the number of survivors of sudden cardiac arrest increased substantially when the victims were helped by community volunteers trained to use CPR and an AED as compared with those aided by volunteers using CPR alone.

EMERGENCY MEDICAL DISPATCHERS

In responding to medical emergencies, EMDs are often the first link in the care continuum. Though they often are not viewed as part of the patient care team, EMDs serve three important medical functions: (1) they perform medical triage by assessing the patient's needs; (2) they dispatch appropriate medical and rescue resources; and (3) as noted above, they sometimes provide prearrival instructions to bystanders, or patients themselves, on how to provide lifesaving first aid on scene.

When responding to calls, EMDs question each caller to determine the type, seriousness, and location of the emergency. They monitor the location of EMS personnel and dispatch the appropriate type and number of units. In a medical emergency, EMDs keep in close touch not only with the dispatched units, but also with the caller. They also give updates on the patient's condition to ambulance personnel who are en route (BLS, 2004a).

Not all emergency dispatchers are trained EMDs. Many are public safety communicators, often fire or police department–based. In many cases, emergency calls are initially fielded by these emergency communicators at a primary call center and then transferred to EMDs at a secondary call center. In many other instances, the primary call center handles all calls, and no EMDs are available.

EMDs are required to undergo education and training to receive their designation. Training for EMDs is conducted mainly by private companies using their own curriculum. NHTSA sought to develop a national standard EMD curriculum in the early 1990s (similar to the curricula for other levels of EMS personnel); however, dispatch protocols for the curriculum were never completed.

Generally, EMDs are poorly paid, and given the stress associated with their jobs, it is not surprising that 9-1-1 call centers experience high rates of turnover. The median annual salary for EMDs in 2003 was below $29,000 (BLS, 2004b). The vast majority of EMDs (85.9 percent) work for local governments (see Figure 4-12). A smaller number (4.7 percent) work for state governments and for private health providers (BLS, 2004a).

A sizable portion of 9-1-1 calls received by public safety answering points (PSAPs) are not emergency calls. One former Philadelphia fire EMS medical director calculated that only 18 percent of calls received by the local PSAP in 1 year could be classified as emergency calls (Davidson, 1995). In Fort Worth, Texas, up to 60 percent of 9-1-1 calls that received an EMS response were later classified as not requiring emergency services (Neely,

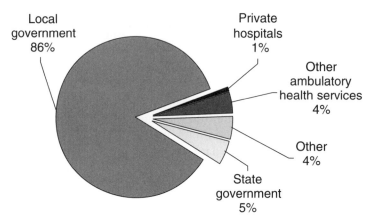

FIGURE 4-12 Employment setting for EMDs, 2002.
SOURCE: BLS, 2004a.

1996). However, these calculations were performed retrospectively, and they mask the difficulty of distinguishing between calls requiring ambulance service and those that could be handled safely through delivery to the hospital in a private vehicle.

Studies in both the United States and the United Kingdom have shown that dispatch criteria can safely identify 9-1-1 calls that do not need an on-scene response (Dale et al., 2000; Smith et al., 2001; Snooks et al., 2002). The successful referral of such calls has the potential to relieve ED and hospital crowding by diffusing demand for care over a wider range of resources. Recent experience in Richmond, Virginia, indicates that, based on a review of dispatch determinants and volume, call referrals can reduce on-scene responses by approximately 15 percent.

EMS MEDICAL DIRECTORS

EMS care has been called "medical care on wheels." Accordingly, nonphysician EMS personnel, whether dispatchers, fire department first responders, EMTs, or paramedics, are required to operate under the orders of a physician medical director. This is especially true of paramedics, who, as detailed earlier, perform the most extensive out-of-hospital medical procedures. In a few communities, such as Seattle, Pittsburgh, Milwaukee, Atlanta, and Houston, highly qualified and experienced EMS physicians provide medical oversight for EMS personnel. In other communities, the medical director is little more than a figurehead.

Anecdotal evidence suggests the importance of strong medical direction in improving outcomes for out-of-hospital emergency care (Davis, 2003b), a view widespread within the field (NRC, 1981; ACEP, 2005). Currently, however, such oversight is minimal in many areas of the country, largely because of funding constraints, but also political and cultural issues (Davis, 2003a). In many cases, medical direction is a contracted service provided through a bid process, with the medical director reporting to the fire chief or the head of the EMS agency. This system forces physicians to compete against each other in terms of cost, and in many cases the rigorousness of the medical direction provided, so that the system is subject to considerable internal conflict. The result is that often there is minimal medical oversight, and physicians face the constant threat of being underbid. Recognizing these limitations, the committee maintains that each EMS system should have highly involved and engaged medical directors who can help ensure that EMS personnel are providing high-quality care based on current standards of evidence.

Medical direction of EMS systems has several components, including on-line (direct) and off-line (indirect) medical oversight. On-line direction involves providing direct orders to EMS field personnel regarding the care of specific patients. Such direction is usually provided over the radio or telephone by a physician at the receiving hospital, although there are other, more centralized models. Off-line medical direction involves providing medical oversight through education, protocol development, and quality assurance. Such direction is typically provided by physicians who are paid or volunteer to serve as the medical director of a local, regional, or state EMS system.

The qualifications for medical directors differ considerably among EMS systems. As a result, the training and experience of EMS medical directors are highly variable. While the National Association of EMS Physicians and the American College of Emergency Physicians have jointly developed guidelines that address the qualifications and role of EMS medical directors, these guidelines are not universally recognized. Over the past decade, an increasing number of residency-trained emergency physicians have completed a 1- or 2-year EMS fellowship program developed by the Society of Academic Emergency Medicine (Marx, 1999). Graduates of these programs are increasingly involved in academic pursuits, including research and direction of EMS systems. Nonetheless, there are currently limited opportunities for emergency physicians to become certified as subspecialists in EMS. While the American Board of Osteopathic Emergency Medicine has established a subspecialty in EMS for its diplomates, the American Board of Emergency Medicine has yet to follow suit.

The 1998 *Emergency Medical Services Agenda for the Future: Implementation Guide* called for the designation of EMS as a physician subspecialty (see Box 4-6). The committee supports this position and recom-

BOX 4-6
EMS Physician Subspecialty Objectives

Short Term: Continue to work to define the specific knowledge and expertise required of physicians who specialize in EMS.
Intermediate Term: Enable the American Board of Emergency Medicine (ABEM) to sponsor an EMS subspecialty.
Long Term: Petition the American Board of Medical Specialties (ABMS) to designate EMS as a physician subspecialty.

SOURCE: NHTSA, 1998.

mends that the American Board of Emergency Medicine create a subspecialty certification in emergency medical services (4.4). The certification would be analogous to those available in toxicology, sports medicine, and pediatric emergency medicine. Creating this type of designation would acknowledge the unique challenges and complexities of the out-of-hospital environment. The certification would ensure that physicians providing medical direction would be trained specifically in prehospital EMS and prepared to meet the challenges likely to be encountered.

SUMMARY OF RECOMMENDATIONS

4.1: State governments should adopt a common scope of practice for emergency medical services personnel, with state licensing reciprocity.

4.2: States should require national accreditation of paramedic education programs.

4.3: States should accept national certification as a prerequisite for state licensure and local credentialing of emergency medical services providers.

4.4: The American Board of Emergency Medicine should create a subspecialty certification in emergency medical services.

REFERENCES

ACEP (American College of Emergency Physicians). 2005. *Medical Direction of Prehospital Emergency Medical Services*. [Online]. Available: http://www.acep.org/webportal/PracticeResources/issues/ems/PREPMedicalDirectionofPrehospitalEmergencyMedicalServices.htm [accessed November 1, 2005].

Beck AH. 2004. STUDENTJAMA. The Flexner report and the standardization of American medical education. *Journal of the American Medical Association* 291(17):2139–2140.

Becker L, Vath J, Eisenberg M, Meischke H. 1999. The impact of television public service announcements on the rate of bystander CPR. *Prehospital Emergency Care* 3(4):353–356.

BLS (Bureau of Labor Statistics). 2004a. *2002 National, State, Metropolitan Area, and Industry-Specific Occupational Employment and Wage Estimates*.

BLS. 2004b. *Occupational Employment Statistics: National Industry-Specific Occupational Employment and Wage Estimates* (NAICS 621900: Other Ambulatory Health Care Services). Washington, DC: U.S. Department of Labor.

BLS. 2006. *Occupational Outlook Handbook, 2006–2007 Edition: Emergency Medical Technicians and Paramedics*. [Online]. Available: http://www.bls.gov/oco/ocos101.htm [accessed March 5, 2006].

Brennan RT, Braslow A. 2000. Video self-instruction for cardiopulmonary resuscitation. *Annals of Emergency Medicine* 36(1):79–80.

Brookoff D, Kellermann AL, Hackman BB, Somes G, Dobyns P. 1994. Do blacks get bystander cardiopulmonary resuscitation as often as whites? *Annals of Emergency Medicine* 24(6):1147–1150.

Brown WE Jr, Dawson D, Levine R. 2003. Compensation, benefits, and satisfaction: The Longitudinal Emergency Medical Technician Demographic Study (LEADS) project. *Prehospital Emergency Care* 7(3):357–362.

Cydulka RK, Emerman CL, Shade B, Kubincanek J. 1997. Stress levels in EMS personnel: A national survey. *Prehospital & Disaster Medicine* 12(2):136–140.

Dale J, Williams S, Foster T, Higgins J, Crouch R, Snooks H, Sharpe C, Glucksman E, George S. 2000. *The Clinical, Organisational and Cost Consequences of Computer-Assisted Telephone Advice to Category C 999 Ambulance Service Callers: Results of a Controlled Trial. Final Report 2000*. [Online]. Available: http://medweb.bham.ac.uk/emerg/ASTAP%20report.pdf [accessed May 24, 2006].

Davidson SJ. 1995. *The Comm Center: Gate Keeper or Access Facilitator?* Presentation at the meeting of the Sand Key II Conference, St. Petersburg Beach, FL.

Davis EA, Mosesso VN Jr. 1998. Performance of police first responders in utilizing automated external defibrillation on victims of sudden cardiac arrest. *Prehospital Emergency Care* 2(2):101–107.

Davis R. 2003a. Doctors in charge rarely call the shots. [Online]. Available: http://www.usatoday.com/news/nation/ems-day2-directors.htm [accessed January 27, 2007].

Davis R. 2003b. Only strong leaders can overhaul EMS. *USA Today*. [Online]. Available: http://www.usatoday.com/news/nation/ems-day3-cover.htm [accessed January 27, 2007].

Delbridge TR, Bailey B, Chew JL Jr, Conn AK, Krakeel JJ, Manz D, Miller DR, O'Malley PJ, Ryan SD, Spaite DW, Stewart RD, Suter RE, Wilson EM. 1998. EMS agenda for the future: Where we are . . . where we want to be. *Prehospital Emergency Care* 2(1):1–12.

DOT (U.S. Department of Transportation). 1998. *EMT-Paramedic: National Standard Curriculum*. [Online]. Available: http://www.nhtsa.dot.gov/people/injury/ems/EMT-P/ [accessed April 24, 2006].

Franks PE, Kocher N, Chapman S. 2004. *Emergency Medical Technicians and Paramedics in California*. San Francisco, CA: University of California, San Francisco Center for the Health Professions.

Garrison HG. 2002. Keeping rescuers safe. *Annals of Emergency Medicine* 40(6):633–635.

Hiatt MD, Stockton CG. 2003. The impact of the Flexner report on the fate of medical schools in North America after 1909. *Journal of American Physicians and Surgeons* 8(2):37–40.

Idris AH, Roppolo L. 2003. Barriers to dispatcher-assisted telephone cardiopulmonary resuscitation. *Annals of Emergency Medicine* 42(6):738–740.

IOM (Institute of Medicine). 2004. *Quality through Collaboration: The Future of Rural Health*. Washington, DC: The National Academies Press.

Lindstrom AM. 2006. 2006 JEMS platinum resource guide. *Journal of Emergency Medical Services* 31(1):42–56, 101.

Maguire BJ, Hunting KL, Smith GS, Levick NR. 2002. Occupational fatalities in emergency medical services: A hidden crisis. *Annals of Emergency Medicine* 40(6):625–632.

Maguire BJ, Hunting KL, Guidotti TL, Smith GS. 2005. Occupational injuries among emergency medical services personnel. *Prehospital Emergency Care* 9(4):405–411.

Marx JA. 1999. SAEM emergency medical services fellowship guidelines. SAEM EMS Task Force. *Academic Emergency Medicine* 6(10):1069–1070.

McGinnis K. 2004. *Rural and Frontier Emergency Medical Services Agenda for the Future*. Kansas City, MO: National Rural Health Association.

Mears G. 2004. *2003 Survey and Analysis of EMS Scope of Practice and Practice Settings Impacting EMS Services in Rural America: Executive Brief and Recommendations*. Chapel Hill, NC: University of North Carolina at Chapel Hill Department of Emergency Medicine.

Monosky KA. 2002. JEMS' 2002 EMS salary and workplace survey: Quantifying the tangible rewards of a career in EMS. *Journal of Emergency Medical Services* 27(10):30–46.

National Center for Education Statistics. 2000. *Integrated Postsecondary Education Data System (IPEDS)*. [Online]. Available: http://nces.ed.gov/ipeds/data.asp [accessed January 12, 2006].

Neely K. 1996. In the starting gates once again, managed care in EMS. *NAEMSP News* 5(4).

NHTSA (National Highway Traffic Safety Administration). 1996. *Emergency Medical Services Agenda for the Future*. Washington, DC: Department of Transportation.

NHTSA. 1998. *Emergency Medical Services Agenda for the Future: Implementation Guide*. Washington, DC: Department of Transportation.

NHTSA. 2000. *Emergency Medical Services Education Agenda for the Future: A Systems Approach*. Washington, DC: Department of Transportation.

NHTSA. 2005. *The National EMS Scope of Practice Model*. Washington, DC: Department of Transportation.

NHTSA. 2006. *National Standard Curricula*. [Online]. Available: http://www.nhtsa.dot.gov/people/injury/ems/nsc.htm [accessed January 25, 2006].

NHTSA, HRSA (NHTSA, Health Resources and Services Administration). 2005. *National EMS Core Content: The Domain of EMS Practice*. Washington, DC: NHTSA, HRSA.

NRC (National Research Council). 1981. *Medical Control in Emergency Medical Services Systems: Report of the Subcommittee on Medical Control in EMS Systems*. Washington, DC: National Academy of Sciences.

NREMT (National Registry of Emergency Medical Technicians). 1993. *National Emergency Medical Services Education and Practice Blueprint*. Columbus, OH: NREMT.

NREMT. 2003. *Longitudinal Emergency Medical Technician Attributes and Demographics Survey (LEADS) Data*. [Online]. Available: http://www.nremt.org/about/lead_survey.asp [accessed February 24, 2006].

NREMT. 2004. *2004 Annual Report*. Columbus, OH: NREMT.

NREMT. 2005. *National EMS Practice Analysis*. Columbus, OH: NREMT.

Patterson PD, Probst JC, Leith KH, Corwin SJ, Powell MP. 2005. Recruitment and retention of emergency medical technicians: A qualitative study. *Journal of Allied Health* 34(3):153–162.

Putnam RD. 2000. *Bowling Alone: The Collapse and Revival of American Community.* New York: Simon & Schuster.

Rea TD, Eisenberg MS, Culley LL, Becker L. 2001. Dispatcher-assisted cardiopulmonary resuscitation and survival in cardiac arrest. *Circulation* 104(21):2513–2516.

Shuster M, Keller JL. 1993. Effect of fire department first-responder automated defibrillation. *Annals of Emergency Medicine* 22(4):721–727.

Smith E, Singh T, Adirim T. 2001. Outstanding outreach: A prehospital notification system makes a difference for special needs children. *Journal of Emergency Medical Services* 26(5):48–55.

Snooks H, Williams S, Crouch R, Foster T, Hartley-Sharpe C, Dale J. 2002. NHS emergency response to 999 calls: Alternatives for cases that are neither life threatening nor serious. *British Medical Journal* 325(7359):330–333.

Todd KH, Heron SL, Thompson M, Dennis R, O'Connor J, Kellermann AL. 1999. Simple CPR: A randomized, controlled trial of video self-instructional cardiopulmonary resuscitation training in an African American church congregation. *Annals of Emergency Medicine* 34(6):730–737.

U.S. Bureau of the Census. 2004. *Annual Estimates of the Population by Sex, Race and Hispanic or Latino Origin for the United States: April 1, 2000 to July 1, 2003.* [Online]. Available: http://www.census.gov/popest/archives/2000s/vintage_2004/ [accessed March 2, 2006].

Wilber DQ. 2005, May 7. D.C. paramedic shortage causes concern. *The Washington Post.* P. B03.

5

Advancing System Infrastructure

Emergency medical services (EMS) personnel rely on many different types of equipment to provide timely and effective treatment to patients requiring emergency care. This equipment ranges from basic transport vehicles, such as ambulances and helicopters; to medical devices, such as defibrillators and heart monitors; to communications equipment that allows for transmission of patient information between ambulance and hospital or among first responders in the case of a significant disaster event. In addition, patients rely on effective communications systems that enable them to summon help when needed and ensure that care is on the way.

Over time, technological advances have led to improvements in the delivery of EMS. Automatic crash notification (ACN) technology enables immediate notification of emergency responders when a car crash has occurred. Devices provide instant, audible warnings to ambulance drivers if their driving becomes unsafe. And systems are under development that may eventually allow prehospital EMS personnel in the field to view complete patient health records and potentially replace paper-based ambulance "run records" with electronic data submissions.

Set against this backdrop of evolving technology, however, is the basic reality that most EMS systems do not have the resources needed to make major system upgrades. A significant percentage of the communications equipment currently in use by ambulances was purchased in the 1970s with federal financial assistance. Revamping EMS voice and data communications capabilities, including the infrastructure required to support an electronic health record (EHR) system, would almost certainly require a significant investment on the part of the federal government. Moreover,

149

not all local EMS providers agree that newer, more sophisticated technology necessarily translates into better or more efficient patient care. The end result is that the infrastructure supporting EMS personnel across the country is highly variable and uneven. In many areas there is a growing gap between the type of equipment now available and that which is actually in use. This chapter details key areas in which technology can play a role in supporting effective EMS response: emergency notification and dispatch, equipment for emergency response, and communications and data systems.

EMERGENCY NOTIFICATION AND DISPATCH

The development and implementation of a single nationwide number to call in emergency situations was a major advance for the U.S. emergency and trauma care system. Before 9-1-1 was fully adopted, states and localities had in place a vast array of 7-digit telephone numbers for citizens to call in the case of an emergency. In the early 1970s, for example, Nebraska had 184 different ambulance service phone numbers in use in various parts of the state (NAS and NRC, 1978; IOM, 1993). Designating a simple 3-digit, standardized number to call in emergencies helped avoid the confusion and delays that inevitably occurred with having so many different numbers for so many different types of emergencies in various parts of the country.

One of the early catalysts for the development of the 9-1-1 system in the United States occurred in 1957 when the National Association of Fire Chiefs recommended the use of a single number for reporting fires. In addition, the 1966 report *Accidental Death and Disability* contained a recommendation that there be "active exploration of the feasibility of designating a single nationwide telephone number to summon an ambulance" (NAS and NRC, 1966).

In 1967, a presidential commission recommended that a uniform number be used to reach emergency response agencies. The following year, AT&T announced that it would establish 9-1-1 as the emergency code throughout the United States. The first 9-1-1 call was placed in February 1968 (NENA, 2004). In 1973, the Department of Transportation recommended that the universal emergency number be 9-1-1 and provided model legislation for states to use in implementing this system (DOT Wireless E9-1-1 Steering Council, 2002). Implementation of the 9-1-1 system occurred very unevenly across the country, however. By 1992, a number of states, including California and Connecticut, had 100 percent of their populations covered by a 9-1-1 system. In that same year, however, other states had less than 50 percent access, while some, including Maine and Vermont, had only 25 percent coverage (IOM, 1993). Such disparities in the management of 9-1-1 systems nationwide persist today.

To improve federal coordination and communication on 9-1-1 activities, the ENHANCE 9-1-1 Act was enacted in 2004. The act established a national 9-1-1 Implementation Coordination Office. In addition to improving federal coordination, this office will develop and disseminate information concerning practices, procedures, and technology used in the implementation of 9-1-1 services and will also administer a grant program to enable 9-1-1 call centers to upgrade their equipment. The National 9-1-1 Office is housed within the National Highway Traffic Safety Administration's (NHTSA) Office of EMS, which will partner with the National Telecommunications and Information Administration, located within the Department of Commerce (NHTSA Office of EMS, 2006).

The Current 9-1-1 System

Americans place an estimated 200 million 9-1-1 calls each year (NENA, 2004). An estimated 85 percent of those calls are directed to the police, while the remaining 15 percent are divided between fire departments and EMS (NENA, 2001). In recent years, the number of EMS calls relative to fire department calls has been increasing. According to the National Fire Protection Association, 80 percent of fire service calls are EMS-related (National Fire Protection Association, 2005).

The 9-1-1 system is locally based and operated, and its structure varies widely across the country. Today there are over 6,000 public safety answering points (PSAPs), or 9-1-1 call centers, nationwide. Various approaches are used to fund these local 9-1-1 systems, including state or local taxes and state or local telephone subscriber fees. Implementation has generally been managed by individual counties or other local governmental units that try to coordinate public resources and work with public safety agencies and telephone companies to help finance and operate the system (IOM, 1993).

While basic 9-1-1 service enables callers to contact an emergency dispatcher, newer, enhanced 9-1-1 (E9-1-1) has the added feature of enabling the dispatcher to identify the telephone number and location of callers using fixed telephone lines (see Table 5-1). This is accomplished through automatic number identification and automatic location identification technologies. These features allow dispatchers to obtain a call-back number in case the call is cut off, as well as immediate access to the caller's location, which speeds ambulance dispatch. Currently, 93 percent of counties that have basic 9-1-1 have E9-1-1; however, there remain 350 counties without automatic location information and access to a call-back number (NENA, 2004).

Impact of Wireless Technology

An estimated one-third of 9-1-1 calls are now made on cell phones (GAO, 2003), and in some jurisdictions that figure is as high as 50 percent

TABLE 5-1 Types of 9-1-1 Call Capacity

Basic 9-1-1	Enhanced 9-1-1	Wireless Phase I	Wireless Phase II	Next-Generation 9-1-1
9-1-1 is dialed, and a public safety answering point (PSAP) dispatcher answers the call.	A 9-1-1 call is selectively routed to the proper PSAP. The PSAP has access to the caller's phone number and address.	The 9-1-1 call taker automatically receives the wireless phone number and the location of the cell tower handling the call, but not the exact location of the caller.	The 9-1-1 call taker receives both the caller's wireless phone number and present location.	Dispatch will be able to receive voice, text, or video transmissions and will have advanced data capabilities.

SOURCE: NENA, 2004.

(DOT Wireless E9-1-1 Steering Council, 2002). The movement toward wireless technology has had a significant impact on 9-1-1 systems because the location of the wireless caller cannot be identified as easily as with a landline phone. This can be medically dangerous because in many emergency situations, callers are incapacitated or unable to speak, or they are unaware of their exact location. The inability to pinpoint the caller's location has resulted in a number of widely reported incidents in which victims have died because rescue workers were not able to arrive in time, even though considerable resources were mobilized to find the caller (DOT Wireless E9-1-1 Steering Council, 2002).

Efforts are under way to ensure that the location of emergency callers can be automatically identified, even if they are using a wireless cell phone. Currently, this capability involves either locating the caller using triangulation of the signal among cell towers or locating the caller by Global Positioning System (GPS) satellite technology. The transition of the telecommunications industry to an E9-1-1 system that is able to detect the location of cellular calls is being directed by the Federal Communications Commission (FCC) and is occurring in two phases. Phase I requires carriers, upon the request of the PSAP, to provide technology that allows the call taker to receive the caller's wireless phone number automatically. This is important in the event that the wireless phone call is dropped, and may allow PSAP employees to work with the wireless company to identify the wireless subscriber. Phase I also delivers the location of the cell tower handling the call. The call is routed to a PSAP based on cell site/sector information. Phase II requires wireless carriers to provide more precise location information in addition to the caller's wireless phone number (DOT Wireless E9-1-1 Steering Council, 2002).

Wireless E9-1-1 capacity is currently being developed nationwide, although its uptake has been sporadic. In 1996, the FCC adopted rules requiring wireless carriers to provide E9-1-1 service. For wireless E9-1-1 to work, however, three parties—the wireless carriers, the PSAPs, and the local exchange carriers (which are the local wireline carriers)—must interconnect and install the equipment necessary to locate wireless callers. These collaborations have been lacking in some areas of the country.

Moreover, the cost of building the required infrastructure is substantial. In 2003, the U.S. Government Accounting Office (GAO; now the Government Accountability Office) estimated the cost of implementation to be at least $8 billion over 5 years. No federal funding has been provided to states or localities to make those upgrades. Wireless carriers have raised funds by charging customers $0.05 to $1.50 more per month for 9-1-1 service, although GAO has reported that states or localities have often appropriated these funds for other purposes, slowing rates of uptake in those jurisdictions (GAO, 2003).

In addition to financial concerns and the difficulties of establishing collaboration among various participants, there is a regulatory vacuum at the federal level. The FCC can regulate carriers, but it has no authority to regulate the PSAPs, which are under state and local jurisdiction. Thus, for example, as of 2005 carriers are required to provide location information for all wireless 9-1-1 calls, but this requirement is contingent on whether the local PSAP is equipped to receive and use that information (Medical Subcommittee of the ITS America Public Safety Advisory Group, 2002). Consequently, the FCC does not have the ability to establish an ultimate nationwide deadline for full implementation of wireless E9-1-1 services (GAO, 2003). Implementation will take place in a piecemeal fashion based on the timeframes established by local entities.

Despite these concerns, however, uptake of wireless E9-1-1 has been proceeding at a fairly rapid pace. Table 5-2 illustrates the gap in wireless E9-1-1 that persists, as well as the degree to which Phase II wireless E9-1-1

TABLE 5-2 Progress Toward Universal Wireless Enhanced 9-1-1 (February 2006)

	Phase I	Phase II
U.S. Population	85 percent	71 percent
Public Safety Access Points (PSAPs)	80 percent	59 percent
Counties	71 percent	45 percent

SOURCE: NENA, 2006.

continues to trail Phase I implementation. Yet the figures also represent a significant increase in the coverage now available as compared with 2 to 3 years ago.

As of October 2003, only 18 percent of PSAPs were receiving Phase II information, compared with 59 percent in 2006. In addition, only 65 percent of PSAPs were receiving Phase I information, as compared with 80 percent in 2006 (GAO, 2003; NENA, 2006). A Department of Transportation survey released in 2003 showed that only 33 of the nation's 3,136 local jurisdictions had wireless call location capability in December 2002, whereas 643 local jurisdictions had that capability in May 2003 (DOT Wireless E9-1-1 Steering Council, 2002). These figures demonstrate substantial growth in wireless E9-1-1 capacity over the past few years.

The committee supports the nationwide adoption of E9-1-1 and wireless E9-1-1. To ensure more rapid adoption, the committee believes that the charges for wireless E9-1-1 services should be bundled with the overall wireless plan rate, rather than allowing 9-1-1 to be listed as a separate option that raises the monthly fee.

Voice over Internet Protocol (VoIP)

Americans are increasingly moving to alternative communications services, and this presents challenges for the 9-1-1 system. VoIP allows customers to make telephone calls using a computer network and the Internet. VoIP converts the voice signal from the telephone into a digital signal that travels over the Internet, then converts it back at the other end so that customers can speak to anyone with a regular phone number. With regard to emergency notification, however, this new type of communications service has limitations similar to those of wireless calls.

In May 2005, the FCC released VoIP E9-1-1 rules. These rules require VoIP providers to (1) deliver all 9-1-1 calls to the customer's local emergency operator, (2) give emergency operators the call-back number and location of their customers if the emergency operator is capable of receiving that information, and (3) inform their customers of their E9-1-1 capabilities and the limitations of the service. The FCC gave VoIP providers 120 days to furnish this information to customers and to receive acknowledgment from customers that they had received the information. The FCC informed VoIP carriers that they would have to disconnect from service those customers who had not provided this acknowledgment (FCC, 2006).

Next-Generation 9-1-1

The 9-1-1 system currently in place was not designed to handle the challenges of multimedia communications in a wireless, mobile society. As

TABLE 5-3 Next-Generation 9-1-1

Today's 9-1-1	Future 9-1-1
Primarily voice calls via telephone	Voice, text, or video from many types of communications devices
Minimal data	Advanced data capabilities
Local access, transfer, and backup	Long-distance access, transfer, and backup
Limited emergency notification	Location-specific emergency alerts possible for any networked device

SOURCE: DOT Intelligent Transportation Systems, 2006.

noted, it is based on 1970s technology and focused on wireline phones. To address this gap, the Department of Transportation is now sponsoring an initiative that would adapt the basic 9-1-1 infrastructure to 21st-century communications technology. The next-generation 9-1-1 initiative, funded by Intelligent Transportation Systems (ITS) and managed by NHTSA's Office of EMS, will establish a 9-1-1 system that is compatible with any communications device and serve as the foundation for public emergency services in a wireless environment (see Table 5-3).

NHTSA's Office of EMS is managing a research initiative that will produce a high-level system architecture and deployment plan for the next-generation 9-1-1 system. The goal of the initiative is to establish the infrastructure for transmission of voice, data, and photographs from different types of communications devices to PSAPs and then to emergency responder networks (NHTSA Office of EMS, 2006).

Automatic Crash Notification

Each year, approximately 5 million Americans are injured in 17 million crashes involving 28 million vehicles (Champion et al., 1999). Of those 28 million vehicle crashes, approximately 250,000 result in serious injuries to passengers and/or drivers. For vehicle occupants who sustain serious injuries in vehicle crashes, the time that elapses between the moment of the crash and the moment medical care arrives is crucial. Over the last decade, ACN has emerged as a new technology that can reduce the time between a crash and initial notification of the local PSAP, thereby reducing likely fatalities. NHTSA has estimated that ACN systems may result in up to a 20 percent reduction in fatalities due to vehicle crashes (Bachman and Preziotti, 2001).

The broad availability of cell phones has helped reduce the time it takes for 9-1-1 to be notified of a vehicle crash. However, many crashes occur at times and in places where there are no witnesses to call 9-1-1. In addition, victims of crashes often do not have cell phones available, or they may be incapacitated and unable to place a 9-1-1 call. ACN technology allows notification of a crash to be sent automatically to ACN call centers, which then notify 9-1-1 dispatchers. This eliminates the need for bystanders or victims themselves to provide notification to the emergency call center.

In 1996, General Motors (GM) introduced ACN technology in a selected number of vehicles through its OnStar program. By 2005, OnStar was available for more than 50 GM models, as well as other vehicle makes such as Saturn and Saab. In addition, ACN programs that use other telematics service providers are available from other car manufacturers, such as Acura, BMW, and Mercedes.

This first-generation ACN technology was able to notify 9-1-1 of the location of a vehicle in which an airbag had been deployed. However, first-generation ACN units were not able to indicate the severity of the accident recorded. GM recently introduced a second-generation technology called advanced ACN (AACN). This more advanced version is able to capture additional information, including speed at impact, occupants' seatbelt status, direction of impact, and whether the vehicle rolled over. This information provides much more detail regarding the severity of the crash and the likely condition of the vehicle occupants. However, the condition of the occupants may still be uncertain (for example, if seatbelts were secured and airbags deployed, but the crash occurred at a fairly high speed).

In recent years, NHTSA has funded the development of URGENCY Decision Assist software, which is able to translate the data collected in the car's event data recorder into information that may be able to improve the triage of crash victims. URGENCY estimates the probability of fatality due to a vehicle crash using telemetric data in a predictive model. In the future, these data may allow dispatch operators to make more informed decisions about deployment of resources and may enhance the EMS provider's ability to make effective triage decisions.

Currently, ACN calls go through a call center, where operators assess the situation and contact emergency personnel if necessary. However, the verbal exchange between the telematics call center and the 9-1-1 call taker is time-consuming and can be prone to information gaps and errors. New technology (recently tested in Minnesota) addresses this issue by allowing electronic data to be transferred directly to PSAPs and then on to EMS responders and emergency department (ED) personnel—providing them with a better picture of the type of incident and possible injuries.

URGENCY software is in the public domain; however, its uptake has been slow, in part because PSAPs would need the technology to receive data transmission, a capability many PSAPS currently lack. In addition, there is no definitive research demonstrating which data elements have clinical utility. Telematics services appear to be moving toward furnishing automatic, instantaneous notification of emergency events to multiple emergency care providers, including EMS ground and air medical services, heavy rescue services, trauma centers, and others. The committee believes evaluations should be conducted to determine whether emergency dispatchers should transmit that information selectively to local emergency providers to enable more efficient allocation of regional assets, or crash scene data should be integrated directly into EMS and hospital ED data systems.

Nonemergency Calls

The 9-1-1 emergency number is familiar to most Americans and is recognized as being highly responsive (NENA, 2001). Because the number is so widely recognized and remembered, however, it is often used in situations that are not true emergencies, such as property crimes no longer in progress, minor vehicle crashes resulting in no injuries, and some situations involving animal control. Use of the 9-1-1 system for questions or concerns that are nonemergent in nature may produce delays in the response provided for true emergencies, which can place victims in danger.

Because of increasing reports of inappropriate 9-1-1 use, some communities have established alternative phone lines for citizens with nonemergency concerns. In some cases, the phone lines devoted to less urgent calls are regular 7-digit telephone numbers. However, these numbers are more difficult for citizens to remember or to access easily. As a result, some communities have established 3-digit numbers—often 3-1-1—that can be used in nonemergency situations. Operators receiving such calls are able to make triage decisions and if necessary refer a call to a 9-1-1 call center; they can also refer calls to other appropriate government agencies. The hope is that this system will improve the processing of both emergency and nonemergency calls.

Because callers cannot always discern which number is most appropriate to call, 9-1-1 call takers and EMS dispatchers may need to exercise the option of transferring callers to a 3-1-1 system, a nonemergency transport service, or a local nurse advice line if they determine that the caller's problem does not require immediate EMS attention. This strategy may help keep the 9-1-1 system open and preserve ambulance capacity for serious or life-threatening calls. However, evaluations are needed to assess the feasibility, impact, and risks of this approach.

EQUIPMENT FOR EMERGENCY RESPONSE

Once a PSAP has been notified that help is needed, the dispatcher can summon an array of equipment and personnel to respond: a fire or rescue vehicle bringing first responders (Key et al., 2003), an ambulance carrying EMTs or paramedics, or an air ambulance bringing additional EMS per-

TABLE 5-4 Fire Department Responses (2003)

Type of Response	Number	Percent Change from 2002
Fire	1,584,500	–6.1
Medical Aid	13,631,500	+5.6
False Alarm	2,189,500	+3.5
Mutual Aid/Assistance	987,000	+11.1
Hazardous Material (hazmat)	349,500	–3.2
Other Hazard (e.g., arcing wires, bomb removal)	660,500	+9.4
Other (e.g., smoke scares, lockouts)	3,003,500	+9.5
Total	22,406,000	+5.2

SOURCE: U.S. Fire Administration, 2005.

sonnel or rescue or other equipment. Using protocols, emergency medical dispatchers must determine whether ground or air ambulance capacity is required for a given emergency call. The default position for dispatchers is to assume that a ground ambulance is needed. Air ambulances are not typically called until an emergency responder on the ground (police, first responder, or emergency medical technician [EMT]) has confirmed the need.

Fire department first responders often provide support for patients before other EMS units can respond. Fire stations are generally well distributed across a given jurisdiction, especially in urban and suburban areas, and are often the first responders able to arrive at the scene of a medical emergency. Although statistics from the U.S. Fire Administration indicate that medical aid calls outnumber fire calls by 9 to 1 (see Table 5-4), fire equipment is typically geared to fighting fires rather than treating sick or injured patients. As a result, it is not uncommon for large fire trucks to carry first responders or EMS personnel to the scene of an incident.

Ground Ambulance Capacity and Safety Issues

Today more than 12,000 ambulance services operate about 24,000 ground ambulance vehicles in the United States (AAA, 2006). Typically, ambulances must be licensed by the state to ensure that they meet specific trained staffing and equipment requirements. Although these requirements vary by state, basic life support (BLS) units typically carry EMS personnel, as well as equipment such as oxygen tanks, equipment to stabilize fractures, airway supplies (including suction devices and manual and automatic ventilators), and often automated external defibrillators (AEDs). Advanced life support (ALS) units carry paramedics, as well as all BLS equipment, plus medications, intravenous fluids, advanced airway adjuncts, portable pulse oximetry, manual heart monitors/defibrillators (some of which are capable of acquiring and transmitting a 12-lead electrocardiogram), and external pacing.

A major function of state EMS offices is ambulance credentialing and inspection. In 2003, 41 state offices were involved in credentialing ambulances, while 42 state offices were engaged in ambulance inspections. Typically, states require EMS vehicles to be recredentialed every 1 to 2 years (Mears et al., 2003). The federal government also requires that all federal agencies—as well as other public and private services that use federal funding to purchase ambulances—comply with what are known as the KKK standards. Some states have adopted these standards as well and require their service to purchase KKK-compliant ambulances. However, these state and federal requirements typically address only basic ambulance capacity, not health and safety issues, which have become an increasingly significant problem.

From the standpoint of the EMS worker, the basic ambulance design is highly problematic. An assessment of EMS working conditions inside ambulances revealed that more than 40 percent of the working postures associated with high-frequency EMS tasks—including oxygen administration, heart monitoring, and blood pressure checks—create excessive musculoskeletal strain that requires corrective measures from an ergonomic perspective (Ferreira and Hignett, 2005). Ambulances are also unsafe for workers because they create an environment in which airborne and blood-borne pathogens can easily be transmitted.

In addition to these dangers, crashes involving ground ambulances are a major concern because of the frequency of high-speed, lights-and-siren driving; the transport of vulnerable patients and family members; and the poor restraint positions of EMS personnel. According to the Centers for Disease Control and Prevention (CDC), 300 fatal crashes involving ambulances occurred in the United States between 1991 and 2000. These crashes resulted in 357 fatalities, 275 of which were occupants of other vehicles or pedestrians (CDC, 2003). These data highlight the major threat posed by ambulances to their crews, their patients, and others on the road.

A number of solutions have been proposed to address these hazards. For example, some ambulances are now equipped with harnesses that allow EMS personnel to work in the back of the ambulance while still providing them with a restraint in the event of a crash or a sudden stop. Newer ambulance designs also include features that prevent patients from being projected through to the main compartment in the event of a crash.

There are also a number of efforts under way to reduce accident rates for ambulances. NHTSA has developed an Emergency Vehicle Operators Course (EVOC) National Standard Curriculum that some states require their providers to complete before being able to drive an ambulance. Other states, local EMS agencies, and even some insurance carriers require their ambulance drivers to complete a driver training course that is often derived from the NHTSA course. EVOC thus represents an important step toward ensuring ambulance safety on the roads. In addition to training improvements, technology has been developed that provides ambulance drivers with automatic, audible feedback when they are not driving according to standards. This technology uses sophisticated on-board computers that are able to monitor speed, revolutions per minute (RPMs), and braking. Other new capabilities, such as "drive cams" and intelligent transportation highway designs (e.g., lane-centering devices in blizzard conditions) can also have a significant impact on safety. The committee supports the exploration of additional technological applications to increase patient and provider safety in ambulances, including the Federal Highway Safety Intelligent Transportation System Public Safety initiative.

Finally, ambulance safety is being addressed through protocols that dictate whether lights and sirens are appropriate to use in given situations. Operating with lights and sirens (i.e., "running hot") can be helpful in navigating through traffic, but numerous studies indicate that doing so leads to increased danger (NAEMSP and NASEMSD, 1994; Hunt et al., 1995; Lacher and Bausher, 1997; Overton, 2001). A central question, then, is whether the use of lights and sirens is justified given the health care needs of the patient. Hunt and colleagues (1995) determined that on average, the use of lights and sirens saved only 43.5 seconds in transporting patients from the scene of an emergency to the hospital. The authors argued that such a small improvement in transport time would be clinically meaningful only in very rare situations. Lacher and Bausher (1997) found that nearly 40 percent of pediatric 9-1-1 responders inappropriately used lights and sirens when the patient was stable. They concluded that limited use of lights and sirens, dictated by strong protocols, could reduce the dangers associated with inappropriate use (Lacher and Bausher, 1997).

Air Medical Services

Air medical operations, including those involving both rotor-wing helicopters and fixed-wing aircraft, have become an increasingly significant component of U.S. medical capabilities (Helicopter Association International, 2005). The air medical industry began in the United States in the early 1970s, following the Vietnam War (Blumen and UCAN Safety Committee, 2002). During the war, the U.S. military used helicopters to transport soldiers from the front lines to mobile army surgical hospitals. After soldiers had been stabilized, the military deployed fixed-wing aircraft to transport them home. In Vietnam, the time it took for soldiers to be transported from the combat theater to a stateside medical hospital averaged approximately 45 days. During the Afghanistan and Iraq wars, transport time for wounded soldiers has been reduced to as little as 36 hours, with medical care provided throughout (Gawande, 2004).

Air ambulance operations for U.S. civilians have traditionally followed the military model of "trauma medevac," which emphasizes speed—moving the patient away from the site of the injury and to definitive care. However, a growing trend in the air medical industry is to bring more of the assets of the trauma center directly to the patient (Judge, 2005). One of the long-recognized goals of EMS is to deliver patients to definitive care within the "golden hour" (Lerner and Moscati, 2001), and in most cases this remains a primary objective. Air ambulance providers play a key role, especially in rural areas, where trauma centers are typically farther away from the scene of an incident. Branas and colleagues (2005) estimated that medical helicopters provide access for 81.4 million Americans who otherwise would not be able to reach a trauma center within an hour.

The Atlas and Database of Air Medical Services (ADAMS)—developed by academic researchers and supported by the Federal Highway Administration and NHTSA—now provides a map of available air medical service areas across the United States. ADAMS indicates that air medical providers have a heavy presence in many urban and suburban areas of the country, but that coverage is sparse in many rural locales. While it is inherently difficult to provide timely care to these remote areas, they have a particular need for greater coverage by air ambulance providers. Data indicate that in 2001, about 39 percent of vehicle-miles traveled were on rural roads, but 61 percent of all crash fatalities occurred on these roads (Flanigan et al., 2005).

In addition to concerns about access, there are concerns regarding safety. As noted earlier, there has recently been an increase in the number of air ambulances involved in crashes and this has prompted greater scrutiny from the media and regulators. The Federal Aviation Administration (FAA) is responsible for certifying the safety of air ambulance programs operating in the United States. However, because of a decrease in the number of FAA inspectors, along with a rapid increase in the number of air medical providers, safety checks have not been sufficiently rigorous in recent years according to print media reports (Davis, 2005; Meier, 2005). This comes at a time when Medicare reimbursements for air medical transport have increased, and competition within the industry has grown substantially (Meier, 2005). In response to growing concerns regarding air ambulance safety, the FAA released guidelines in August 2005 instructing air ambulance firms to implement safety measures, such as using checklists to ensure that maintenance steps have been completed and improving decision making about whether to launch in unsafe weather conditions (Davis, 2005).

The Airline Deregulation Act of 1978 gave the FAA, rather than the states, regulatory authority over the operations of this industry. Court cases between states and the federal government involving air ambulance operations have centered largely on state efforts to control growth in air medical capacity through the certificate-of-need process. However, other questions regarding the federal preemption of state law have not been definitively resolved. Pennsylvania recently established a protocol requiring air ambulance operations to transport patients to the nearest trauma center, rather than to the base hospital. The air medical provider contested the protocol, saying that it was preempted by federal law. However, the FAA acknowledged in a letter to the state that it had never intended to regulate the medical aspects of air medical operations, and the case was never taken to court.

Some states currently have no regulatory framework in place to govern the medical care aspects of air ambulance providers. However, a key objective for state regulatory agencies should be to ensure coordination and improve the allocation of available assets, including air ambulances. Currently, ground EMS and 9-1-1 dispatch centers sometimes call for air medical support without coordination, resulting in more than one air medical provider being dispatched to a scene. This is a problem especially where there are multiple air medical services competing in the same coverage area. These providers typically market their services to EMS agencies, and when multiple EMS agencies are dispatched to the same event, they may each call for the air medical provider best known to them, resulting in multiple responses.

In light of the above issues, the committee recommends that **states assume regulatory oversight of the medical aspects of air medical services, including communications, dispatch, and transport protocols (5.1)**. The regulatory authority of the FAA should extend to helicopters, fixed-wing aircraft, pilots, and company sponsors; however, the state should regulate the medical aspects of the operations, including personnel on board (nurses, paramedics, physicians), medical equipment, and transport protocols regarding hospitals and trauma centers. In addition, states should establish dispatch protocols for air medical response and should incorporate air medical providers into the broader emergency and trauma care system through improved communications. These measures are essential to more coordinated and efficient use of air capacity.

Interfacility Transport

In addition to transport from the scene of an incident directly to a medical facility, air medical helicopters are used extensively to transport patients from a hospital to a definitive care location. This often occurs, for example, with patients suffering a myocardial infarction or stroke, or pediatric patients who are critically ill or injured. This type of interfacility transport is probably the most common use of air medical services today.

Ground and air ambulances may also be used for nonemergency transports, such as those from nursing homes to hospitals for medical treatment or from hospitals to nursing homes following discharge. Unlike emergency calls, these trips can be scheduled in advance. With the aging of the population, these trends are likely to continue and may result in increasing call volumes for such transport operations.

Advances in Medical Technologies

Emerging medical and communications technologies are enabling real-time voice and video links between ambulance crews and emergency physicians. Some cities, such as San Antonio and Seattle, have established systems in which ambulances carry portable computers, video cameras, and microphones to transmit information to physicians. The technology allows physicians to view the patient, assess the extent of the injury, and determine possible treatment options while the patient is still en route (Medical Subcommittee of the ITS America Public Safety Advisory Group, 2002).

Many ambulance units are now equipped with technologies that allow for the direct transmission of patient data to hospital EDs. For example, 12-lead electrocardiograms enable physicians to view a patient's heart readings prior to arrival at the hospital, and this capability has been shown to reduce door-to-treatment intervals significantly (Cannon, 1999; Woollard et al., 2005). In addition, providing this information to the physician allows for the administration of prehospital thrombolytic therapy, which in some studies has been shown to improve outcomes, although relatively few patients are eligible for the treatment (Boersma et al., 2000).

In addition to these emerging technologies, numerous other advances in medical treatment are likely to impact the level of care EMS personnel are able to provide to patients. For example, a study involving 20 level I trauma centers is currently under way to test the efficacy of an experimental oxygen-carrying blood substitute in increasing the survival of critically injured and bleeding trauma patients. Under the study protocol, treatment begins before arrival at the hospital, either at the scene of the injury, in the ambulance, or in an air ambulance. Because blood is not currently carried in ambulances, use of the blood substitute in these settings has the potential to address a critical unmet medical need. The introduction of saline, the current standard of care, helps restore a patient's blood pressure but does not deliver oxygen, which is critical to preventing damage in the brain, heart, lungs, and other organs.

Emerging communications technologies and clinical treatments should be evaluated to determine their impact on treatment cost, quality of care, and patient outcomes. New technologies are often offered at a high cost that is beyond the reach of many EMS systems across the country. Moreover, there is growing evidence that simpler interventions performed effectively in a timely manner may be most important in ensuring good outcomes. Indeed, that was the conclusion of a recent World Health Organization report on prehospital trauma care systems (Sasser et al., 2005). In addition, research, including the Ontario Prehospital Advanced Life Support study, has raised serious questions about the value of ALS beyond early defibrillation and administration of aspirin and oxygen to patients suffering myocardial infarction. Technologies that simplify the job of the prehospital provider, such as AEDs and newly developed airway adjuncts, have been shown to improve outcomes. The appropriate roles of other, more complex technologies have not been well established (Bunn et al., 2001; Sasser et al., 2005).

COMMUNICATIONS AND DATA SYSTEMS

Communications among EMS and other public safety and health care providers are still very limited. Antiquated and incompatible voice communications systems often result in a lack of coordination among emergency personnel as they respond to incidents. As mentioned earlier, many EMS systems rely on voice communications equipment that was purchased in the 1970s with federal financial assistance and has never been upgraded. This equipment frequently suffers from dead spots, interference, and other technical problems (Public Safety Wireless Network Program, 2005) (see Figure 5-1). However, upgrading to new equipment is often prohibitively expensive for local communities.

Advanced data and information systems are now available in the commercial market; however, adoption of these systems has been uneven across the country. Most ambulance systems continue to rely on paper-based run records rather than electronic systems. Similarly, technologies that enable direct transmission of patient information (e.g., vital signs) to hospitals prior to the arrival of an ambulance have not been uniformly adopted. Consequently, there is a growing gap between the types of EMS data and information systems available and those commonly used in the field.

These issues are compounded by the significant variation in EMS operational structures at the local and regional levels. EMS agencies may be operated by local governments, fire departments, private companies, or other entities. This makes communications and data integration difficult, even among EMS providers within a given local area. Communications among EMS, public safety, public health, and other hospital providers are even more problematic given the technical challenges associated with developing interoperable networks. As a result of these challenges and the need for improved coordination, the committee recommends that **hospitals, trauma centers, emergency medical services agencies, public safety departments, emergency management offices, and public health agencies develop integrated and interoperable communications and data systems (5.2). Each**

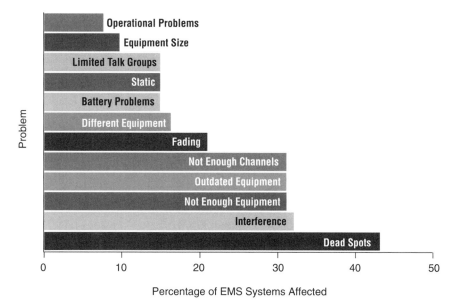

FIGURE 5-1 Problems with existing land mobile radio systems.
SOURCE: Public Safety Wireless Network Program, 2005.

state and local system should have communications plans for EMS that provide for interoperability and interconnectivity with other public service and health providers. A number of states are moving forward in developing wireless interoperable networks with assistance from the National Governors Association (National Governors Association Center for Best Practices, 2005). In addition, Maryland has developed a model communications system, described in Chapter 3. Such efforts need to be expanded nationwide.

Public Safety Communications

Voice communications improvements initiated by the federal government in the aftermath of the terrorist attacks of September 11 have focused on fire and police but have often overlooked EMS (Center for Catastrophe Preparedness and Response NYU, 2005). For example, interoperability of EMS and fire communications systems remains a significant problem. In a survey conducted by the Public Safety Wireless Network Program, 30 percent of responding fire and EMS agencies indicated that the lack of wireless communications interoperability has, at some time in the past, hampered their ability to respond to incidents. EMS agencies were the most adversely affected by this lack of interoperability, with 53 percent indicating that it had limited their response capabilities. In addition, 43 percent of local fire and EMS agencies indicated that a lack of interoperability had affected their ability to communicate with agencies in surrounding jurisdictions (Public Safety Wireless Network Program, 2005).

As with other first responders, there are a number of barriers to improving the EMS system's communications capabilities, including the absence of communications standards, significant technological barriers, and a lack of funding (Center for Catastrophe Preparedness and Response NYU, 2005). In addition, the above survey of EMS and fire agencies identified a number of additional obstacles to communications interoperability (see Figure 5-2). For example, 39 percent of local fire and EMS agencies rated political or turf issues as a severe obstacle. These factors have impeded progress toward a more effective communications system.

GAO reported in 2004 that federal leadership was needed to facilitate interoperable communications between first responders. The report asserted that jurisdictional boundaries and the unique missions of public safety agencies were hindrances to collaboration, and that the federal government should provide the leadership, long-term commitment, and focus to help state and local governments achieve interoperability. Specifically, GAO advised the federal government to assist in this effort by creating a national architecture for interoperable communications, establishing a standard database to coordinate frequencies, and allocating communications spectrum for public safety use (GAO, 2004).

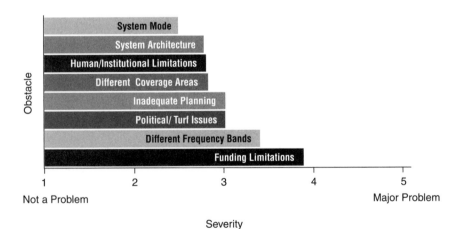

FIGURE 5-2 Obstacles to interoperability.
SOURCE: Public Safety Wireless Network Program, 2005.

The technical challenges to establishing an effective public safety communications system have been a focus of attention for over a decade. In 1996, the Public Safety Wireless Advisory Committee presented a report to the FCC and the National Telecommunications and Information Administration (NTIA) indicating the crucial need to promote interoperability and advocating the allocation of spectrum for the use of public safety agencies (The SAFECOM Project, 2004).

In 1997, Congress instructed the FCC to allocate 24 MHz of spectrum for public safety radio communications operations. However, the spectrum cannot be used in most heavily populated areas until local residents transition to digital television, and no firm date has been set for this transition. In the interim, many public safety agencies are continuing to operate with congested radio systems, and some have postponed the activation of fully interoperable radio networks in their regions (Alliance in Support of America's First Responders, 2005).

To direct the federal government's efforts at establishing an interoperable public safety communications system, the Office of Management and Budget established the Wireless Public Safety Interoperable Communications Program (SAFECOM), housed within the Department of Homeland Security. SAFECOM's purpose is to help local, tribal, state, and federal public safety agencies improve public safety response through more effective and efficient interoperable wireless communications. In 2004, SAFECOM released its Statement of Requirements, focused on the functional needs of public safety first responders to communicate and share information effectively. The document served as a first step toward establishing base-level communications and interoperability standards for all 50,000 public safety agencies across the United States (The SAFECOM Project, 2004). The document describes several scenarios involving first responders, including a future scenario in which an EMS unit responds to a heart attack call. The PSAP responding to the call is equipped with displays indicating likely ambulance response times given current traffic conditions. Computer-activated voice technology assists the ambulance driver in selecting the fastest traffic lanes. On scene, a radio frequency identification (RFID) bracelet worn by the patient allows paramedics to determine the patient's allergies to medicines. Data from the 12-lead electrocardiogram are transmitted wirelessly to the hospital through a public safety communications device (PSCD). All medical monitors are attached wirelessly to the patient, and the encounter is entirely paperless.

Health Care Data Systems

NHTSA's *Emergency Medical Services Agenda for the Future* set forth five goals for the EMS information system of the future: (1) adopt uniform data elements and definitions, and incorporate them into information systems; (2) develop mechanisms for generating and transmitting data that are valid, reliable, and accurate; (3) develop information systems that are able to describe an entire EMS event; (4) develop information systems that are integrated with other health care providers, public safety agencies, and community resources; and (5) provide feedback to those who generate data (NHTSA, 1996). Efforts are under way to achieve each of these objectives through the National EMS Information System (NEMSIS).

The availability of uniform, reliable EMS data has been a long-standing concern that emerged as major priority during the development of the *Emergency Medical Services Agenda for the Future: Implementation Guide* in the late 1990s. The availability of such data was cited as fundamental to a number of the *Agenda's* goals, such as determining the costs and benefits of EMS and improving EMS research. GAO's investigation of state and local EMS agencies in 2001 found unanimous agreement that greater availability of data and improved information systems were needed to monitor the agencies' own performance and to quantify and justify system needs to the local public and decision makers (GAO, 2001).

Federal government efforts to improve EMS data systems date back more than a decade. In 1993, the Department of Health and Human Services, NHTSA, and the U.S. Fire Administration cosponsored a conference that resulted in the development of a model set of EMS data elements and definitions that could be used by states and local systems as the basis for creating their own information systems (GAO, 2001). This Uniform Prehospital EMS Dataset contained a wide array of data elements, including patient characteristics, dispatch and incident data, financial information, EMS system demographic data, and others.

NEMSIS, managed by NHTSA in coordination with the Health Resources and Services Administration, is a continuation of this work. NEMSIS is geared toward improving data standardization and linking disparate EMS databases at the federal, state, and local levels (Mears et al., 2003). It will serve as a national EMS database that can be used to evaluate patient and EMS system outcomes, benchmark performance, facilitate research efforts, develop nationwide EMS training curricula, determine national fee schedules, and address disaster preparedness resource issues. The database will be able to supply information at the national level, such as the total number and types of EMS calls, average response times, and the most widely used medications and procedures. Currently, all of the states except New York and Vermont have elected to participate in the project. By the end of 2006, 6–7 states are expected to be fully operational in the program and will be submitting state-level data to the national EMS database; this number is expected to increase by 17 by the end of 2007. Becoming fully operational means that states are collecting and submitting NEMSIS-compliant data from the individual EMS provider agencies within their respective states. NHTSA houses NEMSIS at its National Center for Statistics and Analysis.

In addition, the American College of Surgeons administers the National Trauma Data Bank (NTDB), the largest single injury database in the country. The NTDB contains over 1.5 million records from 405 trauma centers in the United States and Puerto Rico. Its goal is to inform the medical community, the public, and decision makers about a wide variety of issues that characterize the current state of care for injured persons. The information contained in the NTDB has implications in many areas, including epidemiology, injury control, research, education, acute care, and resource allocation (American College of Surgeons, 2006).

In addition to the development of data systems, new technology now in use by the military has the potential to streamline data collection in the field. The Battlefield Medical Information System Tactical (BMIST) device is a handheld unit that enables military health care providers to record, store, retrieve, and transmit the essential elements of clinical encounters at the point of care (Onley, 2004). The device provides diagnostic and treatment decision aids and has the capability to incorporate new procedures and protocols. In addition, it can retrieve a patient's complete medical records, including drug allergies, immunization status, and dental records. Significant obstacles exist to the adoption of this type of technology in the commercial market, especially with respect to the availability of a patient's complete medical records. However, companies selling to the civilian market are developing formal field tests of similar technology (TeleMedic Systems, 2001).

In addition, the transition to a National Health Information Infrastructure (NHII) for the United States is currently under way. In 2004, the Bush Administration called for widespread adoption of interoperable EHRs within 10 years and designated a National Coordinator for Health Information Technology. Since then, the coordinator has sought to develop common technology standards and broader consensus among the public and private stakeholders involved in this effort. However, discussions regarding the NHII have frequently excluded prehospital emergency care. The initial focus of the effort centered on hospitals, ambulatory care providers, pharmacies, and other more visible components of the health care system. Given the role played by prehospital EMS in providing essential and often lifesaving treatment to patients, this has been a significant oversight. Therefore, the committee recommends that **the Department of Health and Human Services fully involve prehospital emergency medical services leadership in discussions about the design, deployment, and financing of the National Health Information Infrastructure (5.3).**

In addition to this national effort, local areas have moved forward with initiatives to support regional health information sharing. For example, the Santa Barbara County Care Data Exchange project allows for the appropriate sharing of clinical information among medical groups, hospitals, clinics, laboratories, pharmacies, and payers (IOM, 2003; SBCCDE, 2006). Approximately 75 percent of the health care providers in the county are involved in the project. There is also an EMS component to the effort. The Santa Barbara County EMS Information Systems Project has sought to develop accurate EMS information systems that are integrated with other health care providers, public safety agencies, and community resources (Santa Barbara County Public Health Department, 2003). This project has the following objectives: (1) to ensure that the times at which calls are received by the PSAP are recorded; (2) to ensure that all providers have synchronized times based on Coordinated Universal Time (UTC); (3) to integrate information from the various providers into a comprehensive EMS response patient care record; and (4) to provide feedback to individual service providers regarding patient outcomes and provider performance. This project meets a number of the goals established by the *Emergency Medical Services Agenda for the Future* and can serve as a model for other communities across the United States.

Efforts to improve health information technology are aimed at improving the effectiveness, efficiency, and safety of health care interventions. The goal is to link all relevant providers so that communication of vital patient data is smooth, and patient hand-offs are seamless. A key component of that linkage is the hand-off between EMS personnel and hospital-based providers. Therefore, the committee believes there should be improved interface and connectivity between EMS electronic patient records and hospital electronic records, with the goal of transmitting EMS electronic information to EDs in real time.

In addition to patient data, there is often a need for EMS-to-hospital communications regarding the current status of hospital facilities. Ambulance units frequently transport patients to facilities that are on diversion or do not have the necessary subspecialists on call to handle the type of emergency patient they are transporting. Units then must travel to another facility, wasting valuable time in the process. Emerging technology will enable ambulance providers to have ready access to data indicating the current status of hospitals in the local area. Systems in use in Richmond, San Diego, and elsewhere allow ambulance providers to see the diversion status of hospitals throughout the region. This type of information could also assist in detailing recurring diversion patterns at various regional facilities.

SUMMARY OF RECOMMENDATIONS

5.1: States should assume regulatory oversight of the medical aspects of air medical services, including communications, dispatch, and transport protocols.

5.2: Hospitals, trauma centers, emergency medical services agencies, public safety departments, emergency management offices, and public health agencies should develop integrated and interoperable communications and data systems.

5.3: The Department of Health and Human Services should fully involve prehospital emergency medical services leadership in discussions about the design, deployment, and financing of the National Health Information Infrastructure.

REFERENCES

AAA (American Ambulance Association). 2006. *Ambulance Facts.* [Online]. Available: http://www.the-aaa.org/media/AmbulanceFacts.htm [accessed January 5, 2006].

Alliance in Support of America's First Responders. 2005. *Support America's First Responders.* [Online]. Available: http://www.apcointl.com/supportamericasfirstresponders/index.htm [accessed November 1, 2005].

American College of Surgeons. 2006. *National Trauma Data Bank.* [Online]. Available: http://www. facs.org/trauma/ntdb.html [accessed February 7, 2006].

Bachman LR, Preziotti GR. 2001. *Automated Collision Notification (ACN) Field Operational Test (FOT) Evaluation Report.* Springfield, VA: National Technical Information Service.

Blumen IJ, UCAN Safety Committee. 2002. *A Safety Review and Risk Assessment in Air Medical Transport.* Salt Lake City, UT: Air Medical Physician Association.

Boersma E, Akkerhuis M, Simoons ML. 2000. Primary angioplasty versus thrombolysis for acute myocardial infarction. *New England Journal of Medicine* 342(12):890–891; author reply 891–892.

Branas CC, MacKenzie EJ, Williams JC, Schwab CW, Teter HM, Flanigan MC, Blatt AJ, ReVelle CS. 2005. Access to trauma centers in the United States. *Journal of the American Medical Association* 293(21):2626–2633.

Bunn F, Kwan I, Roberts I, Wentz R. 2001. *Effectiveness of Pre-Hospital Trauma Care.* London, England: London School of Hygiene & Tropical Medicine.

Cannon CP. 1999. Advances in the medical management of acute coronary syndromes. *Journal of Thrombosis & Thrombolysis* 7(2):171–189.

CDC (Centers for Disease Control and Prevention). 2003. Ambulance crash-related injuries among emergency medical services workers—United States, 1991–2002. *Morbidity & Mortality Weekly Report* 52(8):154–156.

Center for Catastrophe Preparedness and Response NYU. 2005. *Emergency Medical Services: The Forgotten First Responder: A Report on the Critical Gaps in Organization and Deficits in Resources for America's Medical First Responders.* New York: Center for Catastrophe Preparedness and Response, New York University.

Champion H, Augenstein J, Blatt AJ, Cushing B, Digges KH, Hunt RC, Lombardo LV, Siegel JH. 1999. *Reducing Highway Deaths and Disabilities with Automatic Wireless Transmission of Serious Injury Probability Ratings from Vehicles in Crashes to EMS, Paper 406.* Presentation at the meeting of the Proceedings of the 18th ESV Conference. [Online]. Available: http://www-nrd.nhtsa.dot.gov/pdf/nrd-01/esv/esv18/CD/Files/18ESV-000406.pdf [accessed August 4, 2006].

Davis R. 2005, August 11. Air ambulance firms warned. *USA Today.* P. 1A.

DOT (U.S. Department of Transportation) Intelligent Transportation Systems. 2006, February 10. *Today's 9-1-1 vs. Future 9-1-1.* [Online]. Available: http://www.its.dot.gov/ng911/ng911_future.htm [accessed February 25, 2006].

DOT Wireless E9-1-1 Steering Council. 2002. *Wireless E9-1-1 Priority Action Plan.* Washington, DC: DOT Intelligent Transportation Systems Joint Program Office (HOIT).

FCC (Federal Communications Commission). 2006. *VoIP and 911 Services: VoIP 911 Background.* [Online]. Available: http://www.voip911.gov [accessed February 25, 2006].

Ferreira J, Hignett S. 2005. Reviewing ambulance design for clinical efficiency and paramedic safety. *Applied Ergonomics* 36(1):97–105.

Flanigan M, Blatt A, Lombardo L, Mancuso D, Miller M, Wiles D, Pirson H, Hwang J, Thill J, Majka K. 2005. Assessment of air medical coverage using the atlas and database of air medical services and correlations with reduced highway fatality rates. *Air Medical Journal* 24(4):151–163.

GAO (U.S. Government Accountability Office). 2001. *Emergency Medical Services: Reported Needs Are Wide-Ranging, with a Growing Focus on Lack of Data.* Washington, DC: Government Printing Office.

GAO. 2003. *Uneven Implementation of Wireless Enhanced 911 Raises Prospect of Piecemeal Availability for Years to Come.* Washington, DC: Government Printing Office.

GAO. 2004. *Homeland Security: Federal Leadership Needed to Facilitate Interoperable Communications between First Responders.* Washington, DC: Government Printing Office.

Gawande A. 2004. Casualties of war—military care for the wounded from Iraq and Afghanistan. *New England Journal of Medicine* 351(24):2471–2475.

Helicopter Association International. 2005. *White Paper: Improving Safety in Helicopter Emergency Medical Services (HEMS) Operations.* Alexandria, VA: Helicopter Association International.

Hunt RC, Brown LH, Cabinum ES, Whitley TW, Prasad NH, Owens CF Jr, Mayo CE Jr. 1995. Is ambulance transport time with lights and siren faster than that without? *Annals of Emergency Medicine* 25(4):507–511.

IOM (Institute of Medicine). 1993. *Emergency Medical Services for Children.* Washington, DC: National Academy Press.

IOM. 2003. *Patient Safety: Achieving a New Standard for Care.* Washington, DC: The National Academies Press.

Judge T. 2005, April. *Contemporary Air Medicine in the USA—Briefing for Institute of Medicine.* Unpublished.

Key CB, Pepe PE, Persse DE, Calderon D. 2003. Can first responders be sent to selected 9-1-1 emergency medical services calls without an ambulance? *Academic Emergency Medicine* 10(4):339–346.

Lacher M, Bausher J. 1997. Lights and siren in pediatric 911 ambulance transports: Are they being misused? *Annals of Emergency Medicine* 29(2):223–227.

Lerner EB, Moscati RM. 2001. The golden hour: Scientific fact or medical "urban legend"? *Academic Emergency Medicine* 8(7):758–760.

Mears G, Kagarise J, Raisor C. 2003. *2003 Survey and Analysis of EMS Scope of Practice and Practice Settings Impacting EMS Services in Rural America: Executive Brief and Recommendations.* Chapel Hill, NC: University of North Carolina at Chapel Hill Department of Emergency Medicine.

Medical Subcommittee of the ITS America Public Safety Advisory Group. 2002. *Recommendations for ITS Technology in Emergency Medical Services.* Washington, DC: ITS America.

Meier B. 2005, May 3. Air ambulances are multiplying, and costs rise. *The New York Times.* P. A1.

NAEMSP, NASEMSD (National Association of Emergency Medical Services Physicians, National Association of State EMS Directors). 1994. Use of warning lights and siren in emergency medical vehicle response and patient transport. *Prehospital & Disaster Medicine* 9(2):133–136.

NAS, NRC (National Academy of Sciences, National Research Council). 1966. *Accidental Death and Disability: The Neglected Disease of Modern Society*. Washington, DC: NAS.

NAS, NRC. 1978. *Emergency Medical Services at Midpassage*. Washington, DC: NAS.

National Fire Protection Association. 2005. *Fire Department Calls*. Quincy, MA: National Fire Protection Association.

National Governors Association Center for Best Practices. 2005. *Policy Academy on Wireless Interoperability*. [Online]. Available: http://www.nga.org/portal/site/nga/menuitem. 9123e83a1f6786440ddcbeeb501010a0/?vgnextoid=93d31a37ab8e4010VgnVCM 1000001a01010aRCRD/ [accessed April 20, 2006].

NENA (National Emergency Number Association). 2001. *Report Card to the Nation: The Effectiveness, Accessibility and Future of America's 9-1-1 Service*. Columbus, OH: RCN Commission/NENA.

NENA. 2004. *The Development of 9-1-1*. [Online]. Available: http://www.nena.org/PR_Pubs/ Devel_of_911.htm [accessed September 28, 2004].

NENA. 2006. *9-1-1 Fast Facts*. Arlington, VA: NENA.

NHTSA (National Highway Traffic Safety Administration). 1996. *Emergency Medical Services Agenda for the Future*. Washington, DC: Department of Transportation.

NHTSA Office of EMS. 2006. *EMS Update*. [Online]. Available: http://www.nvfc.org/pdf/2006-ems-upate.pdf [accessed May 1, 2006].

Onley DS. 2004, November 22. Electronic medical records go into combat. *Government Computer News*. [Online]. Available: http://www.gcn.com/print/23_33/27923-1.html [accessed January 27, 2007].

Overton J. 2001. Ambulance design and safety. *Journal of Prehospital and Disaster Medicine* 16(3).

Public Safety Wireless Network Program. 2005. *Information Brief: Fire and EMS Communications Interoperability*. Washington, DC: Department of Justice and Department of the Treasury.

The SAFECOM Project. 2004. *Statement of Requirements for Public Safety Wireless Communications & Interoperability*. Washington, DC: Department of Homeland Security.

Santa Barbara County Public Health Department. 2003. *EMS Information Systems Project*. [Online]. Available: http://www.sbcphd.org/ems/isdisaster.html [accessed December 1, 2005].

Sasser S, Varghese M, Kellermann A, Lormand JD. 2005. *Prehospital Trauma Care Systems*. Geneva, Switzerland: World Health Organization.

SBCCDE (Santa Barbara County Care Data Exchange). 2006. *Background Information & Recent Quotes*. [Online]. Available: http://www.sbccde.org/bginfo.htm [accessed January 5, 2006].

TeleMedic Systems. 2001. *Home Page*. [Online]. Available: http://www.telemedicsystems. com/corpsite/ [accessed February 1, 2006].

U.S. Fire Administration. 2005. *Fire Departments*. [Online]. Available: http://www.usfa.fema. gov/statistics/departments/ [accessed February 1, 2006].

Woollard M, Pitt K, Hayward AJ, Taylor NC. 2005. Limited benefits of ambulance telemetry in delivering early thrombolysis: A randomised controlled trial. *Emergency Medicine Journal* 22(3):209–215.

6

Preparing for Disasters

On August 29, 2005, Hurricane Katrina struck the U.S. Gulf Coast, leaving over 1,300 people dead, countless injured, and over 1 million displaced. The aftermath of the hurricane created a humanitarian crisis unparalleled in the nation's history, with federal disaster declarations covering 90,000 square miles (GAO, 2005). While the scope of Hurricane Katrina extended far beyond typical disaster scenarios, it illustrated the heavy demands that can be placed upon emergency workers in the event of a major crisis.

The term "disaster" denotes a low-probability but high-impact event that causes a large number of individuals to become ill or injured. The International Federation of Red Cross and Red Crescent Societies defines a disaster as an event that causes more than 10 deaths, affects more than 100 people, or leads to an appeal for assistance by those affected (Bravata et al., 2004). Disaster events overwhelm a community's emergency response capacity (Waeckerle et al., 1994) and create an imbalance between the supply of available resources and the need for those resources (Noji, 1996).

Even in responding to day-to-day demands, however, the emergency and trauma care system in the United States is often stretched beyond its capacity. This is evidenced by the frequency with which hospitals are placed on diversion and ambulances are required to find alternative receiving hospitals (GAO, 2003a). The capacity shortages that are observable on a day-to-day basis in many areas of the country are magnified considerably in the event of a disaster. Given the existing challenges, there is substantial evidence that the emergency and trauma care system is not well prepared for larger-scale disaster events (Schur et al., 2004).

Emergency medical services (EMS) personnel are always among the first to respond in the event of a disaster. However, they are also the least supported in fulfilling this role among all public safety personnel nationwide, lacking both adequate training and proper equipment for disaster response. According to New York University's Center for Catastrophe Preparedness and Response, more than half of emergency medical technicians (EMTs) and paramedics have received less than 1 hour of training in dealing with biological and chemical agents and explosives since the terrorist attacks of September 11, and 20 percent have received no such training. In 25 states, moreover, fewer than 50 percent of EMTs and paramedics have adequate equipment to respond to a biological or chemical attack (Center for Catastrophe Preparedness and Response NYU, 2005).

In the aftermath of September 11, President Bush promulgated a set of Homeland Security Presidential Directives designed to ensure a coordinated response to a national emergency. But the absence of effective federal, state, and local coordination following Hurricane Katrina demonstrated just how far we have to go in this regard. The integration of emergency care, trauma systems, and EMS into the overall disaster planning process has proven even more problematic. EMS providers and state and local EMS directors are often excluded from critical disaster planning efforts (Center for Catastrophe Preparedness and Response NYU, 2005). Federal programs dealing with medical aspects of disaster preparedness are dispersed among multiple agencies, including the Department of Homeland Security (DHS), the National Highway Traffic Safety Administration (NHTSA), and the Department of Health and Human Services (DHHS). And there are no EMS-specific standards and guidelines for the training and equipment necessary to respond effectively to a terrorist attack or disaster (Center for Catastrophe Preparedness and Response NYU, 2005).

This lack of coordination is reflected in the haphazard funding of preparedness initiatives. EMS and trauma systems have consistently been underfunded relative to their presence and role in the field (Rudman et al., 2003; Center for Catastrophe Preparedness and Response NYU, 2005). Recent audits have found that EMS systems have received only 4–6 percent of federal disaster preparedness funds from DHS and DHHS (GAO, 2003b; Center for Catastrophe Preparedness and Response NYU, 2005). One recent survey revealed that 58 percent of responding ambulance agencies had not been allocated any federal funding for terrorism preparedness. Nearly 60 percent stated that their organization had not benefited from indirect access to items purchased with federal funds. Fully 82.8 percent of respondents had encountered either extreme difficulty or difficulty in obtaining federal funding and access to items purchased with federal funding (AAA, 2004).

This chapter reviews the array of threats faced by the United States and describes the medical responses to recent disasters both here and abroad.

Against this background, the committee details measures that can be taken to improve the nation's EMS-related disaster preparedness.

THE ARRAY OF THREATS

Worldwide, disasters occur almost daily; in the past 20 years, they have claimed nearly 3 million lives and adversely affected 800 million more (Waeckerle, 2000; Chan et al., 2004). Such events can be either naturally occurring catastrophes or, increasingly, intentional (terrorist) or unintentional man-made disasters (see Table 6-1). Recent experience demonstrates the frequency with which disasters can strike and the tremendous impact they can have on the residents of stricken areas.

TABLE 6-1 Recent Disaster Events (United States and Worldwide)

Type	Category	Location	Deaths
Naturally Occurring	Hurricane (Katrina)	Louisiana (especially New Orleans), Mississippi, Alabama (2005–2006)	1,326
	Avian influenza	6 countries (2005–2006)	118 (as of 10/20/05)
	Earthquake	Kashmir (2005)	73,000 (69,000 injured)
	Tsunami	12 countries (2004)	212,611
	Severe acute respiratory syndrome (SARS)	25 countries (2002–2003)	774
	Earthquake	Northridge, California (1994)	57 (5,000+ injured)
Man-made, Intentional (Terrorist) or Unintentional	Train bombings	London (2005)	52 (700 injured)
		Madrid (2004)	191 (2,000 injured)
	Nightclub fire	Rhode Island (2003)	100 (200+ injured)
	Nightclub bombing	Bali (2002)	202
	Anthrax attacks	Washington, D.C. (2001)	5 (13 injured)
	Terrorist attacks of September 11	New York/Washington, D.C. (2001)	2,752
	Embassy bombings	Nairobi and Tanzania (1998)	224 (4,000+ injured)
	Sarin gas attack	Tokyo, Japan (1995)	12 (5,000 injured)

SOURCE: Accountability Review Boards on the Embassy Bombings in Nairobi and Dar es Salaam, 1999; CNN.com, 2003, 2005a,b; Hirschkorn, 2003; Gutierrez de Ceballos et al., 2004; IOM, 2004; Rand Corporation, 2004; BBC News, 2005, 2006a,b; Times Foundation, 2005; Associated Press, 2006a,b; Insurance Information Network of California, 2006.

Naturally Occurring Disasters

The nation is vulnerable to a wide range of natural disasters, including earthquakes, extreme heat, forest fires, wildfires, floods, hurricanes, mudslides, thunderstorms, tornadoes, tsunamis, volcanoes, and winter storms/extreme cold (DHS READYAmerica, 2005). Responders in areas that are prone to certain types of disasters (e.g., search and rescue teams in cities along the San Andreas Fault in California) are generally well prepared and cognizant of the risks involved. As with Hurricane Katrina, however, responders may be unprepared for the magnitude of the crisis in a worst-case scenario. Such events can overwhelm local resources and require additional help from neighboring areas, adjoining states, or, in many cases, the federal government.

Historically, flooding has been the nation's most common natural disaster, having occurred in every state (DHS READYAmerica, 2005). Earthquakes, regarded as a West Coast phenomenon, in fact pose a moderate to high risk to the majority of states. Tornados are focused primarily in states located in "tornado alley" in the Midwest. Hurricanes form in the southern Atlantic Ocean, Caribbean Sea, Gulf of Mexico, and eastern Pacific Ocean and affect coastal states in those areas (DHS READYAmerica, 2005).

Disease outbreaks also pose a significant risk to the United States. In 2003, severe acute respiratory syndrome (SARS) spread quickly from China to several countries in Asia and to Toronto, Canada, representing a potential threat to the United States (Augustine et al., 2004). Infected travelers spread the disease before public health officials in China were able to recognize its significance. SARS is highly infectious and is transmitted through close personal contact. The outbreak illustrated how quickly such an event can get out of control when health care workers themselves become not only victims, but also transmitters of the disease. The spread of SARS was contained in 2003; however, public health officials in the United States have warned that the possibility of another outbreak remains.

In addition to the threat posed by SARS, world health officials continue to issue warnings about the potential for avian influenza (H5N1) to mutate and become transmissible from human to human, potentially resulting in a global pandemic. There are widespread fears that this strain of influenza could result in deaths of the magnitude experienced during the 1918–1919 Spanish flu pandemic, which by some estimates claimed the lives of 500,000 Americans and more than 20 million people worldwide (Fee and Parry, 2005; IOM, 2005).

The United States is seeking to stockpile sufficient quantities of vaccines and antivirals to protect against the threat of pandemic influenza, but a scenario in which the government is unable to stop the spread of the disease remains highly plausible. Currently, common influenza causes the deaths of approximately 36,000 Americans each year. A pandemic occurs when there is a major change in the influenza virus such that most or all of the world's population has never been exposed to and therefore is vulnerable to the virus (IOM, 2005). Vaccine manufacturers are ramping up capacity to produce a vaccine that will be effective against H5N1, but it will take 6–9 months to produce an adequate supply, and the effectiveness of a vaccine will depend on how the virus mutates.

In the event of an outbreak of pandemic influenza, emergency medical responders will potentially be called upon to treat and transport thousands of afflicted individuals. However, there are a number of concerns regarding the nation's preparedness for and potential response to such an event, including (1) the overwhelming number of afflicted individuals who would require hospitalization or outpatient medical care, stretching an already overburdened emergency and trauma care system; (2) the fact that communities across the country would be affected simultaneously, limiting the ability of any jurisdiction to provide support and assistance to other areas; and (3) disruptions that would occur in public safety and emergency and trauma care systems as their personnel fell ill and even succumbed to the disease (IOM, 2005). These challenges call into question U.S. readiness for a catastrophic public health emergency.

Unintentional Man-Made Disasters

While terrorist attacks are a constant concern, an array of other man-made disasters threaten communities and have the potential to strain or exceed the capacity of local emergency and trauma care resources. These include train wrecks, plane crashes, and fires (which may also be intentionally set). For example, the 2003 nightclub fire in West Warwick, Rhode Island, killed 100 people and injured 200 others, placing a strain on the local emergency care system, as well as area firefighters. This type of incident illustrates the need for effective surge capacity in the emergency and trauma care system and the value of an "all hazards" approach to disaster preparedness.

Terrorist Threats

Concerns regarding the likelihood of terrorist attacks increased dramatically in the wake of September 11, 2001. Recent terrorist events overseas, including the Madrid train bombings in 2004 and the London transit bombings of 2005, have added to those concerns. Terrorist attacks on the United States could take a number of different forms (see Box 6-1). Threats emanate from chemical, biological, radiological, nuclear, and explosive (CBRNE) sources and could be directed against a range of targets, includ-

---

BOX 6-1
Examples of Major Terrorist Threats to the United States

Explosives
- Suicide bomber
- Truck bomb
- Subway bomb

Chemical
- Ricin
- Sarin gas
- Sulfur
- Mustard gas

Biological
- Smallpox
- Anthrax
- Plague

Radiological
- Dirty bomb

Nuclear
- Nuclear bomb

SOURCE: CDC, 2006a.

---

ing our transportation systems, government institutions, and food supplies, among others.

Explosions are by far the most common cause of casualties associated with terrorism. From 1991 to 2000, 93 reported terrorist attacks resulted in more than 30 casualties, and 88 percent of those attacks involved explosions (Arnold et al., 2004). Over the past 25 years, explosives or firearms have been used to commit countless acts of terrorism in Israel, Egypt, Kenya, Argentina, Colombia, Bali, Yemen, Russia, the United Kingdom, Germany, France, Italy, the United States, and many other countries. Every week, if not every day, another suicide bombing, car bombing, or improvised explosive device claims the lives of innocent victims. This threat of terrorism involving conventional weapons is especially prevalent in large urban areas. Yet even though traumatic injury is likely to be the primary result of these types of explosive attacks, the federal government recently eliminated the Health Resources and Service Administration's (HRSA) Trauma-EMS Systems Program and the grants it provided to states to develop and maintain trauma systems. There are presently 52 Centers for Public Health Preparedness supported by federal funding that focus on various aspects of bioterrorism, but not one federally funded center is focused on the civilian consequences of terrorist bombings (CDC, 2006b).

Although explosive devices are the most commonly used terrorist weapon, there is evidence that terrorists have also sought to develop chemical, biological, and radiological weapons, such as the following:

- **Mustard gas** is a blister agent that poses a threat through direct contact or inhalation. Inhalation of mustard gas damages the lungs, causes breathing difficulties, and leads to death by suffocation in severe cases as a result of water in the lungs (DHS, 2003).
- **Sarin** disrupts a victim's nervous system by blocking the transmission of nerve signals. Exposure to nerve agents causes constriction of the pupils, salivation, and convulsions that can lead to death (DHS, 2003).
- **Ricin** is a plant toxin that is 30 times more potent than the nerve agent VX. There is no treatment for ricin poisoning once the agent has entered the bloodstream (DHS, 2003).
- Inhaled **anthrax** is usually fatal unless antibiotic treatment is started prior to the onset of symptoms. Anthrax can be disseminated in aerosol form or used to contaminate food or water. The anthrax attacks in the United States in 2001 involved placing aerosolized anthrax in letters sent to U.S. Congressmen and impacted postal workers near the nation's capitol (DHS, 2003).
- **Smallpox** is a contagious and often fatal infectious disease. Although it was eradicated from human populations through a globally coordinated program of vaccination, there are concerns that the virus could still be used in a terrorist attack. Stockpiles of the virus exist in the United States and Russia, and some fear that they could be stolen by terrorists. One study showed that if 100 people were initially infected with smallpox, a 15-day delay in control measures could result in over 15,000 excess cases after 1 year (Henning, 2003; CDC, 2004).
- A **dirty bomb** is designed to disperse radioactive material. While unlikely to cause mass casualties or extensive destruction, such a device would lead to fear, injuries, and possibly levels of contamination requiring costly and time-consuming cleanup (DHS, 2003).

In addition to these and other well-known threats, an increasing number of "next-generation" bioterrorist agents are emerging. A recent National Academy of Sciences report, *Global Effort Needed to Anticipate and Prevent Potential Misuse of Advances in Life Sciences*, asserted that intelligence agencies are too focused on specific lists of bacteria and viruses and should place more emphasis on dangerous emerging threats, such as RNA interference, synthetic biology, and nanotechnology (IOM and NRC, 2006). Nevertheless, more basic weapons, including conventional bombs and improvised explosive devices, appear to be the primary terrorist threats facing the United States today.

RESPONSES TO RECENT DISASTERS

Responding to a disaster requires preparation and also adaptability on the part of emergency responders. In many crisis situations, such as a natural disaster or terrorist incident, communications equipment may become inoperable, leaving rescue workers and emergency managers without any effective means of transmitting information. The chaotic flow of events in an evolving disaster can produce an effect that has been likened to "the fog of war" (Horwitz and Davenport, 2005; U.S. House of Representatives, 2006).

Emergency workers themselves may be victims of the catastrophic event and unable to respond. Some may be among the wounded, killed, or infected; others may have to respond to the needs of their own families. Those who are able to respond confront an array of challenges. During Hurricane Katrina, many roads were flooded and impassable, leaving personnel without an adequate means to reach those in need. In the case of Katrina, as well as other past catastrophes, working situations became unsafe as law and order began to break down. While serving as an EMT or paramedic typically involves a number of dangers, such as transporting patients at high speeds and entering scenes of recent violence (see Chapter 4), these dangers are amplified during a large-scale disaster.

Managing patients in a large-scale disaster is also extremely challenging. Although disaster planners frequently assume that casualties will be transported to hospitals by ambulance, research shows that most arrive by other means, including private cars, police vehicles, buses, taxis, or on foot (Auf der Heide, 2006). This frequently results in the crowding of nearby hospitals and reduced system efficiency since patients are not immediately directed to facilities that are open and ready. In most instances, the patients first arriving, who have "self-triaged" themselves from the scene, are often less seriously ill or injured than those that follow. This contributes to the chaos and confusion that mass casualty incidents typically produce.

Following a mass-casualty incident, there are often calls for policy changes that will produce more effective means of dealing with crisis events. Such changes may involve restructuring government bureaucracy or improving the way help from neighboring cities and states is utilized. These types of reforms have been introduced subsequent to a number of major disaster events in U.S. history, including September 11 and the Oklahoma City bombing, as well as disasters that have taken place in foreign countries.

Terrorist Attacks of September 11

The terrorist attacks on the World Trade Center and the Pentagon on September 11, 2001, represented a seminal event in U.S. history. The damage suffered that day increased awareness of the threat posed by terrorist groups and the potential for future attacks. The crisis spawned a series of actions on the part of the U.S. government to mitigate the possibility of such a disaster happening again.

EMS played a vital role in the emergency response to the attacks. Along with fire, police, and other rescue workers, EMS personnel were among the first to respond. According to the New York State Department of Health, 2,500 EMS personnel from 345 ambulance services responded to the World Trade Center attack, and 8 EMS workers were killed (Hall, 2005).

In addition to the bombing victims who were treated on scene by EMS personnel and transported to area hospitals, a large number of the injured either walked or were transported by other means to nearby hospitals. Two affiliated hospitals in lower Manhattan reported that 85 percent of the patients they received were "walking wounded" (Cushman et al., 2003). Beekman Hospital, a 170-bed facility 4 blocks from the disaster site, was overwhelmed with more than 500 patients in the first 24 hours, in addition to approximately 1,000 walk-ins seeking shelter from the dust (Pesola et al., 2002). This situation illustrates the challenge regarding overutilization of the most proximate hospitals in the event of a crisis.

In addition to direct transports from ground zero to area hospitals, ambulances were called upon to transport patients from overburdened local hospitals to other area hospitals with more available capacity. Following initial triage, patients were transported to other hospitals on the basis of their condition (e.g., burn victims, head trauma patients, and orthopedic patients). Because communications systems were disabled, however, ambulances had to transport the patients without advance communication with the destination hospitals (Pesola et al., 2002). As was the case with other first responders who participated in ground zero rescue efforts, EMS personnel struggled with faulty communications systems during the peak hours of the crisis.

Experience with the 1993 World Trade Center bombing provided some of the basis for New York City's response to the attack of September 11. A review of that incident conducted by the U.S. Fire Administration concluded with a recommendation that hospital transport decisions be made on an incident-wide basis, rather than by individuals on a case-by-case basis (Fire

Engineering, 2004). However, the number of "self-referred" victims, as well as communications challenges, made this approach extremely problematic on September 11. The U.S. Fire Administration report also concluded that "the need for a medical incident command system cannot be overstated" and that both medical and fire operations required extensive management. The report suggested that "fire departments that have EMS responsibility should closely examine their medical management procedures to ensure their ability to manage both major elements simultaneously" (Fire Engineering, 2004).

In response to the attacks of September 11, the U.S. government initiated a massive restructuring of the federal bureaucracy by establishing DHS. This restructuring involved the consolidation of dozens of federal agencies involved in homeland security functions (The White House, 2002). Agencies such as the Transportation Security Administration, the Federal Emergency Management Agency (FEMA), the National Disaster Medical System (NDMS), the U.S. Coast Guard, and many others were consolidated under DHS. The development of this new department coincided with a significant increase in homeland security spending.

In addition, in February 2003 President Bush issued Homeland Security Presidential Directive (HSPD)-5, which directed the Secretary of Homeland Security to develop and administer the National Incident Management System (NIMS). NIMS, released in March 2004, was intended to establish a more coherent incident command structure to handle all potential hazards facing the United States. It represented a significant shift in the nation's approach to incident management—from event- and discipline-specific incident response to an all-hazards, cooperative, multiagency approach (Walsh and Christen, 2005). In addition, the NIMS Integration Center (NIC) was established to provide strategic direction and oversight for NIMS. The NIC, which operates with FEMA as lead, aims to ensure that the all-hazards approach is an integral part of response training. It is also working to develop and facilitate national standards for NIMS education and training and to refine the system over time.

HSPD-5 also directed DHS to develop a National Response Plan (NRP) that builds on the basic framework provided by NIMS. Released in December 2004, the NRP represents "a concerted national effort to prevent terrorist attacks within the United States; reduce America's vulnerability to terrorism, major disasters, and other emergencies; and minimize the damage and recover from attacks, major disasters, and other emergencies that occur" (DHS, 2004).

One central premise of the NRP is that incidents should be handled at the lowest possible jurisdictional level. However, incidents of national significance—such as situations in which the resources of state and local authorities have been overwhelmed and federal assistance has been requested—would result in a full federal response. In such cases, federal actions would be taken in conjunction with state, local, tribal, nongovernmental, and private-sector entities (DHS, 2004).

The NRP identifies specific emergency support functions (ESFs) that are required in a crisis event. ESF-8 is the health and medical component of the plan, which is overseen by DHHS. ESF-8 identifies four major necessities for a medical response effort: (1) facilities in which to provide care (which may require building field hospitals since other facilities may have been damaged); (2) personnel to provide the care (which involves licensure issues for those coming from outside areas to help); (3) supplies and medications (including chronic care medications); and (4) the ability to move victims away from the impacted area (Alson, 2005). Disputes regarding the authority provided by ESF-8 hindered relief efforts during Hurricane Katrina (see below).

Hurricane Katrina

Hurricane Katrina was the first major disaster handled by FEMA after its relocation within DHS. The agency was severely criticized for its slow response to the crisis, and the director of relief operations at FEMA subsequently resigned from office. State and city managers also received a significant share of criticism. Local government officials were taken to task for having no effective incident command system in place to handle the crisis that ensued following the hurricane (Lindstrom and Losavio, 2005).

Although planners had anticipated that the city of New Orleans would be particularly vulnerable to a major hurricane, the magnitude of the crisis overwhelmed emergency responders and government officials at the federal, state, and local levels. Years prior to Katrina, FEMA had developed a disaster simulation, referred to as Hurricane Pam, illustrating the significant potential for damage from a major hurricane in New Orleans (CNN, 2005c; U.S. House of Representatives, 2006). However, this preparation did not result in an effective disaster operation. Instead, extreme chaos descended upon New Orleans, as well as some of the other affected areas in Louisiana, Mississippi, and Alabama.

A central criticism of the federal government was its failure to act proactively as weather reports indicated that a category 4 hurricane was headed for the Gulf Coast. The result was the loss of several critical days vital to the response effort and additional hardships for hurricane victims. In addition, while considerable federal resources were eventually brought to bear, these resources were not adequately coordinated, resulting in added confusion. Despite the tremendous organizational failures that occurred at each level of government, care providers on scene did the best they could to supply adequate care. The U.S. House of Representatives report on Katrina concluded that "ultimately, public health and medical support services were effectively but inefficiently delivered" (U.S. House of Representatives, 2006).

FEMA was essentially created as a disaster recovery agency that could coordinate the efforts of various federal departments. Its focus historically was on logistics and recovery distribution. However, Hurricane Katrina presented a number of additional challenges, including major evacuations and search and rescue operations, as well as issues of health care delivery and public health. The NDMS, housed within FEMA, took a primary role in mobilizing medical care for hurricane victims. According to FEMA testimony, the agency's Disaster Medical Assistance Teams (DMATs) treated over 100,000 patients during the crisis (Burris, 2005). The various disaster response teams within the NDMS are detailed in Box 6-2.

DMATs are medical units designed to complement state and local medical resources. They consist of approximately 35 individuals with a range of health care skills, as well as support personnel serving communications, logistics, and security functions. Fully operational DMATs have the ability

---

BOX 6-2
National Disaster Medical System (NDMS) Assets

- **DMATs:** 55 Disaster Medical Assistance Teams, which include federal, state, local, and private medical professionals. In addition, there are specialized teams to handle burns, pediatric patients, crush injuries, surgery, and mental health.
- **DMORTs:** 11 Disaster Mortuary Operational Response Teams, which consist of private citizens with specialized training and experience to help in the recovery, identification, and processing of deceased victims.
- **NMRTs:** 4 National Medical Response Teams to deal with the medical consequences of incidents potentially involving chemical, biological, or nuclear materials.
- **VMATs:** 4 Veterinary Medical Assistance Teams, which include clinician veterinarians, pathologists, animal health technicians, microbiologists, and others who assist animal disaster victims and provide care to search dogs.
- **IMSuRTs:** 3 International Medical Surgical Teams—1 operational and 2 under development. These teams are highly specialized and trained and equipped to establish a fully capable free-standing field surgical facility anywhere in the world.

SOURCE: FEMA, 2005.

to triage and treat up to 250 patients per day for up to 3 days without re-supply. DMAT team members are community-based volunteers and can be federalized upon the team's activation. This provides the team members with licensure and certification anywhere in the federal domain and addresses liability and compensation issues (Mediccom.org, 2006). In addition, DMATs may be used by states for emergencies within their borders. Thus there is a need for close coordination between the federal government and the states when the teams are deployed. During Katrina, many DMAT teams were moved around the country multiple times without ever setting up operations and seeing patients. Teams that did set up had difficulty being resupplied or being integrated within the local health care system. These problems limited the effectiveness of the teams in responding to the crisis.

Along with FEMA, the NDMS was moved from DHHS to DHS in 2003. According to the U.S. House of Representatives report on Katrina, however, some DHHS officials believe their agency assumes functional jurisdiction over the NDMS in the event of a disaster, based on authority provided under ESF-8 (U.S. House of Representatives, 2006). This uncertainty regarding appropriate authority contributed to confusion during the Katrina crisis. Following a review of the events, the White House report on Katrina, released in 2006, recommended that the NDMS be moved from DHS back to DHHS (The White House, 2006). Also in 2006, a congressional committee proposed a major restructuring of FEMA to expand its responsibilities while keeping it within DHS (Lipton, 2006).

In Hancock County, Mississippi, identified as Katrina's epicenter, a medical assistance team supported by HRSA Hospital Preparedness grants set up a 120-bed mobile hospital in the parking lot of a large shopping center. Beds, medical equipment, and provider training were made available through the HRSA grant program. As of early October 2005, the 450 medical personnel who staffed the unit on a rotating basis had treated 7,000 local residents (HRSA, 2005).

In addition to federal support, New Orleans and the other affected areas received assistance from states through the Emergency Management Assistance Compact (EMAC), an arrangement for interstate mutual aid that is managed by the National Emergency Management Association (NGA Center for Best Practices, 2005). Currently, 49 states participate in the arrangement. Through EMAC, states undergoing a disaster can immediately request assistance from other member states without the need for a federal disaster declaration. Issues related to licensure, liability, and reimbursement are resolved in advance. States that are prepared to provide assistance must wait for a formal request from a state in need. Including civilian personnel (19,481) and National Guard troops (48,477), Hurricanes Katrina and Rita resulted in the largest deployment of mutual aid through EMAC to date (Emergency Management Assistance Compact, 2005). The 2006 report of the U.S. House of Representatives concluded that EMAC "successfully provided unprecedented levels of response and recovery personnel and assets to the Gulf coast in record time following Hurricane Katrina" (U.S. House of Representatives, 2006). However, the system also suffered from significant disorganization during the crisis. In many cases, physicians were brought in and never used, while in others, physicians were used but not provided with any relief.

One of the significant challenges presented by a disaster of Katrina's magnitude is managing the flood of volunteers who arrive on scene wanting to provide help. Authorities are often unable to distinguish those who are qualified to provide care from who are unqualified but well intentioned. HRSA was charged by Congress with establishing a national system for identifying, authenticating, and credentialing responders under a program called Emergency Systems for Advance Registration of Volunteer Health Professionals (ESAR-VHP); however, this system had not been sufficiently developed to provide help during Hurricane Katrina.

During Katrina, air ambulance crews also played an important role, assisting in evacuating survivors from flooded areas. Overall, 27 civilian EMS helicopters were involved in evacuating Tulane Medical Center, Charity Hospital, and other facilities (Lindstrom and Losavio, 2005). In many cases, the helicopters used the roof of the hospital parking garage as a landing zone, and patients were brought upstairs to meet them. Despite these efforts, however, which took place largely without the aid of FEMA (U.S. House of Representatives, 2006), evacuations from these facilities were highly disorganized and agonizingly slow.

Patients who survived the evacuation were treated initially and then transported via buses and airplanes to hospitals in other cities for definitive care. However, this process also suffered from significant disorganization and delays. Many patients were evacuated to the airport but were left there for hours or days before being transported. Others were sent to distant cities with little or no information about where they were going or how they could find out about the location of their families. The NDMS did a poor job of allocating the patient load. Some cities, such as Houston and Atlanta, were inundated with patients, while others, such as Winston Salem, North Carolina, and Augusta, Georgia, received very few.

In Houston and Dallas, the Metropolitan Medical Response System (MMRS) was activated to coordinate the provision of shelter and medical care to evacuees. The MMRS was founded in 1996 by DHHS in response to the increased terrorist threat demonstrated by the Tokyo subway sarin attack in March 1995 and the Oklahoma City bombing in April 1995. The program was designed to enhance and coordinate local and regional response capabilities for highly populated areas that could be targeted by a terrorist attack using weapons of mass destruction. The MMRS concept and resources can also be applied to the management of large-scale incidents such as accidents involving hazardous materials, epidemic disease outbreaks, and natural disasters requiring specialized and carefully coordinated medical preparation and response. The MMRS became part of the new DHS in 2003 (DHS, 2005).

Following Katrina, both the Dallas Convention Center and the Reunion Arena were transformed into makeshift shelters for evacuees. Medical teams established a field hospital in the basement of the Dallas Convention Center and triaged individuals as they exited buses arriving from New Orleans. This helped ease the burden on local trauma centers. However, hospitals receiving large numbers of NDMS evacuees likely were filled to capacity, causing crowding in hospital emergency rooms, ambulance diversions, and reductions in access to emergency and trauma care.

After the initial blow and immediate aftermath of Hurricane Katrina, emergency health workers increasingly shifted their focus to the treatment of chronic illnesses. Patients suffering from conditions such as congestive heart failure and asthma required treatment, and patients with diabetes needed glucose monitors, syringes, insulin, and other medications. Emergency response teams were unequipped for these needs in many cases (Lindstrom and Losavio, 2005). In addition to a lack of adequate supplies and medications, no system was in place to verify the prescriptions of these patients. Moreoever, acute health issues unrelated to the hurricane, such as heart attacks and high-risk pregnancies, had to be addressed as well as possible by the emergency workers on the ground.

Terrorist Bombings in London and Madrid

On July 7, 2005, three bombs were detonated nearly simultaneously in London's Underground subway system. A short time later, a fourth bomb exploded on a double-decker bus at street level. Together, these explosions killed more than 50 people and injured more than 700.

In response to the September 11 terrorist attacks in the United States, London had planned for a possible mass casualty incident on its own soil, and EMS personnel had been trained accordingly. On the day of the bombings, emergency services set up a command structure and a triage area in the concourse of the rail station to determine the type of care required by each victim.

The London Ambulance Service (LAS) called for mutual aid from neighboring ambulance services and from voluntary agencies, which staged at previously agreed-upon locations. In total, more than 250 EMS personnel and 100 ambulances were mobilized to provide assistance (Hines et al., 2005). Altogether, LAS treated 45 patients for serious and critical injuries (e.g., burns, amputations, and chest and blast injuries) and approximately

300 patients for minor injuries (e.g., lacerations, smoke inhalation, and bruises). An additional 300 people went on their own to local London hospitals (Hines et al., 2005).

On March 11, 2004, Madrid experienced a similar but even more deadly terrorist attack. Ten bombs exploded nearly simultaneously in four commuter trains during rush hour, killing 191 people and injuring 2,000. Spain launched a massive emergency operation, mobilizing (according to government information) over 70,000 health personnel, 291 ambulances, 200 firemen, and 500 volunteers to assist in rescue and recovery operations and subsequent treatment (Gutierrez de Ceballos et al., 2004). According to one analysis, overtriage to the closest hospital was likely the largest problem with the rescue operations, making it more difficult to ensure that all patients were triaged appropriately.

Rhode Island Nightclub Fire

In February 2003, a fire erupted in a West Warwick, Rhode Island, nightclub when a band attempted to light pyrotechnics inside the club. The fire killed 100 people and injured more than 200 others. At the scene, two senior EMS officers provided triage. Victims were first assigned to one of two categories: dead or not dead. The fatalities were moved to a separate mass fatality management area. The remaining victims were brought by various means (e.g., walking or through the use of a backboard) to the primary triage site 100 feet from the nightclub. A captain scanned patients for signs of severe smoke inhalation and burns to the face, neck, torso, and upper extremities and directed the most critically injured to the next available EMS vehicle. Ambulances were lined up nearby, and pickups occurred in less than 5 minutes according to reports. Less critical patients were directed to a second triage area where another captain reassessed and retriaged them as necessary. EMS personnel reportedly transported 186 seriously injured persons from the incident site to 10 Rhode Island hospitals in less than 2 hours (CNN.com, 2003; Suburban Emergency Management Project, 2005).

Israeli Building Collapse

Israel frequently confronts mass casualty incidents, including suicide bombings and other incidents involving improvised explosive devices. One of its most serious recent mass casualty events occurred in May 2001 at a wedding celebration involving 700 participants, when the third floor of the wedding hall suddenly collapsed, causing 23 fatalities and 315 injuries (Avitzour et al., 2004).

In response to this disaster, more than 30 ambulances from the Jerusalem region were dispatched immediately to the scene, and additional units from other regions were mobilized. Approximately 600 EMTs, 40 paramedics, and 15 physicians operating 97 basic life support (BLS) ambulances, 18 mobile intensive care vehicles, and 6 mobile first aid stations were mobilized. On site, the senior paramedic assumed command of all medical teams and established a triage and resuscitation center. Casualties were dispatched to hospitals after receiving immediate necessary life support on site. The distribution of casualties to hospitals was controlled by the medical commander on site and coordinated by the area dispatch center, given that citywide communications were still in operation. The ambulances had a turnover time of 30 minutes and evacuated 42 percent of the victims within the first hour and an additional 33 percent in the next hour. Avitzour and colleagues (2004) found that a unified medical command system facilitated rapid response on scene, full utilization of all medical resources, and early evacuation and triage of casualties to nearby hospitals. Because of the crowding caused at the scene, however, the authors concluded that the automatic dispatching of a large number of ambulances to the incident site was ill advised (Avitzour et al., 2004).

Additional Experience from the Iraq War

Experience from the Iraq war and previous conflicts has led to improvements in the delivery of health care services to wounded American soldiers. The U.S. military is now able to provide high levels of medical care to soldiers much more quickly than was possible in the past. Medical assets are closer to the front lines, and air medical capabilities have been improved (Miles, 2005). The U.S. Marine Corps and Navy introduced forward resuscitative surgery systems (FRSSs)—small, mobile trauma surgical teams of eight individuals (including two surgeons and support staff) designed to provide tactical surgical intervention for combat casualties in the forward area (Chambers et al., 2005). The units can erect a battlefield hospital with two operating tables and four ventilator-equipped beds in less than 1 hour (Gawande, 2004). New medical technologies, such as compact ultrasound and x-ray machines, generators that extract pure oxygen from the air, and computerized diagnostic equipment, have allowed the teams to provide fairly sophisticated care (Barnes et al., 2005). With these new surgical teams, the U.S. military's strategy is to conduct damage control in the field (e.g., stopping bleeding and keeping patients warm), leaving definitive care to physicians at a hospital. Surgeons in the forward areas provide intermediate treatment, limiting surgery to 2 hours or less and sending the patient off to the next level of care.

Air medical evacuation procedures and equipment have improved to allow rapid transport of a critically injured solider. Because of those advances, the Air Force is transporting patients that never would have been moved in previous wars (Miles, 2005). From the field surgery teams, patients are brought by helicopter to a larger combat support hospital in Iraq. Air medical evacuations are now lighter and more adaptable; patient support pallets can be moved from one aircraft to another, and medical teams carry much of their equipment in backpacks. If a soldier is critically wounded, a critical care air transport (CCAT) team joins the air medical evacuation to help transport the patient to a combat hospital in Iraq with additional equipment.

Lessons Learned

Experience gained from recent domestic and international incidents such as those described above demonstrates that many commonly held assumptions about disasters do not correspond to the research evidence (Auf der Heide, 2006). Typically, events unfolding in the aftermath of a disaster are likely to be much more chaotic than what is optimal from an emergency management standpoint. In disaster events, emergency response units from neighboring communities and states often self-dispatch, which can overwhelm the ability of local managers to process them; casualties at the scene of the disaster are likely to self-triage and self-transport; and nearby hospitals are likely to be overwhelmed with patients arriving at their doors (see Table 6-2). Although emergency responders play an essential role in caring for victims at the scene of a disaster, previous experience shows that the overall response is likely to be more disorganized than planners would hope.

IMPROVING EMS-RELATED DISASTER PREPAREDNESS IN THE UNITED STATES

The array of threats facing the United States is substantial. Existing dangers, such as natural calamities and the potential for disease outbreaks, are now compounded by the threat of terrorism. Many disaster scenarios involve the disruption or destruction of local emergency care assets and institutions and the need for immediate help from outside the affected area. Other scenarios involve broader threats that potentially could challenge emergency systems throughout the country.

Since September 11, considerable resources have been devoted to preparing for large-scale disasters. Homeland security spending, which is estimated to have been below $10 billion in the mid-1990s, rose to nearly $50 billion subsequent to September 11 and the establishment of DHS in 2002 (see Figure 6-1). These homeland security funds were directed to a number of different areas, including border security, aviation security, and bioterrorism. However, very little funding has been directed to strengthen-

TABLE 6-2 Commonly Held Misconceptions About Disasters

Assumption	Research Observation
Dispatchers will hear of the disaster and send response units to the scene.	Emergency response units, both local and distant, will often self-dispatch.
Trained emergency personnel will carry out field search and rescue.	Most initial search and rescue is carried out by the survivors themselves.
Trained EMS personnel will carry out triage, provide first aid or stabilizing medical care, and decontaminate casualties before patient transport.	Casualties are likely to bypass on-site triage, first-aid, and decontamination stations and go directly to hospitals.
Casualties will be transported to hospitals by ambulance.	Most casualties are not transported by ambulance. They arrive by private car, police vehicle, bus, taxi, on foot, etc.
Casualties will be transported to hospitals appropriate to their needs, and no hospital will receive a disproportionate share.	Most casualties are transported to the closest or most familiar hospitals.
Authorities in the field will ensure that area hospitals are promptly notified of the disaster and the numbers, types, and severities of casualties they will receive.	Hospitals may be notified by the first arriving victims or the news media rather than authorities in the field. Often, information and updates about incoming casualties are insufficient or lacking.
The most serious casualties will be the first to be transported to hospitals.	The least serious casualties often arrive first.

SOURCE: Auf der Heide, 2006.

ing the nation's trauma care system or its capacity to respond to terrorism involving conventional weapons. In fiscal year 2003, just 9 percent of homeland security spending was directed to first responders, including fire, police, and EMS (see Figure 6-2). Programs through which EMS providers received preparedness funding included the Urban Area Security Initiative Grant, Assistance to Firefighters Grant, and Homeland Security Grant programs. (The issue of funding for EMS in disaster planning is discussed further below.)

In some limited respects, the nation may be better prepared for disasters now than it was in the past (e.g., in the case of aviation security). However, these gains have been extremely uneven. For example, federal disaster planning has focused much more on biological and chemical threats than on explosive attacks by terrorists. And prior to Hurricane Katrina, much more attention had been focused on terrorism than on natural disasters (Arkin, 2005; Kellermann, 2005). Of the 15 national planning scenarios introduced

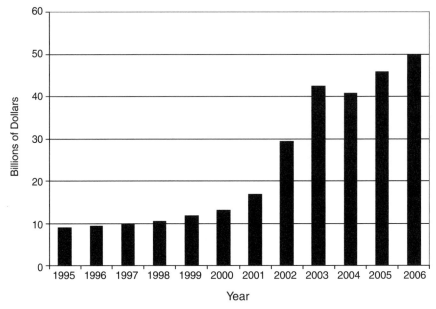

FIGURE 6-1 Trend in homeland security spending, fiscal years 1995 through 2006.
SOURCE: Reprinted, with permission, from de Rugy, 2005.

by DHS to guide disaster preparation efforts, only two involve natural disasters and only one attack uses explosives (see Box 6-3).

Following Hurricane Katrina, DHS did alter the selection criteria for its Urban Area Security Initiatives grants to ensure that the program would give as much weight to cities under threat from natural disasters as those that are likely targets of terrorism (Jordan, 2006). This shift reflected an effort on the part of the Secretary of Homeland Security to increase the emphasis on the department's all-hazards mission.

Local Capacity and Day-to-Day Readiness

The challenges facing the federal government in improving preparedness are matched by those facing local communities that provide the immediate response to disaster events. In the field of emergency management, it is axiomatic that all response is local and that state and federal governments assist only as needed. However, local emergency and trauma care systems across the country face sizable day-to-day challenges, even without the additional responsibilities that might be placed upon them in the event of a

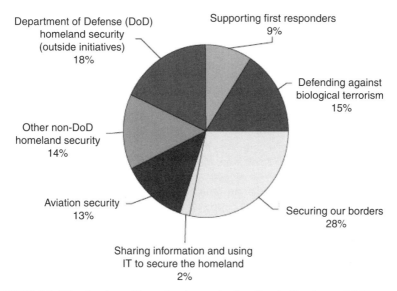

FIGURE 6-2 Distribution of homeland security funding in fiscal year 2003 request by activity.
NOTE: IT = information technology.
SOURCE: The White House, 2003.

major crisis. As described earlier, ED crowding is common in most cities and ambulance diversions occur regularly, even under normal operating conditions (GAO, 2003a). In terms of physical capacity, EMS, hospital EDs, and trauma centers in most cities have limited or no surge capacity, especially for pediatric and critical patients. Even multivehicle highway crashes can stretch local systems to their limit. The committee maintains that to be adequately prepared for disaster events, it is necessary first to establish strong and highly efficient emergency and trauma care systems that work smoothly on a day-to-day basis.

In addition, local systems should be prepared and equipped for specific potential disaster events. The training and equipment and emergency planning currently under way in most areas are inadequate. Few EMS personnel have any training or experience in assessing the scene of a terrorist bombing or evaluating casualties for a range of potential injuries. A serious natural or man-made biological threat—one that required sophisticated surveillance, highly coordinated communications and planning, decontamination, negative pressure suites, and staff equipped and trained in the use of personal protective equipment—would seriously challenge even the most well-

---

BOX 6-3
The Department of Homeland Security's 15 National
Planning Scenarios

1. Nuclear Detonation: 10-Kiloton Improvised Nuclear Device
2. Biological Attack: Aerosol Anthrax
3. Biological Disease Outbreak: Pandemic Influenza
4. Biological Attack: Plague
5. Chemical Attack: Blister Agent
6. Chemical Attack: Toxic Industrial Chemical
7. Chemical Attack: Nerve Agent
8. Chemical Attack: Chlorine Tank Explosion
9. Natural Disaster: Major Earthquake
10. Natural Disaster: Major Hurricane
11. Radiological Attack: Radiological Dispersal Device
12. Explosives Attack: Bombing Using Improvised Explosive Devices
13. Biological Attack: Food Contamination
14. Biological Attack: Foreign Animal Disease (Foot and Mouth Disease)
15. Cyber Attack

SOURCE: Homeland Security Council, 2004.

---

prepared community today. Given the enormous deficiencies in preparation for disasters in communities throughout the United States, the committee maintains that DHS and other agencies should enhance the equipment, training, and surge capacity of local emergency and trauma care systems in order to prepare for both day-to-day spikes in demand and mass-casualty disaster events. Mass-casualty preparations should heavily emphasize the most likely disaster scenarios.

Recognizing EMS as an Equal Partner in Disaster Planning and Funding

EMS and trauma systems have to a large extent been overlooked in disaster preparedness planning at both the state and federal levels (NASEMSD, 2003). This is due in part to the fact that EMS is often regarded as a subset of fire response, though the medical role that would be undertaken by EMS personnel in the event of a major emergency is distinct from the role of fire suppression teams (Fire Engineering, 2004). Given the specific homeland security threats that confront the United States, most of which have a heavy medical component, the committee recommends that the Department of Health and Human Services, the Department of Transportation, the Department of Homeland Security, and the states elevate emergency and trauma care to a position of parity with other public safety entities in disaster planning and operations (6.1). These care providers represent a critical component of the broader, multiagency response to a major crisis, whether a natural disaster, terrorist incident, or other public health emergency, and should be included in all preparedness activities.

The fact that EMS has not been adequately included in disaster preparations is evidenced by the small share of disaster-related funding received by EMS from the federal government since September 11. Although they represent a third of the nation's first responders, EMS providers received only 4 percent of the $3.38 billion distributed for emergency preparedness by DHS in 2002 and 2003 (see Figure 6-3). Similarly, EMS received only 5 percent of the Bioterrorism Hospital Preparedness Grant, a program administered by DHHS (Center for Catastrophe Preparedness and Response NYU, 2005). To date, the vast majority of these federal resources have been directed at law enforcement, fire response, hospitals, and public health systems. Few resources have been directed at EMS except through these means (NASEMSD, 2004).

The final version of the fiscal year 2006 Homeland Security Appropriations report included language calling for greater recognition of EMS

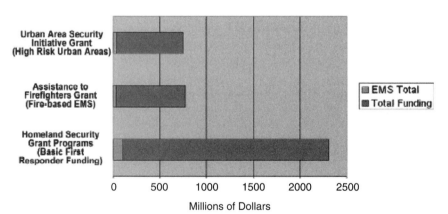

FIGURE 6-3 EMS receives only 4 percent of first responder funding.
SOURCE: Reprinted, with permission, from the Center for Catastrophe Preparedness and Response. 2005. Emergency Medical Services: The Forgotten First Responder—A Report on the Critical Gaps in Organization and Deficits in Resources for America's Medical First Responders. New York, NY: Center for Catastrophe Preparedness and Response, New York University.

in homeland security funding distributions. The report stated that "the conferees are very concerned with the lack of first responder grant funding being provided to the Emergency Medical Services (EMS) community." The conferees directed DHS's Office of Domestic Preparedness (ODP) to require state and local governments to include EMS representatives in planning committees as an equal partner and to facilitate a nationwide needs assessment. While the conferees did not mandate that a specific percentage of grant funds be allocated to each type of first responder, they directed ODP to evaluate how much money goes to EMS. The conferees also inserted a requirement that a state provide an explanation if it does not award at least 10 percent of its grant funding to EMS providers to enhance training and equipment (Advocates for EMS, 2006).

While significant federal funds are available to states and localities for disaster preparedness, emergency care in general has not been able to secure a meaningful share of these funds because they have been folded into other pubic safety functions in which emergency medical care is considered a low priority. To address the serious deficits in health-related disaster preparedness, the committee recommends that **Congress substantially increase funding for emergency medical services–related disaster preparedness through dedicated funding streams (6.2)**. These funding streams could be directed through the states to regional systems and localities based on priorities established through the regional planning process, thus ensuring that resources would be allocated according to the real needs identified by communities.

In budgeting for disaster preparedness, the committee believes it critical to separate medical functions from other public safety functions by establishing them as a separate line item. Without this separation, politics and culture will always pose a threat to the commitment to the medical component.

Finally, changes in the disaster preparedness grant process should also be considered. A 2003 survey conducted by the National Association of State EMS Directors (NASEMSD) found that its membership believed the federal grant process needs to be simplified and state EMS offices to have more support and involvement in the process. In addition, NASEMSD advocated the identification of specific funding streams for EMS, including non-fire-related EMS (NASEMSD, 2004).

Equipment, Education, and Training

One consistent challenge for disaster responders is communication and information management. Effective response requires the transmission of real-time information to assess needs and available resources, which can change suddenly and unexpectedly (Chan et al., 2004). On September 11, communications failures led to chaos and confusion, and by one estimate resulted in more problems than all other factors combined (Simon and Teperman, 2001; Martinez and Gonzalez, 2001). The U.S. House of Representatives report on Hurricane Katrina likewise concluded that destruction of communications capability hindered command and control and severely limited situational awareness. The report concluded that "one of the most common and pervasive themes in the response to Hurricane Katrina has been a systematic failure of communications at the local, state, and federal levels" (U.S. House of Representatives, 2006).

Current disaster preparedness efforts have focused on creating interoperable communications systems among first responders, which is an urgent priority for EMS providers. This type of system will be essential in avoiding a repeat of the experience of September 11, as well as other disaster events in which communications links have been a central problem. However, the systems now being developed are primarily public safety communications networks; they are not designed to meet medical communication needs. The committee recommends that a greater focus be placed on developing an effective interoperable medical communications system that works efficiently on a day-to-day basis and can be employed in the event of a major disaster. In addition to voice communications systems, DHS could contribute to emergency preparedness by providing financial support for improving the nation's health information technology infrastructure.

The International Association of Fire Chiefs, the International Association of Chiefs of Police, and the National League of Cities have pointed to congested radio communications systems as a key problem and have advocated a consumer transition to digital television to free up additional spectrum for public safety agencies. They have called for the creation of a single command and control center that would coordinate federal, state, and local officials in times of emergency. However, these recommendations are focused on public safety emergencies that are distinct from the provision of health care, including the transmission of medical data.

In addition to the central challenge of ensuring effective communications, providers currently lack appropriate equipment for specific disaster events, such as chemical and biological attacks. The use of personal protective equipment (PPE) is one method of protecting providers from biological or chemical hazards, but very few emergency medical professionals have been provided with such equipment or trained in its proper use. As mentioned above, in 25 states fewer than 50 percent of EMTs and paramedics have reported having adequate equipment to respond to these types of attacks. Only 1 state has reported that adequate personal protective equipment would be immediately available for all EMS personnel statewide in the event of a biological or chemical event (Center for Catastrophe Preparedness and Response NYU, 2005). These deficiencies must be addressed to prevent emergency responders from becoming victims themselves and to enable a meaningful response in the event of a major terrorist attack.

Ultimately, disasters are characterized by many people trying to do quickly what they do not ordinarily do, in an environment with which they are not familiar (Chan et al., 2004). Regardless of the quality of disaster plans, efforts will be ineffective if personnel are not well trained in executing them. Currently, the lack of this type of training is a serious deficiency of the national disaster preparedness effort. Most hospitals have disaster plans, but providers have not been adequately instructed in how to execute those plans. Disaster training has been equally deficient among EMS professionals, as evidenced by the following facts:

- During the past year, fewer than 33 percent of EMTs and paramedics have participated in a drill simulating a radiological, biological, or chemical attack.
- Fire department EMTs and paramedics have received an average of 4.5 hours of training in homeland security and disaster management since September 11, 2001. EMTs and paramedics not affiliated with fire departments have received an average of less than 1 hour of such training.
- EMTs and paramedics in urban areas have received less than 3.5 hours of training in homeland security and disaster management since September 11 (Center for Catastrophe Preparedness and Response NYU, 2005).

Moreover, in rural areas, training for more commonly occurring disasters (including weather-related incidents and unintentional man-made disasters) has declined over the past few years in favor of terrorism preparedness (Furbee et al., in press). These findings indicate that U.S. EMS personnel are not well prepared to handle a catastrophic emergency such as a major earthquake, bioterrorist attack, or pandemic influenza outbreak. Adequate funding directed specifically to emergency medical personnel is required to address this deficiency.

Establishing effective training in disaster preparedness for EMS personnel will require a coordinated and well-funded national effort that involves both professional and continuing education. The committee therefore recommends that **professional training, continuing education, and credentialing and certification programs for all the relevant professional categories of emergency medical services personnel incorporate disaster preparedness into their curricula and require the maintenance of competency in these skills (6.3).** These changes would ensure that emergency personnel would remain up to date on essential disaster skills and would bolster preparedness efforts.

Finally, state and federal response to a national disaster is hindered by inconsistent standards for the licensure of all emergency care providers and a lack of adequate reciprocity agreements between states. For example, state EMS scope of practice and professional licensure standards, designations, and educational requirements vary widely (Center for Catastrophe Preparedness and Response NYU, 2005). To facilitate improved response to a disaster, each state should adopt consistent standards for the licensure of all emergency care providers and enter into reciprocity agreements with all other states. The adoption by states of the National EMS Scope of Practice Model, a component of NHTSA's *Emergency Medical Services Education Agenda for the Future*, would be a major step in this direction (see Chapter 4). This would enable state and federal agencies to quickly identify and deploy EMS personnel, physicians, nurses, and other critical professionals across state lines in the event of a major disaster.

Coordination of Government Disaster Response

Hurricane Katrina illustrated the breakdowns that can occur among local, state, and federal governments in a time of crisis. Critical delays in bringing relief supplies to stranded New Orleans residents, an extremely faulty incident command structure, and a breakdown in law and order resulted in the exchange of blame among officials involved at each level of government. Criticisms often centered on how and when requests for help were made by local officials and why help did not arrive sooner. These conflicts demonstrate the challenge of delineating the roles and responsibilities of each level of government given the right of local self-determination and the need to ensure that sufficient resources are brought to bear in the event of a major catastrophe.

In the aftermath of Hurricane Katrina, the federal government moved to assert more control over future disaster situations, proposing greater utilization of the U.S. military and other federal resources (NEMA, 2005). In October 2005, however, the National Governors Association (NGA) responded with a position statement calling for continued respect for the central role of the state. NGA stated that "following the tragedies inflicted on the citizens of the gulf coast by hurricanes Katrina and Rita, local, state and federal government must examine the way the three levels of government communicate and coordinate their response. The possibility of the federal government pre-empting the authority of states or governors in emergencies, however, is opposed by the nation's governors." NGA indicated that "governors are responsible for the safety and welfare of their citizens and are in the best position to coordinate all resources to prepare for, respond to and recover from disasters." At the same time, NGA acknowledged that federal aid and assistance are sometimes necessary, and said that a dialogue between state and federal officials about how best to achieve these goals should continue (NGA Center for Best Practices, 2005).

Managing large-scale disasters continues to be a challenge for officials at each level of government. The responses to September 11 and Hurricane Katrina demonstrate that there is a significant gap between the dangers that now present themselves and the nation's readiness to address them effectively. From the EMS perspective, significant deficiencies in education, training, and equipment reflect a lack of funding directed to preparing for the emergency medical component of likely disaster events. These deficiencies will need to be addressed if the nation is to be well prepared for the next major disaster.

SUMMARY OF RECOMMENDATIONS

6.1: The Department of Health and Human Services, the Department of Transportation, the Department of Homeland Security, and the states should elevate emergency and trauma care to a position of parity with other public safety entities in disaster planning and operations.

6.2: Congress should substantially increase funding for emergency medical services–related disaster preparedness through dedicated funding streams.

6.3: Professional training, continuing education, and credentialing and certification programs for all the relevant professional categories of emergency medical services personnel should incorporate disaster preparedness into their curricula and require the maintenance of competency in these skills.

REFERENCES

AAA (American Ambulance Association). 2004. AAA Terrorism Preparedness Survey. [Online]. Available: http://64.233.161.104/search?q=cache:yCdVtVqLUTIJ:www.the-aaa.org/Members_Only/Oncapitolhill/4%2520Summary%2520AAA%2520Terrorism%2520Prep%2520Survey.doc+AAA+Terrorism+Preparedness+Survey&hl=en&gl=us&ct=clnk&cd=1[accessed May 2, 2006].

Accountability Review Boards on the Embassy Bombings in Nairobi and Dar es Salaam. 1999. *Report of the Accountability Review Boards on the Embassy Bombings in Nairobi and Dar es Salaam on August 7, 1998.* Washington, DC.

Advocates for EMS. 2006. *Language Included in the Final FY 2006 Homeland Security Appropriations Report.* [Online]. Available: http://www.advocatesforems.org/Library/upload/EMS_HS_conference_ report_language.pdf [accessed May 25, 2006].

Alson RL. 2005. *Medical Response to Catastrophic Events.* Statement at the October 20, 2005, Hearing of the Subcommittee on Subcommittee on Prevention of Nuclear and Biological Attack, Committee on Committee on House Homeland Security, Washington, DC.

Arkin WM. 2005. *Michael Brown Was Set Up: It's All in the Numbers.* [Online]. Available: http://blogs.washingtonpost.com/earlywarning/2005/09/michael_brown_w.html [accessed November 1, 2005].

Arnold JL, Halpern P, Tsai MC, Smithline H. 2004. Mass casualty terrorist bombings: A comparison of outcomes by bombing type. *Annals of Emergency Medicine* 43(2):263–273.

Associated Press. 2006a. *Four Bodies Found Since Dec. 21; Katrina Death Toll Now 1,326.* [Online]. Available: http://www.katc.com/global/story.asp?s=4317545&ClientType=Prin table [accessed May 1, 2006].

Associated Press. 2006b. *Band Ex-Manager Sentenced to Four Years in R.I. Club Fire Case.* [Online]. Available: http://www.usatoday.com/news/nation/2006-05-09-fire-hearing_x.htm [accessed May 11, 2006].

Auf der Heide E. 2006. The importance of evidence-based disaster planning. *Annals of Emergency Medicine* 47(1):34–49.

Augustine J, Kellermann A, Koplan J. 2004. America's emergency care system and severe acute respiratory syndrome: Are we ready? *Annals of Emergency Medicine* 43(1):23–26.

Avitzour M, Libergal M, Assaf J, Adler J, Beyth S, Mosheiff R, Rubin A, Feigenberg Z, Slatnikovitz R, Gofin R, Shapira SC. 2004. A multicasualty event: Out-of-hospital and in-hospital organizational aspects. *Academic Emergency Medicine* 11(10):1102–1104.

Barnes J, Roane K, Szegedy-Maszak M. 2005, April. 5. Stemming the fatalities with a modern touch. *Sydney Morning Herald.* [Online]. Available: http://www.smh.com.au/articles/2003/04/04/1048962935279.html?oneclick=true [accessed January 29, 2007].

BBC News. 2005. *Sarin Attack Remembered in Tokyo.* [Online]. Available: http://news.bbc.co.uk/2/hi/asia-pacific/4365417.stm [accessed May 1, 2006].

BBC News. 2006a. *Bali Death Toll Set at 202.* [Online]. Available: http://news.bbc.co.uk/1/hi/in_depth/asia_pacific/2002/bali/default.stm [accessed May 1, 2006].

BBC News. 2006b. *Q&A: Bird Flu.* [Online]. Available: http://news.bbc.co.uk/2/hi/health/3422839.stm [accessed May 1, 2006].

Bravata DM, McDonald K, Owens DK. 2004. *Regionalization of Bioterrorism Preparedness and Response.* [Online]. Available: http://www.ahrq.gov/clinic/epcsums/bioregsum.pdf [accessed May 25, 2006].

Burris K. 2005. *Legislative Proposals in Response to Hurricane Katrina.* Statement at the October 3, 2005, Hearing of the Subcommittee on Economic Development, Public Buildings and Emergency Management, Committee on House Transportation and Infrastructure, Washington, DC.

CDC (Centers for Disease Control and Prevention). 2004. *Smallpox Fact Sheet.* [Online]. Available: http://www.bt.cdc.gov/agent/smallpox/overview/disease-facts.asp [accessed January 29, 2007].

CDC. 2006a. *Emergency Preparedness and Response: Agents, Disease, & Other Threats.* [Online]. Available: http://www.bt.cdc.gov [accessed February 1, 2006].

CDC. 2006b. *Emergency Preparedness & Response: Training, Centers for Public Health Preparedness (CPHP) Program.* [Online]. Available: http://www.bt.cdc.gov/training/cphp/ [accessed February 1, 2006].

Center for Catastrophe Preparedness and Response NYU. 2005. *Emergency Medical Services: The Forgotten First Responder—A Report on the Critical Gaps in Organization and Deficits in Resources for America's Medical First Responders.* New York: Center for Catastrophe Preparedness and Response, New York University.

Chambers LW, Rhee P, Baker BC, Perciballi J, Cubano M, Compeggie M, Nace M, Bohman HR. 2005. Initial experience of US Marine Corps forward resuscitative surgical system during Operation Iraqi Freedom. *Archives of Surgery* 140(1):26–32.

Chan TC, Killeen J, Griswold W, Lenert L. 2004. Information technology and emergency medical care during disasters. *Academic Emergency Medicine* 11(11):1229–1236.

CNN.com. 2003. *At Least 96 Killed in Nightclub Inferno, Governor: DNA Might Be Only Clue to Identity of Some Victims.* [Online]. Available: http://www.cnn.com/2003/US/Northeast/02/21/deadly.nightclub.fire [accessed May 1, 2006].

CNN.com. 2005a. *Tsunami Deaths Soar Past 212,000.* [Online]. Available: http://www.cnn.com/2005/WORLD/asiapcf/01/19/asia.tsunami [accessed May 1, 2005].

CNN.com. 2005b. *Four Sought in Attempted Attacks: Police Say Man Shot and Killed in Underground Not One of Four.* [Online]. Available: http://www.cnn.com/2005/WORLD/europe/07/22/london.tube/index.html [accessed May 1, 2006].

CNN.com. 2005c. *Chertoff: Katrina Scenario Did Not Exist.* [Online]. Available: http://www.cnn.com/2005/US/09/03/katrina.chertoff [accessed January 7, 2006].

Cushman JG, Pachter HL, Beaton HL. 2003. Two New York city hospitals' surgical response to the September 11, 2001, terrorist attack in New York City. *Journal of Trauma-Injury Infection & Critical Care* 54(1):147–154; discussion 154–155.

de Rugy V. 2005. *What Does Homeland Security Spending Buy?* Washington, DC: American Enterprise Institute for Public Policy Research.

DHS (U.S. Department of Homeland Security). 2003. *Homeland Security Information Bulletin: Chemical, Biological, Radiological and Nuclear (CBRN) Materials and Effects.* [Online]. Available: http://www.iwar.org.uk/homesec/resources/dhs-bulletin/cbrn.htm [accessed May 25, 2006].

DHS. 2004. *National Response Plan.* [Online]. Available: http://www.dhs.gov/interweb/assetlibrary/NRP_FullText.pdf [accessed March 2, 2006].

DHS. 2005. Metropolitan Medical Response System (MMRS) the First Decade (1995–2005). [Online]. Available: http://mmrs.fema.gov/press/2005/pr2005-07-05.aspx [accessed February 10, 2006].

DHS READYAmerica. 2005. *Be Informed: Natural Disasters.* [Online]. Available: http://www.ready.gov/america/natural_disasters.html [accessed January 15, 2006].

Emergency Management Assistance Compact. 2005. *EMAC Home Page.* [Online]. Available: http://www.emacweb.org [accessed January 7, 2006].

Fee E, Parry M. 2005. Dangerous illusions: Cautionary tales in the history of medicine. *Health Affairs* 24(4):1178–1179.

FEMA (Federal Emergency Management Agency). 2005. *FEMA News: FEMA Disaster Medical Assistance Teams Hard at Work; Federal Teams Have Treated More Than 100,000 Patients.* [Online]. Available: http://www.fema.gov/news/newsrelease.fema?id=19304 [accessed November 1, 2005].

Fire Engineering. 2004. *The World Trade Center Bombing: Report and Analysis.* Emmitsburg, MD: Federal Emergency Management Agency/U.S. Fire Administration National Fire Data Center.

Furbee PM, Coben JH, Smyth SK, Manley WG, Summers DE, Sanddal ND, Sanddal TL, Helmkamp JC, Kimble RL, Althouse RC, Kocsis AT. In press. Realities of rural emergency medical services disaster preparedness. *Prehospital and Disaster Medicine* 21.

GAO (U.S. Government Accountability Office). 2003a. *Hospital Emergency Departments: Crowded Conditions Vary among Hospitals and Communities.* Washington, DC: GAO.

GAO. 2003b. *Hospital Preparedness: Most Urban Hospitals Have Emergency Plans but Lack Certain Capacities for Bioterrorism Response.* Washington, DC: GAO.

GAO. 2005. *Hurricane Katrina: Providing Oversight of the Nation's Preparedness, Response, and Recovery Activities.* [Online]. Available: http://www.gao.gov/new.items/d051053t.pdf [accessed March 29, 2006].

Gawande A. 2004. Casualties of war—military care for the wounded from Iraq and Afghanistan. *New England Journal of Medicine* 351(24):2471–2475.

Gutierrez de Ceballos JP, Turegano-Fuentes F, Perez–Diaz D, Sanz-Sanchez M, Martin-Llorente C, Guerrero-Sanz JE. 2004. 11 March 2004: The terrorist bomb explosions in Madrid, Spain: An analysis of the logistics, injuries sustained and clinical management of casualties treated at the closest hospital. *Critical Care* 8.

Hall M. 2005, March 10. Report: EMS lacks terrorism training, equipment. *USA Today.* Nation.

Henning KJ. 2003. Syndromic surveillance. In: *Microbial Threats to Health: Emergence, Detection, and Response.* Washington, DC: The National Academies Press.

Hines S, Payne A, Edmondson J, Heightman AJ. 2005. Bombs under London: The EMS response plan that worked. *Journal of Emergency Medical Services* 23(8).

Hirschkorn P. 2003. *New York Reduces 9/11 Death Toll by 40.* [Online]. Available: http://www.cnn.com/2003/US/Northeast/10/29/wtc.deaths [accessed May 1, 2006].

Homeland Security Council. 2004. *Planning Scenarios: Executive Summaries.* [Online]. Available: http://www.globalsecurity.org/security/library/report/2004/hsc-planning-scenarios-jul04_exec-sum.pdf [accessed May 1, 2006].

Horwitz S, Davenport C. 2005, September 11. Terrorism could hurl D.C. area into turmoil: Despite efforts since 9/11, response plans incomplete. *The Washington Post.* P. A01.

HRSA. 2005. *HRSA Hospital Preparedness Grantee in N.C. Takes Mobile Hospital, Staff to Miss. to Help Hurricane Victims.* [Online]. Available: http://www.hrsa.gov/katrina/updatehrsa1011/htm [accessed January 7, 2006].

Insurance Information Network of California. 2006. *Earthquakes.* [Online]. Available: http://iinc.org/pdf/EQ percent20Kit percent20final.updated.pdf [accessed May 1, 2006].

IOM (Institute of Medicine). 2004. *Learning from SARS: Preparing for the Next Disease Outbreak. Workshop Summary.* Washington, DC: The National Academies Press.

IOM. 2005. *The Threat of Pandemic Influenza: Are We Ready? Workshop Summary.* Washington, DC: The National Academies Press.

IOM, NRC (Institute of Medicine, National Research Council). 2006. *Globalization, Biosecurity, and the Future of the Life Sciences.* Washington, DC: The National Academies Press.

Jordan LJ. 2006, January 2. Homeland security to re-prioritize grants. *Washington Dateline.*

Kellermann A. 2005, August 5. Still not ready in the ER. *The Washington Post.* P. A15.

Lindstrom A-M, Losavio K. 2005. Chaos of Katrina: EMS maintains composure in the midst of anarchy. *Journal of Emergency Medical Services* 23(11).

Lipton, E. 2006, April 27. Senate panel urges FEMA dismantling. *The New York Times.* P. A22.

Martinez C, Gonzalez D. 2001. The World Trade Center attack. Doctors in the fire and police services. *Critical Care* 5(6):304–306.

Mediccom.org. 2006. *The NDMS Disaster Medical Assistance Teams.* [Online]. Available: http://mediccom.org/public/tadmat/ndms/dmat.html [accessed January 7, 2006].

Miles D. 2005, August 10. Aeromedical evacuation improvements saving lives. *DefenseLink News.* [Online]. Available: http://www.defenselink.mil/news/Aug2005/20050810_2386.html [accessed January 30, 2007].

NASEMSD (National Association of State EMS Directors). 2003. *Linkages of Acute Care and EMS with State and Local Prevention Programs, Part 3: Status of State EMS System Funding.* Falls Church, VA: NASEMSD.

NASEMSD. 2004. *NASEMSD Survey: Identification of Obstacles to EMS Terrorism Preparedness.* Falls Church, VA: NASEMSD.

NEMA (National Emergency Management Association). 2005. *NEMA Policy Position on the Role of the Military in Disaster Response.* Lexington, KY: NEMA.

NGA Center for Best Practices. 2005. *Beyond EMAC: Legal Issues in Mutual Aid Agreements for Public Health Practice.* Issue Brief, Washington, DC.

Noji EK. 1996. Disaster epidemiology. *Emergency Medical Clinics of North America* 14(2):289–300.

Pesola GR, Dujar A, Wilson S. 2002. Emergency preparedness: The World Trade Center and Singapore airline disasters. *Academic Emergency Medicine* 9(3):220–222.

Rand Corporation. 2004. *Rand Study Shows Compensation for 9/11 Terror Attacks Tops $38 Billion; Businesses Receive Biggest Share.* [Online]. Available: http://www.rand.org/news/press.04/11.08b.html [accessed May 1, 2006].

Rudman WB, Clarke RA, Metzl JF. 2003. *Emergency Responders: Drastically Underfunded, Dangerously Unprepared.* New York, NY: Council on Foreign Relations.

Schur CL, Berk ML, Mueller CD. 2004. *Perspectives of Rural Hospitals on Bioterrorism Preparedness Planning.* Bethesda, MD: NORC Walsh Center for Rural Health Analysis.

Simon R, Teperman S. 2001. The World Trade Center attack. Lessons for disaster management. *Critical Care (London)* 5(6):318–320.

Suburban Emergency Management Project. 2005. *SEMP Biot #250: What Is "Graceful Degradation"?* [Online]. Available: http://www.semp.us/biots/biot_250.html [accessed February 1, 2006].

Times Foundation. 2005. *Kashmir Earthquake—A Situation Report.* India: The Times Group.

U.S. House of Representatives. 2006. *A Failure of Initiative: Final Report of the Select Bipartisan Committee to Investigate the Preparation for and Response to Hurricane Katrina.* Washington, DC: Government Printing Office.

Waeckerle JF. 2000. Domestic preparedness for events involving weapons of mass destruction. *Journal of the American Medical Association* 283(2):252–254.

Waeckerle J, Lillibridge S, Burkle F, Noji E. 1994. Disaster medicine: Challenges for today. *Annals of Emergency Medicine* 23(4):715–718.

Walsh DW, Christen H. 2005. The National Incident Management System fully interfaces EMS operations in disaster and MCI responses. *Journal of Emergency Medical Services* 23(4).

The White House. 2003. *Securing the Homeland, Strengthening the Nation.* [Online]. Available: http://www.whitehouse.gov/homeland/homeland_security_book.pdf [accessed May 25, 2006].

The White House. 2006. *Federal Response to Hurricane Katrina: Lessons Learned.* [Online]. Available: http://www.whitehouse.gov/reports/katrina-lessons-learned.pdf [accessed May 25, 2006].

7

Optimizing Prehospital Care
Through Research

The aim of prehospital emergency medical services (EMS) research is to guide the field with respect to clinical interventions and system designs. Research provides an evidence base to support the application of particular medical treatments and raises red flags when interventions are demonstrated to cause harm to patients. Systems-related research seeks to address operational and structural questions such as the optimum configuration of EMS personnel and the impact of medical direction in EMS systems.

Most of the evidence base that exists to support EMS has been generated by researchers at a small number of medical schools, generally in midsized cities, who have ongoing relationships with municipal EMS systems (NHTSA, 1996). The preponderance of published EMS research is component-based, focusing on a single intervention or health problem rather than broader system-level issues.

Prehospital EMS research is often categorized under emergency medicine research, which encompasses hospital-based emergency care. Unlike medical research that is defined by specific diseases or organ systems, emergency medicine research is defined by time and place. It addresses conditions and interventions common to the prehospital EMS and hospital emergency department (ED) settings, and its focus is on the acute management of patients. It is often conducted by emergency physicians in collaboration with specialists in other fields, such as pediatrics and cardiology. In addition, there has been a growing contribution to the EMS literature by nonphysicians. Trauma care research is a parallel field of study that is also defined by time and place. Trauma care deals principally with the acute management of patients with traumatic injuries. Like emergency medicine research, trauma care research is concerned with the treatment of these patients in the prehospital and hospital settings, but it reaches further into the inpatient setting, particularly the intensive care unit (ICU) and surgical departments. This chapter focuses primarily on research in the area of prehospital EMS, including prehospital trauma care.

Currently, a range of federal government agencies each contribute relatively small amounts of funding to prehospital EMS research. The National Institutes of Health (NIH), the Agency for Healthcare Research and Quality (AHRQ), the National Highway Traffic Safety Administration (NHTSA), the Health Resources and Services Administration (HRSA), and the Centers for Disease Control and Prevention (CDC) all have programs in place to support research in this area. But while the federal government dedicates tens of billions of dollars each year to health-related research, a tiny percentage of that funding is directed to emergency care research in general and prehospital emergency care in particular. The primary foundation-based supporters of emergency care research training are the Emergency Medicine Foundation (EMF), affiliated with the American College of Emergency Physicians (ACEP), and the Society for Academic Emergency Medicine (SAEM). However, both of these programs are quite small, allocating less than $1 million per year combined, and only part of that to EMS.

AN INADEQUATE RESEARCH BASE TO SUPPORT EMS

Despite the size, scope, sophistication, and critical role of EMS in the United States, the evidence base to support EMS-related clinical and system design decisions is much less well developed than that in other areas of medicine (NHTSA, 1996). Consequently, EMS has for years operated without a sufficient scientific basis to support many of its actions (NHTSA, 2001a; McLean et al., 2002; Sayre et al., 2003).

Policy makers and experts in the field have long recognized the paucity of information relating to EMS, and there have been numerous efforts to expand this research base. The 1996 *Emergency Medical Services Agenda for the Future*, developed by NHTSA's Office of EMS together with HRSA, focused on the importance of research and evaluation and the need for robust data and information systems (NHTSA, 1996). The 1998 *Emergency Medical Services Agenda for the Future: Implementation Guide* identified the creation of a national EMS research agenda as a key priority (NHTSA, 1998). The *Implementation Guide* also stressed the importance of developing academic institutional commitments to EMS-related research and forming collaborative relationships among EMS systems, private foundations, medical schools, and other academic institutions.

In 2001, NHTSA and the Maternal and Child Health Bureau within HRSA released the *National EMS Research Agenda*. The report presented eight recommendations: (1) career EMS investigators should be developed and supported; (2) centers of excellence should be created to facilitate EMS research; (3) federal agencies should commit to supporting EMS research; (4) other public and private institutions should be encouraged to support EMS research; (5) results of this research should be applied by EMS professionals and others; (6) EMS providers should require that evidence be available before implementing new procedures, devices, or drugs; (7) standardized data collection methods should be established; and (8) exceptions from informed consent rules should be adopted (NHTSA, 2001a).

The above efforts have helped draw attention to the lack of a research base for EMS and spurred some development in the area. Despite these efforts, however, large gaps in information remain. Patients in the prehospital setting often receive services that have not been proven to work or for which the evidence base is very limited. In many situations, emergency diagnostic and therapeutic strategies have been adapted from patient populations and settings that differ substantially from those of the prehospital environment. Major new programs have been launched with little or no evidence for their cost-effectiveness. Consequently, many treatment strategies employed in the field are of questionable benefit and in some cases may even be harmful.

Questions related to core aspects of current clinical practice—for example, the value of field intubation, fluid resuscitation, and advanced life support (ALS) interventions for cardiac arrest—remain unresolved. Rather than being based on scientific evidence, practices are often based on tradition or convention. And because EMS is slow to adopt a current standard of care, the care that is delivered is highly variable. Nonetheless, advancing the science base to determine what constitutes effective care in the prehospital setting would allow for improvements in EMS care over time.

Not infrequently, treatments that have established effectiveness and safety profiles when used in hospital- or office-based settings are now implemented in the out-of-hospital setting without adequate examination of patient outcomes. For example, the use of endotracheal intubation to provide ventilation and oxygenation for critically ill or injured children is a well-established and highly effective technique when employed in the relatively controlled environment of the operating room, the pediatric ICU, or even the ED. This technique, however, has been widely incorporated into the practice of paramedics in the out-of-hospital setting without sufficient evidence for its efficacy or safety. Gausche-Hill and colleagues conducted a prospective controlled evaluation of this technique compared with simple bag-valve-mask ventilation to determine its effect on survival and neurological outcomes in critically ill and injured children (Gausche-Hill, 2000; Gausche et al., 2000). The study found no evidence for the benefit of endotracheal intubation in the out-of-hospital setting but did show a substantial incidence of complications. Based on these findings, the Los Angeles and

Orange County EMS agencies in California eliminated pediatric intubation from the scope of paramedic practice.

To counter the considerable lack of data available to support specific medical interventions conducted in the field by EMS personnel, EMS professionals and policy makers at all levels should work to establish a culture of science-based decision making. In addition to specific clinical interventions, scientific evidence should be used to support systems-level decisions such as the appropriate level of training of responders, the proper deployment of new technologies, the utilization of EMS resources, and the optimal use of medical direction within EMS systems.

KEY BARRIERS TO EMS RESEARCH

The capacity to investigate key clinical and systems issues in EMS is limited by a variety of factors, including a lack of trained investigators having elected to focus their work on this area of medicine, legal and regulatory barriers that limit the number of qualified research subjects and the sharing of research-related information, and a lack of funding directed specifically to support EMS research. In addition, the infrastructure to support EMS research is lacking in many ways. Existing information systems present a number of problems related to data storage and retrieval (NHTSA, 2001a). For example, data definitions used by different EMS agencies and hospitals often differ, which makes compiling research data more difficult. In addition, most EMS programs continue to use pen-and-paper records, which introduces problems such as illegibility, gaps in information, and estimated data (e.g., time points). This problem may be exacerbated because most EMS personnel in the field do not consider themselves part of the research process and may resent any added paperwork requirements. The move to electronic data collection and more passive forms of data gathering might help alleviate this problem.

Even before the enactment of the Health Insurance Portability and Accountability Act (HIPAA; see below), researchers had difficulty in obtaining patient-level data from hospitals and other health care facilities. In general, hospitals have been reluctant to provide such information, in part because of the resources required to organize and collect the data, and more important because of fear of how the information might be used. With or without the restrictions HIPAA places on data sharing, EMS agencies would need to build trust with hospitals to facilitate this type of research work.

The complexity of the various agencies and personnel that deliver out-of-hospital care also hinders EMS research. Spaite and colleagues (1995) noted that component research, the cornerstone of "traditional" medical research, is characterized by focused, directed questions, with small numbers of data points that are easily obtained by small numbers of data collectors representing a single agency or institution, working in a tightly controlled environment. The out-of-hospital environment lacks all of these characteristics; rather, it involves complex interrelated questions, with diverse data points collected by many data collectors representing multiple agencies and disciplines in a complex, uncontrolled environment. The authors observed that there are very few examples of successful systems research in EMS, the best of these being the work done on trauma systems (Mullins et al., 1998; Mullins, 1999) and the "chain of survival" concept for out-of-hospital cardiac arrest (Becker and Pepe, 1993; Larsen et al., 1993; Swor et al., 1995).

As suggested above, moreover, successful EMS research that has been completed and published in peer-reviewed journals may not be applied in the field until years later. While this problem is not unique to EMS, it presents a significant barrier to ensuring that patients receive prehospital medical services that are supported by a strong evidence base. Accordingly, the *National EMS Research Agenda* recommended that "EMS professionals of all levels should hold themselves to higher standards of requiring evidence before implementing new procedures, devices, or drugs" (NHTSA, 2001a; Sayre et al., 2002).

Limited Research Capacity

Research related to EMS is hindered by both the small number of people who decide to pursue such research as a career and institutional factors that limit opportunities for potential EMS researchers. Interest in EMS research and opportunities for formally developing EMS research skills have been promoted in the *National EMS Research Agenda* and elsewhere (NHTSA, 2001a).

Emergency medical technicians (EMTs) and paramedics currently receive little or no formal training in research methodologies, biostatistics, or informed consent and are not instructed in how to perform a critical reading of the literature (Delbridge et al., 1998). A fairly small number of such field personnel have become accomplished EMS researchers (Brown et al., 1996; Lerner et al., 1999; Neely et al., 2000a,b; Brown et al., 2003) by pursuing formal coursework and advanced degrees that were not part of their initial training. A number of EMS physician researchers have backgrounds as field providers, and it appears likely that this experience has contributed to the success and relevance of their projects (Cone and Wydro, 2001; Persse et al., 2003; Key et al., 2003). However, professional training for EMTs and paramedics typically does not encourage future careers in EMS-related research.

The *National EMS Research Agenda* recommended that EMS investigators be developed and supported in the initial stages of their careers and that highly structured training programs with content focused on EMS research methodologies be developed (NHTSA, 2001a). The report noted that many colleges and universities have existing programs that could provide training to interested EMS professionals. For example, graduate degree programs in research and public health could be tailored to meet the specific needs of students with an interest in EMS. The report also supported the development of federally funded research fellowship training programs capable of producing at least five EMS researchers per year.

Existing postgraduate fellowships fall into two groups: those that are dedicated research training fellowships and those that are primarily clinical but include a research component. The latter category, which typically includes EMS, is frequently funded by institutional resources and for this reason necessarily includes a substantial patient care component, limiting the fellow's opportunities to develop research skills. Frequently, this clinical care component provides the financial support for the fellowship. It is generally accepted, however, that a research training program that fails to include 2 years of dedicated research training and at least 80 percent research time is unlikely to result in long-term success in today's research climate (NIH, 2003). As a result, it is unlikely that postgraduate fellowship programs with a primarily clinical focus are or ever will be an effective tool for improving EMS research capacity. Establishing federally funded fellowship training programs that are research-focused would promote the development of a larger cadre of highly qualified EMS researchers.

Regulatory Barriers

A number of regulations are in place at the federal and state levels to ensure that patient interests are protected with respect to prospective research work. While these regulations have maintained important patient rights, such as privacy and informed consent, they have also had the effect of reducing the number of patients who participate in research investigations and limiting the ability of researchers to gain access to clinical data. Their ultimate effect is to limit the evidence base available to providers who treat similar patients in the future.

Waiver of Informed Consent in Emergency Circumstances

The out-of-hospital environment is generally a difficult place to obtain informed consent from patients and/or their families, and EMS personnel typically have no training or experience in doing so (Hsieh et al., 2001; Valenzuela and Copass, 2001; Moscati, 2002). Moreover, patients treated in the emergency and trauma care setting frequently suffer acute, debilitating illnesses or injuries that affect their capacity to make informed decisions. Thus, potential research subjects frequently cannot participate in the informed consent process prior to taking part in an interventional clinical trial, even when the therapy being investigated holds the prospect of benefiting them directly. Moreover, it is almost impossible to withhold the current standards of care from potential research subjects even if those standards have not been demonstrated through research to be effective (Spaite et al., 1997).

Health Insurance Portability and Accountability Act

To investigate patient outcomes resulting from out-of-hospital interventions, it is necessary to obtain outcome information from each of the facilities in which patients were subsequently treated. Out-of-hospital and ED records must be linked with hospital records, vital statistics, and coroner's records when appropriate. The patient identifiers required to effect such linkages, even when probabilistic record linkage is employed, are subject to the confidentiality provisions of the HIPAA legislation. Because of greater scrutiny of privacy provisions related to HIPAA, it is increasingly difficult for EMS agencies, even when performing quality assurance work, to obtain patient-specific outcome data.

Federalwide Assurance Program

Another regulatory barrier concerns the Federalwide Assurance (FWA) program. An FWA is an agreement between the federal government, represented by the Office for Human Research Protections (OHRP) within the Department of Health and Human Services (DHHS), and a research organization. The agreement provides assurance that the research organization intends to comply with applicable federal laws and standards for the protection of human research subjects (Newgard and Lewis, 2002). The FWA program, established in 2000, is intended to streamline the previous, more cumbersome system of single-project and multiple-project assurances. An FWA must be in place for an organization to participate in federally funded research that involves human subjects.

The FWA regulations have become a significant barrier to obtaining population-based outcome data from patients treated in the emergency and trauma care setting (Newgard and Lewis, 2002). Many patients treated in this setting, either those initially treated by EMS or those treated in community EDs, produce important health care utilization and outcome data that are stored at nonacademic community-based medical facilities. These facilities are unlikely to participate in federally supported research in general and therefore usually do not have an FWA in place. Illustrating the problem, Newgard and Lewis (2002) reported difficulties associated with obtaining

FWAs with community hospitals to procure patient-level outcome data from a low-risk EMS study.

Limited Federal Research Funding

The U.S. federal government expends tens of billions of dollars each year on health-related research, including clinical trials and other research examining health care services and treatment guidelines. However, a small share of available research dollars is directed to emergency and trauma care, and even less to prehospital care in particular. This situation has contributed to a dearth of evidence regarding which interventions produce positive outcomes in the prehospital environment.

National Institutes of Health

NIH is the largest single source of support for biomedical research in the world, with a budget of over $27 billion in 2004 (IOM, 2004). NIH includes 20 Institutes, 7 Centers, and 4 Program Offices contained within the Office of the Director. All Institutes but only some of the Centers provide research funding, while several other Centers provide general support (e.g., the Center on Scientific Review). All Institutes and 4 of the Centers receive individual congressional appropriations.

The NIH Institutes are organized into five categories: disease, organ system, stage of life, scientific discipline, and profession or technology (IOM, 2003). None of the current Institutes or Centers are defined either by the site of care or the timing or urgency of care, which are the defining characteristics of emergency and trauma care research. NIH does not have an Institute or Center focused specifically on emergency services. Thus, many important emergency care–related clinical questions extend beyond the domains of single NIH Institutes or Centers. Although both a 2003 Institute of Medicine report (IOM, 2003) and the NIH Roadmap Initiative (Zerhouni, 2003) emphasized the importance of stimulating and funding trans-NIH research, the fact that EMS and emergency care research questions naturally span the domains of multiple Institutes and Centers has not been effectively addressed.

Agency for Healthcare Research and Quality

AHRQ is another federal agency charged with supporting health services research, though on a much smaller scale than NIH. It is estimated that NIH spends approximately $800 million annually on health services research, while the entire AHRQ budget is only approximately $300 million (IOM, 2003).

Because funding provided to AHRQ is increasingly tied to specific activities, such as patient safety research, progressively fewer funds have been available for investigator-initiated research and research training. Nonetheless, AHRQ remains a major source of funds for health services and outcomes research, with a specific focus on translating research into practice. The development of methods for effectively translating new research findings into clinical practice is particularly important in emergency care, and it is not surprising that AHRQ has funded a number of important studies in this area, including early research on treatment for cardiac arrest (Eisenberg et al., 1990), studies of first responder defibrillation and prehospital cardiac arrest outcomes in Memphis (Kellermann et al., 1993), and the Pediatric Airway Management project of Gausche-Hill and colleagues mentioned previously (Gausche et al., 2000).

National Highway Traffic Safety Administration

The Office of EMS within NHTSA plays a lead role in coordinating activities related to EMS system development and research. As mentioned above, the Office of EMS together with HRSA sponsored the development of the *National EMS Research Agenda* (NHTSA, 2001b). This report highlighted the lack of evidence available to support many clinical practices in the field and detailed an agenda for building the research base. NHTSA's Office of EMS also currently funds two key research initiatives: the Emergency Medical Services Outcomes Project (EMSOP), a study to develop metrics for use in EMS-related outcomes research (see Box 7-1), and the Emergency Medical Services Cost Analysis Project (EMSCAP), a study to develop metrics for assessing the costs and benefits of EMS.

NHTSA and HRSA also cosponsor the National EMS Information System (NEMSIS), the national database on EMS systems and outcomes. NHTSA's Office of Human-Centered Research sponsors the Crash Injury Research and Engineering Network (CIREN), which collects and shares detailed research data on automobile crashes and patient outcomes (see Box 7-2).

Though not specifically research related, NHTSA's Office of EMS also supports the National EMS Scope of Practice Model project, a joint initiative of the National Association of State EMS Officials and the National Council of State EMS Training Coordinators (see Chapter 4). In addition, the Longitudinal Emergency Medical Technician Attribute and Demographics Study (LEADS) is a project of the National Registry of EMTs partially funded by NHTSA. An annual LEADS survey collects information on the EMS workforce.

BOX 7-1
Emergency Medical Services Outcomes Project (EMSOP)

EMSOP was designed to develop a foundation and framework for out-of-hospital outcomes research—a branch of clinical research that focuses on determining whether interventions performed in clinical practice actually work (Maio et al., 1999). Given the rate of growth in health care expenditures and the uncertainty regarding the effectiveness of EMS practices, increased emphasis has been placed on demonstrating which clinical interventions can be shown to improve patient outcomes in the out-of-hospital setting (Maio et al.,1999; Spaite et al., 2001). EMSOP resulted in a series of four journal articles outlining the key components of the framework for outcomes research: (1) specific patient conditions that should take precedence in EMS outcomes research; (2) methodologically acceptable outcome models, including the Episode of Care model; (3) core risk-adjustment measures; and (4) specific issues related to pain measurement (Maio et al., 1999, 2002; Spaite et al., 2001; Garrison et al., 2002).

BOX 7-2
Crash Injury Research and Engineering Network (CIREN)

CIREN is a multicenter research program focused on improving the prevention, treatment, and rehabilitation of motor vehicle crash injuries, with the aim of reducing deaths, disabilities, and economic costs. The program supports a linked computer network of seven level I trauma centers and the collaboration of clinicians and engineers in academia, industry, and government who perform in-depth studies of crashes, injuries, and treatments to improve processes and patient outcomes. The CIREN database, which extends back to 1996, consists of multiple data fields related to severe motor vehicle crashes, including medical injury profiles and crash reconstructions. More than 250 common data elements are standardized across all CIREN sites.

Health Resources and Services Administration

The Emergency Medical Services for Children (EMS-C) program, jointly funded by HRSA and NHTSA, is one of the largest grant programs supporting EMS research. The EMS-C program also sponsors the Pediatric Emer-

---

BOX 7-3
National EMSC Data Analysis Resource Center (NEDARC)

NEDARC is a technical resource for EMS-C grantees and state EMS offices, focused on assisting them in developing their capabilities to collect, analyze, and utilize EMS and other health care data, with the ultimate goal of improving the quality of care provided by state EMS and trauma systems. Established in 1995 through the EMS-C program, NEDARC assists EMS offices in establishing research designs, determining what data to collect, selecting a collection tool, storing the data, overcoming barriers to collection, coordinating data from other systems or agencies, converting data to a standard dictionary, formatting them to conform to a data model, and cleaning or standardizing and aggregating them (NEDARC, 2006). NEDARC also assists in disseminating model data systems from states that have developed such systems.

---

gency Care Applied Research Network (PECARN), the first federally funded multi-institutional network for research in pediatric emergency medicine (PECARN, 2004), as well as the National EMSC Data Analysis Resource Center (NEDARC), which helps states collect and analyze data on pediatric EMS systems and populate the pediatric trauma registry (see Box 7-3). HRSA's Trauma-EMS Systems Program and Office of Rural Health Policy have also supported research efforts in emergency care.

Centers for Disease Control and Prevention

The National Center for Injury Prevention and Control (NCIPC) was established at CDC in 1992 as the lead federal agency for injury prevention. Its extramural research program funds and monitors research in all three phases of injury control: prevention, acute care, and rehabilitation. Research supported by the program focuses on the broad-based need to control morbidity, disability, death, and costs associated with injury. CDC's recently completed *Acute Injury Care Research Agenda* (CDC, 2005) was developed with extensive input from academic research centers, national nonprofit organizations, and other federal agencies with a stake in injury prevention. The report included seven recommendations for research areas, including the components of trauma systems and disaster preparedness. In addition, CDC's National Center for Chronic Disease Prevention is funding the Cardiac Arrest Registry to Enhance Survival (CARES) project (discussed in Chapter 3).

RESEARCH CONDUCTED IN THE PREHOSPITAL SETTING

Despite the limitations of prehospital EMS research enumerated above, there have been a number of important, highly successful EMS studies that have helped inform practice. The Ontario Prehospital Advanced Life Support (OPALS) study, for example, funded by the Canadian government, is systematically examining a series of prehospital treatments using a sequential before/after design. The first major OPALS study examined the impact of adding automated external defibrillators (AEDs) to improve treatment for cardiac arrest. A subsequent study compared outcomes achieved by rapid defibrillation programs versus the addition of ALS (primarily endotracheal intubation and administration of cardiac medications). This study, conducted in the Canadian province of Ontario, was the largest multicenter controlled clinical trial ever conducted in a prehospital setting. OPALS examined 5,638 Toronto-area patients who had out-of-hospital cardiac arrest—1,391 when the area had only a rapid defibrillation program and 4,247 after it had instituted full ALS care. The researchers reported that "the addition of [ALS] interventions did not improve the rate of survival after out-of-hospital cardiac arrest in a previously optimized emergency-medical-services system with rapid defibrillation" (Stiell et al., 2004). The OPALS research study also assessed the incremental benefits for survival, morbidity, and processes of care that resulted from the introduction of prehospital ALS programs for patients with major trauma and respiratory distress. In addition, researchers conducted an economic evaluation of ALS programs by estimating the incremental cost per life saved and per quality-adjusted life year.

The largest EMS clinical study completed in the United States to date is the Public Access Defibrillation (PAD) trial, which involved 19,000 volunteer responders from 993 community units in 24 North American (U.S. and Canadian) regions. The primary objective of the study was to determine whether the use of AEDs by response teams composed of volunteer laypersons who were also trained in cardiopulmonary resuscitation (CPR) would increase the number of survivors among patients with out-of-hospital cardiac arrest. The study was supported by approximately $16 million in funding, with $10.5 million from the National Heart, Lung, and Blood Institute; $3.5 million from the American Heart Association; and roughly $3 million in donated AEDs, supplies, training mannequins, and other equipment from several manufacturers. This strategy of funding from a variety of sources is common in EMS studies. The PAD trial found that the rate of successful cardiac resuscitation from witnessed out-of-hospital cardiac arrest due to ventricular fibrillation was higher when the victim received treatment by community volunteers trained to perform CPR and also equipped with an AED as opposed to similarly trained volunteers who did not have an AED.

Over an average of 21.5 months, there were 29 cardiac arrest survivors to hospital discharge in the group assigned to CPR plus AED compared with 15 survivors in the group assigned to CPR only.

The above-cited study conducted by Gausche-Hill and colleagues in southern California is likely the second-largest externally funded EMS study in the United States. As described above, this study examined survival and neurological outcomes in children whose airways were managed with bag-valve-mask ventilation versus those who were managed with endotracheal intubation (Gausche-Hill, 2000; Gausche et al., 2000). The project involved the training of over 2,500 paramedics from 56 different EMS agencies in Los Angeles and Orange Counties, as well as 500 paramedic students. A total of 830 patients were enrolled, and no differences in either survival or neurological outcomes were found. The authors concluded that the addition of pediatric intubation to the scope of practice of a paramedic system that was already using bag-valve-mask ventilation did not improve outcomes.

The out-of-hospital pediatric intubation study was funded in several phases by four California EMS Authority Special Projects Grants (totaling $377,648), three grants from the Maternal and Child Health Bureau and NHTSA through the EMS-C Targeted Issues program (totaling $860,536), and an ACEP Section Grant ($8,910). Equipment and supplies were also donated by a number of medical equipment manufacturers.

Another recent landmark study involved randomizing 9-1-1 callers to receive instructions on providing CPR that involved chest compressions only or chest compressions with mouth-to-mouth ventilation. This trial was supported by the Seattle Medic I Foundation for about 1 year, by the Washington State Affiliate of the American Heart Association for 1–2 years, and by a grant from AHRQ for the remainder of the 12-year project. Total funding was approximately $600,000 (Hallstrom et al., 2000). Based primarily on this study, with support from several studies suggesting that any interruption in chest compression is detrimental, a number of large U.S. cities have changed the way their 9-1-1 dispatchers provide CPR prearrival instructions.

A 1993 AHRQ-funded study of first responder defibrillation in Memphis, Tennessee, employing a quasi-experimental design revealed that AED-equipped firefighters did not achieve significantly higher rates of successful cardiac resuscitation compared with firefighters performing CPR alone. This was the first AED study to employ a control group rather than "historical controls." It revealed that both groups did better than historical performance, indicating a "Hawthorne effect" in which performance improves when it is studied (a common flaw in EMS studies that use before/after designs) (Kellermann et al., 1993).

Some research in prehospital EMS has centered on issues related to the design and structure of EMS systems. For example, a study by Eisenberg and colleagues (1990) examined rates of survival from out-of-hospital cardiac arrest in 29 cities. The authors found that the chance of survival ranged from 2 percent to more than 25 percent depending on the locality. They concluded that survivability appeared to reflect how rapidly and effectively the system could provide CPR, defibrillation, medication, and intubation, and noted that survival was highest in "double-response" (more often referred to as "two-tiered") systems in which a first responder EMT arrives to begin CPR, followed by the arrival of a paramedic. Although this appears counterintuitive compared with systems in which all EMS units are staffed by paramedics, the advantage may derive from the fact that a smaller number of paramedic units results in more frequent practice of ALS skills, which may result in better care.

Another example is a study conducted by Hunt and colleagues (1995), which showed that on average, the use of lights and sirens saved 43.5 seconds in transporting patients from the scene of an emergency to the hospital, which they concluded was clinically meaningful only in very rare situations. Another systems-related question that has not been adequately addressed by the literature is the impact of medical directors on EMS system performance. Although there is widespread belief in the EMS community that strong medical direction is needed to improve performance, this view has never been conclusively demonstrated. Likewise, data on the cost-effectiveness of specific prehospital medical interventions are almost completely lacking.

EXPANDING THE EVIDENCE BASE

While prehospital and hospital-based emergency care research focuses on topics of significant public interest and public health importance and has achieved some notable successes, it lacks support within the broader scientific community. As described above, the cross-cutting nature of emergency care means that it overlaps with many other medical disciplines, making it difficult to establish a unique funding home for such research within NIH and other agencies that tend to have a traditional disease or body part orientation. As a result, funding for EMS and emergency and trauma care research is not proportionate to its importance to the nation.

Thus there is a need for a broad national commitment to expanding emergency and trauma care research in general and prehospital EMS research in particular. The development of this commitment will require increased recognition of EMS research successes, broader understanding of the need for and value of prehospital EMS research, and enhanced federal support for EMS researchers throughout the relevant federal agencies. The committee recommends that **federal agencies that fund emergency and trauma care research target additional funding at prehospital emergency medical services research, with an emphasis on systems and outcomes** research (7.1). This increased funding should reflect the benefits likely to accrue from advancing the science of emergency care.

Funding devoted to prehospital emergency care research should be aimed at addressing a number of needs that must be met if research in the field is to advance. These include developing a cadre of career researchers, helping to develop routes for prehospital EMS professionals to transition into careers in research, providing research training, funding centers of excellence, and developing multicenter/multisystem research consortiums. For example, a prehospital research network might be established to examine low-volume prehospital events. Meeting each of these needs would develop and strengthen the science base for enhancing the quality, safety, and impact of EMS.

With regard to funding, there are critical ties between emergency and trauma care research and disaster preparedness. Because of the current political climate, there is widespread recognition of the importance of improving our understanding of optimal disaster preparedness and management, whether in response to natural or man-made incidents. As discussed in Chapter 6, although current antiterrorism funding is to a large extent focused on combating bioterrorism, the vast majority of terrorist events have involved conventional explosives and nonbiological agents (DePalma et al., 2005). Likewise, natural disasters such as hurricanes and earthquakes continue to occur, and constantly challenge our ability to provide emergency care and effective disaster relief (Schultz et al., 2003). Greater emphasis should be placed on these other, high-probability disaster events, including an increased volume of research supported through disaster preparedness funding.

Expanding the Role of Emergency and Trauma Care Researchers in the Grant Review Process

One of the greatest impediments to grant funding for emergency and trauma care research at NIH and other agencies is the dearth of researchers in the field involved in developing intramural and extramural research strategies and serving on grant review panels. This is due in part to the cross-cutting nature of the discipline, the relative youth of the field, and the small number of mature investigators. But the exclusion of emergency and trauma care researchers creates a "catch-22": unless experienced advocates for emergency and trauma care research are involved in the grant development and review processes, junior researchers in the field are unlikely to be successful with their proposals, but without successful proposals, it is unlikely that emergency and trauma care researchers will be asked to participate in the grant development and review processes. While the development of investigators is a critical imperative for the field, the number of mature investigators is growing, and these researchers should be afforded more visibility and authority in grant funding. To address this need, the committee believes that all federal agencies should expand the role of emergency and trauma care researchers in the grant review process. This involvement should encompass any areas of research—including basic, clinical, and systems research—that could have significant application to emergency and trauma care settings, including prehospital, hospital-based emergency, and trauma care.

Removing Regulatory Barriers

As described above, conducting research in the out-of-hospital environment is unusually challenging. Patients may not be able to make informed consent decisions because they are unconscious or otherwise incapacitated, and paperwork may be prohibitively time-consuming if a patient requires urgent attention. Emergency care already has some flexibility with regard to research, but the rules continue to be problematic in many situations (NHTSA, 2001a).

Adherence to federal rules governing the protection of human subjects is ensured by institutional review boards (IRBs). Additional provisions to protect the privacy of human subjects are defined by the HIPAA privacy rule. OHRP is the agency assigned to ensure human subject protections. The rules attempt to balance the value of important research against the potential harm to patients resulting from that research. Some have argued that the current rules overly restrict critically important research, particularly in emergency and trauma care (Newgard et al., 2002).

Informed consent requirements are important in ensuring that evaluations of new and promising therapies are conducted in an ethical and publicly transparent manner. However, complying with these requirements can be overly burdensome for emergency and trauma care researchers given the condition of many such patients and the circumstances of their treatment (as discussed earlier). Currently, federal regulations (21 Code of Federal Regulations §50.24) allow a narrow exception to the general requirement for prospective, written informed consent for participation in research studies in the setting of an acute, debilitating illness or injury for which there is no accepted effective therapy (Biros et al., 1995, 1998, 1999; Baren et al., 1999; Sloan et al., 1999; Lewis et al., 2001). Under this exception, some flexibility in the informed consent requirements is allowed in emergency situations, but it remains difficult to comply with the rules in many cases (NHTSA, 2001). As noted by Mann and colleagues (2005), ". . . the logistical application of these ethical standards across institutions or among different research studies remains complex and variable." Furthermore, state regulations occasionally preempt the federal exception for emergency care research. Active guidance from OHRP to states and individual IRBs could eliminate some of the current obstacles that discourage innovation in treatment approaches with the potential to benefit critically ill or injured patients.

In addition, the FWA program was designed to simplify informed consent for research institutions, but sometimes makes it more difficult to conduct emergency and trauma care research that involves nonacademic institutions in the continuum of care. Therefore, the committee recommends that **Congress modify Federalwide Assurance program regulations to allow the acquisition of limited, linked, patient outcome data without the existence of a Federalwide Assurance program (7.2).**

Finally, HIPAA regulations can deter systems research by inhibiting the flow of information across settings—from dispatch to EMS to hospital or trauma center—that constitute an episode of care. To address this issue, specific regulatory language would be required to allow EMS systems or other emergency and trauma care providers to obtain specific outcome data when needed for the assessment of quality of care or effectiveness or for research purposes. Such access would have to be subject to strict confidentiality provisions, with penalties for inappropriate use. The committee therefore believes that Congress and state governments should amend patient confidentiality regulations to allow, under strictly defined circumstances, out-of-hospital and ED records to be linked with longitudinal data on patient outcomes. A working group should be established to consider the specific changes required to address the dampening effect of these regulations on emergency and trauma care research while maintaining their original patient protection goals.

Establishing a Research Agenda

Until recently, little attention had been paid to the issue of research priorities in EMS. In the past few years, three projects have attempted to disseminate opinions regarding priorities in EMS research. The first, a consensus conference sponsored by the National EMS for Children Resource Alliance, focused on out-of-hospital treatment of children (Seidel et al., 1999). The second was EMSOP, described earlier, which examined needs in EMS outcomes research (Maio et al., 1999). The third is a continuation of the *National EMS Research Agenda* (Sayre et al., 2002, 2005).

In 2002, the *National EMS Research Agenda* identified the need for a strategic plan for EMS research to concentrate the efforts of EMS researchers, policy makers, and funders, with the ultimate goal of improving clinical outcomes (Sayre et al., 2005). The strategic plan was developed by a multidisciplinary team of EMS personnel, administrators, policy makers, and researchers who participated in a structured consensus-building process. The group has now identified priority topics in EMS research, which include clinical issues in the categories of airway and breathing, cardiovascular disease and stroke, general medical, pediatrics, and trauma, as well as systems and broader medical science issues, including EMS provider education, EMS system design and operation, improving global outcomes, and research and evaluation methods.

In addition to these key research areas determined through the strategic planning effort, the committee identified a number of research topics that have not been adequately addressed in the literature to date. These include both clinical and systems issues that are centrally important to the delivery of effective EMS (see Box 7-4).

As the largest federal funder of health research, NIH should also take a greater role in facilitating the development of a research agenda for the field. As described above, EMS and emergency and trauma care research is dispersed across many disciplines and funding agencies. The *National EMS Research Agenda* and other recent efforts have documented evidence gaps and research opportunities across the many fields of emergency and trauma care (NHTSA, 2001a). Except for the recent efforts described above, however, the field has lacked an integrated research strategy prioritizing the critical areas of neglect and establishing a systematic plan for addressing those areas. As a result, NIH and other agencies have continued to pursue a haphazard approach to funding emergency and trauma care research. To address this problem, the committee recommends that **the Secretary of the Department of Health and Human Services conduct a study to examine the research gaps and opportunities in emergency and trauma care research, and recommend a strategy for the optimal organization and funding of the research effort. This study should include consideration of the training of new investigators, the development of multicenter research networks, the involvement of emergency medical services researchers in the grant review and research advisory processes, and improved research coordination through a dedicated center or institute. Congress and federal agencies involved in emergency and trauma care research (including the Department of Transportation, the Department of Health and Human Services, the Department of Homeland Security, and the Department of Defense) should implement the study's recommendations (7.3).**

SUMMARY OF RECOMMENDATIONS

7.1: Federal agencies that fund emergency and trauma care research should target additional funding at prehospital emergency medical services research, with an emphasis on systems and outcomes research.

BOX 7-4
Research Topics Identified by the Committee

Clinical Research
- Impact of prehospital ventilation and intubation on patients with head injuries
- Identification of the safest and most effective technique for managing respiratory insufficiency in the prehospital setting
- Testing of the administration of intravenous (IV) fluid to correct hypotension prior to surgery for trauma
- Performance of new CPR techniques, including chest compression–only CPR
- Impact on outcomes of performing prehospital 12-lead electrocardiograms (ECGs) for patients with acute (ST) segment elevation myocardial infarction
- Impact on outcomes of prehospital administration of medications for selected medical conditions (e.g., asthma, congestive heart failure, diabetes, acute myocardial infarction)

Systems Research
- Impact of level of training (e.g., EMT-Basic, EMT-Paramedic) on condition upon arrival and long-term outcome
- Cost and effectiveness of EMS systems, in particular how they are impacted by the characteristics of the system
- Time interval modeling identifying what changes outcomes, and when and where, in the prehospital setting
- Cost-effectiveness of procedures needed for a range of conditions in a range of settings, including nonemergent care
- Safety and impact of routing nonemergency 9-1-1 calls to nurse advice lines
- Safety and impact of treat and release policies versus EMS transport
- Impact of medical direction on the performance of EMS systems
- Effectiveness of EMS with respect to injury and acute disease
- Incremental value of advanced life support over basic techniques in trauma care
- Effectiveness of new communication techniques (e.g., streaming video) and information technology
- Impact of technology on error reduction or improved decision making (e.g., electronic algorithms, electronic monitor, patient video, and smart implanted chips)
- Impact of prearrival instructions by dispatchers on the condition of patients upon arrival at the hospital and long-term outcome

7.2: Congress should modify Federalwide Assurance program regulations to allow the acquisition of limited, linked patient outcome data without the existence of a Federalwide Assurance program.

7.3: The Secretary of the Department of Health and Human Services should conduct a study to examine the research gaps and opportunities in emergency and trauma care research, and recommend a strategy for the optimal organization and funding of the research effort. This study should include consideration of the training of new investigators, the development of multicenter research networks, the involvement of emergency medical services researchers in the grant review and research advisory processes, and improved research coordination through a dedicated center or institute. Congress and federal agencies involved in emergency and trauma care research (including the Department of Transportation, the Department of Health and Human Services, the Department of Homeland Security, and the Department of Defense) should implement the study's recommendations.

REFERENCES

Baren JM, Anicetti JP, Ledesma S, Biros MH, Mahabee-Gittens M, Lewis RJ. 1999. An approach to community consultation prior to initiating an emergency research study incorporating a waiver of informed consent. *Academic Emergency Medicine* 6(12):1210–1215.

Becker LB, Pepe PE. 1993. Ensuring the effectiveness of community-wide emergency cardiac care. *Annals of Emergency Medicine* 22(2 Pt. 2):354–365.

Biros MH, Lewis RJ, Olson CM, Runge JW, Cummins RO, Fost N. 1995. Informed consent in emergency research. Consensus statement from the coalition conference of acute resuscitation and critical care researchers. *Journal of the American Medical Association* 273(16):1283–1287.

Biros M, Barsan W, Lewis R, Sanders A. 1998. Supporting emergency medicine research: Developing the infrastructure. *Academic Emergency Medicine* 5(2):177–184.

Biros MH, Fish SS, Lewis RJ. 1999. Implementing the Food and Drug Administration's final rule for waiver of informed consent in certain emergency research circumstances. *Academic Emergency Medicine* 6(12):1272–1282.

Brown LH, Owens CF Jr, March JA, Archino EA. 1996. Does ambulance crew size affect on-scene time or number of prehospital interventions? *Prehospital Disaster Medicine* 11(3):214–217; discussion 217–218.

Brown LH, Bailey LC, Medwick T, Okeke CC, Krumperman K, Tran CD. 2003. Medication storage on US ambulances: A prospective multi-center observational study. *Pharmacopeia Forum* 29:540–547.

CDC (Centers for Disease Control). 2005. *Acute Injury Care Research Agenda: Guiding Research for the Future*. Atlanta, GA: CDC.

Cone DC, Wydro GC. 2001. Can basic life support personnel safely determine that advanced life support is not needed? *Prehospital Emergency Care* 5(4):360–365.

Delbridge TR, Bailey B, Chew JL Jr, Conn AK, Krakeel JJ, Manz D, Miller DR, O'Malley PJ, Ryan SD, Spaite DW, Stewart RD, Suter RE, Wilson EM. 1998. EMS agenda for the future: Where we are . . . where we want to be. *Prehospital Emergency Care* 2(1):1–12.

DePalma RG, Burris DG, Champion HR, Hodgson MJ. 2005. Blast injuries. *New England Journal of Medicine* 352(13):1335–1342.

Eisenberg MS, Horwood BT, Cummins RO, Reynolds-Haertle R, Hearne TR. 1990. Cardiac arrest and resuscitation: A tale of 29 cities. *Annals of Emergency Medicine* 19(2):179–186.

Garrison HG, Maio RF, Spaite DW, Desmond JS, Gregor MA, O'Malley PJ, Stiell IG, Cayten CG, Chew JL Jr, Mackenzie EJ, Miller DR. 2002. Emergency Medical Services Outcomes Project III (EMSOP III): The role of risk adjustment in out-of-hospital outcomes research. *Annals of Emergency Medicine* 40(1):79–88.

Gausche M, Lewis RJ, Stratton SJ, Haynes BE, Gunter CS, Goodrich SM, Poore PD, McCollough MD, Henderson DP, Pratt FD, Seidel JS. 2000. Effect of out-of-hospital pediatric endotracheal intubation on survival and neurologic outcome: A controlled clinical trial. *Journal of the American Medical Association* 283(6):783–790.

Gausche-Hill M. 2000. Pediatric continuing education for out-of-hospital providers: Is it time to mandate review of pediatric knowledge and skills? *Annals of Emergency Medicine* 36(1):72–74.

Hallstrom A, Cobb L, Johnson E, Copass M. 2000. Cardiopulmonary resuscitation by chest compression alone or with mouth-to-mouth ventilation. *New England Journal of Medicine* 342(21):1546–1453.

Hsieh M, Dailey MW, Callaway CW. 2001. Surrogate consent by family members for out-of-hospital cardiac arrest research. *Academic Emergency Medicine* 8(8):851–853.

Hunt RC, Brown LH, Cabinum ES, Whitley TW, Prasad NH, Owens CF Jr, Mayo CE Jr. 1995. Is ambulance transport time with lights and siren faster than that without? *Annals of Emergency Medicine* 25(4):507–511.

IOM (Institute of Medicine). 2003. *Enhancing the Vitality of the National Institutes of Health: Organizational Change to Meet New Challenges*. Washington, DC: The National Academies Press.

IOM. 2004. *NIH Extramural Center Programs: Criteria for Initiation and Evaluation*. Washington, DC: The National Academies Press.

Kellermann AL, Hackman BB, Somes G, Kreth TK, Nail L, Dobyns P. 1993. Impact of first-responder defibrillation in an urban emergency medical services system. *Journal of the American Medical Association* 270(14):1708–1713.

Key CB, Pepe PE, Persse DE, Calderon D. 2003. Can first responders be sent to selected 9-1-1 emergency medical services calls without an ambulance? *Academic Emergency Medicine* 10(4):339–346.

Larsen MP, Eisenberg MS, Cummins RO, Hallstrom AP. 1993. Predicting survival from out-of-hospital cardiac arrest: A graphic model. *Annals of Emergency Medicine* 22(11):1652–1658.

Lerner EB, Billittier AJt, Sikora J, Moscati RM. 1999. Use of a geographic information system to determine appropriate means of trauma patient transport. *Academic Emergency Medicine* 6(11):1127–1133.

Lewis RJ, Berry DA, Cryer H III, Fost N, Krome R, Washington GR, Houghton J, Blue JW, Bechhofer R, Cook T, Fisher M. 2001. Monitoring a clinical trial conducted under the Food and Drug Administration regulations allowing a waiver of prospective informed consent: The diaspirin cross-linked hemoglobin traumatic hemorrhagic shock efficacy trial. *Annals of Emergency Medicine* 38(4):397–404.

Maio RF, Garrison HG, Spaite DW, Desmond JS, Gregor MA, Cayten CG, Chew JL Jr, Hill EM, Joyce SM, MacKenzie EJ, Miller DR, O'Malley PJ, Stiell IG. 1999. Emergency Medical Services Outcomes Project I (EMSOP I): Prioritizing conditions for outcomes research. *Annals of Emergency Medicine* 33(4):423–432.

Maio RF, Garrison HG, Spaite DW, Desmond JS, Gregor MA, Stiell IG, Cayten CG, Chew JL Jr, Mackenzie EJ, Miller DR, O' Malley PJ. 2002. Emergency Medical Services Outcomes Project (EMSOP) IV: Pain measurement in out-of-hospital outcomes research. *Annals of Emergency Medicine* 40(2):172–179.

Mann NC, Schmidt TA, Richardson LD. 2005. Confronting the ethical conduct of resuscitation research: A consensus opinion. *Academic Emergency Medicine* 12(11):1078–1081.

McLean SA, Maio RF, Spaite DW, Garrison HG. 2002. Emergency medical services outcomes research: Evaluating the effectiveness of prehospital care. *Prehospital Emergency Care* 6(Suppl. 2):S52–S56.

Moscati R. 2002. Protection of human subjects in prehospital research. *Prehospital Emergency Care* 6(Suppl. 2):S18–S23.

Mullins RJ. 1999. A historical perspective of trauma system development in the United States. *Journal of Trauma-Injury Infection & Critical Care* 47(Suppl. 3):S8–S14.

Mullins RJ, Mann NC, Hedges JR, Worrall W, Jurkovich GJ. 1998. Preferential benefit of implementation of a statewide trauma system in one of two adjacent states. *The Journal of Trauma* 44(4):609–616; discussion 617.

NEDARC (National EMSC Data Analysis Resource Center). 2006. *Data Collection.* [Online]. Available: http://www.nedarc.org/data_coll/Default.htm [accessed January 13, 2006].

Neely KW, Eldurkar JA, Drake ME. 2000a. Do emergency medical services dispatch nature and severity codes agree with paramedic field findings? *Academic Emergency Medicine* 7(2):174–180.

Neely KW, Norton RL, Schmidt TA. 2000b. The strength of specific EMS dispatcher questions for identifying patients with important clinical field findings. *Prehospital Emergency Care* 4(4):322–326.

Newgard CD, Lewis RJ. 2002. The paradox of human subjects protection in research: Some thoughts on and experiences with the federalwide assurance program. *Academic Emergency Medicine* 9(12):1426–1429.

NHTSA (National Highway Traffic Safety Administration). 1996. *Emergency Medical Services Agenda for the Future.* Washington, DC: Department of Transportation.

NHTSA. 1998. *Emergency Medical Services Agenda for the Future: Implementation Guide.* Washington, DC: Department of Transportation.

NHTSA. 2001a. *National EMS Research Agenda.* Washington, DC: Department of Transportation.

NHTSA. 2001b. *Trauma System Agenda for the Future.* Washington, DC: Department of Transportation.

NIH (National Institutes of Health). 2003. *Ruth L. Kirschstein National Research Service Awards for Individual Postdoctoral Fellows (F32).* [Online]. Available: http://grants1.nih.gov/grants/guide/pa–files/PA-03-067.html [accessed February 1, 2006].

PECARN (Pediatric Emergency Care Applied Research Network). 2004. *About PECARN.* [Online]. Available: http://www.pecarn.org/about_pecarn.htm [accessed August 2, 2004].

Persse DE, Key CB, Bradley RN, Miller CC, Dhingra A. 2003. Cardiac arrest survival as a function of ambulance deployment strategy in a large urban emergency medical services system. *Resuscitation* 59(1):97–104.

Sayre MR, White LJ, Brown LH, McHenry SD. 2002. National EMS research agenda. *Prehospital Emergency Care* 6(Suppl. 3):S1–S43.

Sayre MR, White LJ, Brown LH, McHenry SD, Implementation Symposium Participants. 2003. National EMS research agenda: Proceedings of the implementation symposium. *Academic Emergency Medicine* 10(10):1100–1108.

Sayre MR, White LJ, Brown LH, McHenry SD, National EMS Research Strategic Plan Writing Team. 2005. The national EMS research strategic plan. *Prehospital Emergency Care* 9(3):255–266.

Schultz CH, Koenig KL, Lewis RJ. 2003. Implications of hospital evacuation after the Northridge, California, Earthquake. *New England Journal of Medicine* 348(14):1349–1355.

Seidel J, Henderson D, Tittle S, Jaffe D, Spaite D, Dean J, Gausche M, Lewis R, Cooper A, Zaritsky A, Espisito T, Maederis D. 1999. Priorities for research in emergency medical services for children: Results of a consensus conference. *Annals of Emergency Medicine* 33(2):206–210.

Sloan EP, Koenigsberg M, Houghton J, Gens D, Cipolle M, Runge J, Mallory MN, Rodman G Jr. 1999. The informed consent process and the use of the exception to informed consent in the clinical trial of diaspirin cross-linked hemoglobin (DCLHB) in severe traumatic hemorrhagic shock. DCLHB Traumatic Hemorrhagic Shock Study Group. *Academic Emergency Medicine* 6(12):1203–1209.

Spaite DW, Criss EA, Valenzuela TD, Guisto J. 1995. Emergency medical service systems research: Problems of the past, challenges of the future. *Annals of Emergency Medicine* 26(2):146–152.

Spaite DW, Criss EA, Valenzuela TD, Meislin HW. 1997. Developing a foundation for the evaluation of expanded-scope EMS: A window of opportunity that cannot be ignored. *Annals of Emergency Medicine* 30(6):791–796.

Spaite DW, Maio R, Garrison HG, Desmond JS, Gregor MA, Stiell IG, Cayten CG, Chew JL Jr, Mackenzie EJ, Miller DR, O'Malley PJ. 2001. Emergency Medical Services Outcomes Project (EMSOP) II: Developing the foundation and conceptual models for out-of-hospital outcomes research. *Annals of Emergency Medicine* 37(6):657–663.

Stiell IG, Wells GA, Field B, Spaite DW, Nesbitt LP, De Maio VJ, Nichol G, Cousineau D, Blackburn J, Munkley D, Luinstra-Toohey L, Campeau T, Dagnone E, Lyver M, the Ontario Prehospital Advanced Life Support Study Group. 2004. Advanced cardiac life support in out-of-hospital cardiac arrest. *New England Journal of Medicine* 351(7):647–656.

Swor RA, Jackson RE, Cynar M, Sadler E, Basse E, Boji B, Rivera-Rivera EJ, Jacobson R, et al. 1995. Bystander CPR, ventricular fibrillation, and survival in witnessed, unmonitored out-of-hospital cardiac arrest. *Annals of Emergency Medicine* 25(6):780–784.

Valenzuela TD, Copass MK. 2001. Clinical research on out-of-hospital emergency care. *New England Journal of Medicine* 345(9):689–690.

Zerhouni E. 2003. Medicine. The NIH roadmap. *Science* 302(5642):63–72.

APPENDIX
A

Committee and Subcommittee Membership

Gail Warden, MHA, *Chair*

SUBCOMMITTEES			MAIN COMMITTEE	SUBCOMMITTEE ONLY
Pediatric Emergency Care (PEDS)	Prehospital Emergency Medical Services (EMS)	Hospital-Based Emergency Care (ED)		
David Sundwall, MD (Chair)	Shirley Gamble, MBA (Chair)	Benjamin Chu, MD, MPH (Chair)	Thomas Babor, PhD, MPH	
George Foltin, MD	Robert Bass, MD	Stuart Altman, PhD	Robert Gates, MPA	
Darrell Gaskin, PhD	Brent Eastman, MD	Brent Asplin, MD, MPH	William Kelley, MD	
Marianne Gausche-Hill, MD, MPH	Arthur Kellermann, MD, MPH	John Halamka, MD	Mark Smith, MD, MBA	
Richard Orr, MD	Jerry Overton, MA	Mary Jagim, RN		
	Nels Sanddal, MS, REMT-B	Peter Layde, MD, MSc		
		Eugene Litvak, PhD		
		John Prescott, MD		
		William Schwab, MD		
Rosalyn Baker	Kaye Bender, PhD, RN	Kenneth Kizer, MD		
Mary Fallat, MD	Herbert Garrison, MD	John Lumpkin, MD		
Jane Knapp, MD	Mary Beth Michos, RN	Daniel Manz, EMT		
Thomas Loyacono, EMT-P	Fred Neis, RN	Joseph Wright, MD		
Milap Nahata, PharmD	Daniel Spaite, MD			
Donna Ojanen Thomas, RN				

APPENDIX
B

Biographical Information for Main Committee and Prehospital Emergency Medical Services Subcommittee

Gail L. Warden, M.H.A., F.A.C.H.E., *Main Committee Chair,* is president emeritus of Henry Ford Health System in Detroit, Michigan, one of the nation's leading vertically integrated health care systems. He is an elected member of the Institute of Medicine (IOM) of the National Academy of Sciences and served on its Board of Health Care Services and Committee on Quality Health Care in America, as well as serving its two terms on its Governing Council. He chairs the board of the National Quality Forum, the Healthcare Research and Development Institute, and the newly created National Center for Healthcare Leadership. Mr. Warden cochairs the National Advisory Committee on Pursuing Perfection: Raising the Bar for Health Care Performance. He is a member of The Robert Wood Johnson Foundation Board of Trustees, the Institute for Healthcare Improvement Board, and the RAND Health Board of Advisors. He is director emeritus and past chair of the Board of the National Committee on Quality Assurance. In 1997 President Clinton appointed him to the Federal Advisory Commission on Consumer Protection and Quality in the Health Care Industry. In 1995 Mr. Warden served as chair of the American Hospital Association Board of Trustees. He served as a member of the Pew Health Professions Commission and the National Commission on Civic Renewal, and is past chair of the Health Research and Education Trust Board of Directors. Mr. Warden served as president and chief executive officer of Henry Ford Health System from April 1988 until June 2003. Previously, he served as president and chief executive officer of Group Health Cooperative of Puget Sound in Seattle from 1981 to 1988. Prior to that he was executive vice president of the American Hospital Association from 1976 to 1981, and from 1965 to 1976 he served as executive vice president and chief operating officer of Rush-Presbyterian-St. Luke's Medical Center in Chicago. Mr. Warden is a graduate of Dartmouth College and holds an M.H.A. from the University of Michigan. He has an honorary doctorate in public administration from Central Michigan University and is a member of the faculty of the University of Michigan School of Public Health.

Shirley Gamble, M.B.A., *EMS Subcommittee Chair,* served as senior advisor to The Robert Wood Johnson Foundation's Urgent Matters initiative, which is working to help hospitals eliminate emergency department crowding and help communities understand the challenges facing the health care safety net. Ms. Gamble has over 20 years of experience in the health care industry, serving as an executive with Incarnate Word Health Services, Texas Health Plans HMO, and Tampa General Hospital. As partner of Phase 2 Consulting, a health care management and economic consulting firm, Ms. Gamble led performance improvement and strategic planning initiatives for major hospital systems, managed care entities, and university faculty practice plans. She currently is chief operating officer for the United Way Capital Area in Austin, Texas. She holds an M.B.A. and B.A. from the University of Texas at Austin.

Stuart H. Altman, Ph.D., is Sol C. Chaikin Professor of National Health Policy at the Heller Graduate School for Social Policy and Management. He served as dean of the Heller School from 1977 to a 1993. In August 2005 he again assumed the deanship of the Heller School. Dr. Altman has had extensive experience with the federal government, serving as deputy assistant secretary for planning and evaluation/health in the U.S. Department of Health, Education, and Welfare, 1971–1976; chair of the congressionally mandated Prospective Payment Assessment Commission, 1983–1996; and a member of the Bipartisan Commission on the Future of Medicare, 1999–2001. In addition, from 1973 to 1974 he served as deputy director for health of the President's Cost-of-Living Council and was responsible for developing the council's program on health care cost containment. Dr. Altman has testified before various congressional committees on the problems of rising health care costs, Medicare reform, and the need to create a national health insurance program for the United States. He chaired the IOM's Committee on the Changing Market, Managed Care, and the Future Viability of Safety Net Providers. His research activities include several studies concerning the factors responsible for the recent increases in the use of emergency departments. He holds a Ph.D. in economics from the University of California, Los Angeles, and has taught at Brown University and the University of California, Berkeley.

Brent R. Asplin, M.D., M.P.H., F.A.C.E.P., is department head of emergency medicine at Regions Hospital and HealthPartners Research Foundation in St. Paul, Minnesota, and is an associate professor and vice chair of the Department of Emergency Medicine at the University of Minnesota. After receiving his degree from Mayo Medical School, he completed the University of Pittsburgh's Affiliated Residency in Emergency Medicine. To develop his interests in research and health care policy, Dr. Asplin completed the Robert Wood Johnson Clinical Scholars Program at the University of Michigan, where he obtained an M.P.H. in health management and policy. He is currently studying methods for enhancing the reliability and efficiency of health care operations, particularly strategies for improving patient flow in hospital settings.

Thomas F. Babor, Ph.D., M.P.H., spent several years in postdoctoral research training in social psychiatry at Harvard Medical School, and subsequently served as head of social science research at McLean Hospital's Alcohol and Drug Abuse Research Center in Belmont, Massachusetts. In 1982 he moved to the University of Connecticut School of Medicine, where he has served as scientific director at the Alcohol Research Center and interim chair of the Psychiatry Department. Dr. Babor's primary interests are psychiatric epidemiology and alcohol and drug abuse. In 1998 he became chair of the Department of Community Medicine and Health Care at the University of Connecticut School of Medicine, where he directs an active research program. Dr. Babor is regional editor of the international journal *Addiction*. He previously served on two IOM committees—Prevention and Treatment of Alcohol-Related Problems: An Update on Research Opportunities, and Treatment of Alcohol Problems.

Robert R. Bass, M.D., F.A.C.E.P., received his undergraduate and medical degrees from the University of North Carolina at Chapel Hill in 1972 and 1975, respectively. Prior to completing his undergraduate education, he was employed as a police officer in Chapel Hill, North Carolina, and served as a volunteer member of the South Orange Rescue Squad. Dr. Bass completed an internship and residency in the navy and is currently board certified in both emergency medicine and family medicine. He has served as a medical director for emergency medical services (EMS) systems in Charleston, South Carolina; Houston, Texas; Norfolk, Virginia; and Washington, DC. Since 1994, Dr. Bass has been executive director of the Maryland Institute for EMS Systems, the state agency responsible for the oversight of Maryland's EMS and trauma system. He is clinical associate professor of surgery (emergency medicine) at the University of Maryland at Baltimore and is associate professor in the Emergency Health Services Program at the University of Maryland, Baltimore County. Dr. Bass is currently president of the National

Association of State EMS Officials and a founding member and the immediate past president of the National Association of EMS Physicians. Additionally, he serves on the board of directors of the American Trauma Society and the University of Maryland Medical System, and is past chair of the EMS Committee of the American College of Emergency Physicians.

Kaye Bender, R.N., Ph.D., F.A.A.N., is dean and professor at the School of Nursing and associate vice chancellor for Nursing at the University of Mississippi Medical Center. Prior to assuming that position, she was deputy state health officer for the Mississippi State Department of Health for 5 years and chief of staff for the Mississippi State Department of Health for 10 years. Dr. Bender holds a B.S.N. from the University of Mississippi; an M.S. in Community Health Nursing from the University of Southern Mississippi; and a Ph.D. in Clinical Health Sciences from the University of Mississippi Medical Center. She is a fellow of the American Academy of Nursing and is a graduate of the Centers for Disease Control and Prevention (CDC)/Western Consortium Public Health Leadership Institute. Dr. Bender has served on a number of local, state, and national public health and nursing committees and has held several offices in public health and nursing organizations. She currently chairs the Steering Committee of the Exploring Accreditation Project for the National Association of County and City Health Officials and the Association of State and Territorial Health Officials. She serves on the Education Board of the American Public Health Association and on the Government Affairs Committee for the Association of Colleges of Nursing. She has served on two IOM study committees: The Future of the Public's Health in the 21st Century and Who Will Keep the Public Healthy? Dr. Bender has published several articles and book chapters and has provided numerous presentations on public health and nursing topics. Her area of research interest is public health policy and health systems.

Benjamin K. Chu, M.D., M.P.H., was appointed president, Kaiser Foundation Health Plan, Inc. and Kaiser Foundation Hospitals, Southern California Region, in February 2005. Before joining Kaiser Permanente, Dr. Chu was president of the New York City Health and Hospitals Corporation, with primary responsibility for management and policy implementation. Prior to that, he was senior associate dean at Columbia University College of Physicians and Surgeons. He has also served as associate dean and vice president for clinical affairs at the New York University Medical Center, managing and developing the clinical academic hospital network. Dr. Chu is a primary care internist by training, with extensive experience as a clinician, administrator, and policy advocate for the public hospital sector. He was senior vice president for medical and professional affairs at the New

York City Health and Hospitals Corporation from 1990 to 1994. During that period, he also served as acting commissioner of health for the New York City Department of Health and acting executive director for Kings County Hospital Center. Dr. Chu has extensive experience in crafting public policy. He served as legislative assistant for health for Senator Bill Bradley as a 1989–1990 Robert Wood Johnson Health Policy Fellow. Earlier in his career, he served as acting director of the Kings County Hospital Adult Emergency Department. His areas of interests include health care access and insurance, graduate medical education policy, primary care, and public health issues. He has served on numerous advisory and not-for-profit boards focused on health care policy issues. Dr. Chu received a masters in public health from the Mailman School at Columbia University and his doctorate of medicine at New York University School of Medicine.

A. Brent Eastman, M.D., joined Scripps Memorial Hospital La Jolla in 1984 as director of trauma services and was appointed chief medical officer in 1998. He continues to serve in the role of director of trauma. Dr. Eastman received his medical degree from the University of California, San Francisco, where he also did his general surgical residency and served as chief surgical resident. He spent a year abroad in surgical training in England at Norfolk and Norwich Hospitals. Dr. Eastman served as chair of the Committee on Trauma for the American College of Surgeons from 1990 to 1994. This organization sets the standards for trauma care in the United States and abroad. The position led to his involvement nationally and internationally in the development of trauma systems in the United States, Canada, England, Ireland, Australia, Brazil, Argentina, Mexico, and South Africa. Dr. Eastman has authored or coauthored more than 25 publications and chapters relating principally to trauma. He has held numerous appointments and chairmanships over the last two decades, including chair, Trauma Systems Committee, for the U.S. Department of Health and Human Services; member of the board of directors, American Association for the Surgery of Trauma; and chair, Grant Review Committee, Center for Injury Prevention and Control at the U.S. Centers for Disease Control and Prevention.

George L. Foltin, M.D., F.A.A.P., F.A.C.E.P., began his involvement with the Emergency Medical Services for Children (EMS-C) Program of the Health Resources and Services Administration in 1985. He is board certified in pediatrics, emergency medicine, and pediatric emergency medicine. Dr. Foltin served on the Medical Oversight Committee for the EMT-Basic National Standard Curriculum project and was a subject expert for the Project to Revise EMT-Intermediate and Paramedic National Standard Curriculum. He is a former board member of the National Association of EMS Physicians and served on the Committee on Pediatric Emergency Medicine of the American

Academy of Pediatrics (AAP). Currently Dr. Foltin cochairs the Statewide AAP Committee on Pediatric Emergency Medicine and sits on the Regional Medical Advisory Committee of New York City. He has published extensively in the field of EMS for children, has been principal investigator for several federal grants, and serves as a consultant to the New York City and State departments of health, as well as to federal programs such as those of the Maternal and Child Health Bureau, the Agency for Healthcare Research and Quality, and the National Highway Traffic Safety Administration.

Herbert G. Garrison, M.D., M.P.H., F.A.C.E.P., is professor of emergency medicine at the Brody School of Medicine of East Carolina University. He also serves as director of the Eastern Carolina Injury Prevention Program. Dr. Garrison earned his M.D. and M.P.H. from the University of North Carolina at Chapel Hill, and has completed residencies in emergency medicine and preventive medicine and a fellowship in prehospital emergency medical services. He also served as a Robert Wood Johnson Clinical Scholar from 1990–1992. Dr. Garrison's clinical and research interests include injury prevention and prehospital EMS.

Darrell J. Gaskin, Ph.D., M.S., is associate professor of health policy and management at The Johns Hopkins Bloomberg School of Public Health and deputy director of the Morgan-Hopkins Center for Health Disparities Solutions. Dr. Gaskin's research focuses on health care disparities and access to care for vulnerable populations. Dr. Gaskin was awarded the Academy Health 2002 Article-of-the-Year Award for his *Health Services Research* article entitled "Are Urban Safety-Net Hospitals Losing Low-Risk Medicaid Maternity Patients?" Dr. Gaskin is active in professional organizations. He is a member of Academy Health, the American Economic Association, the National Economics Association (NEA), the International Health Economics Association, the American Society of Health Economists, and the American Public Health Association (APHA). He has served as a member of the board of directors of the NEA. He has been a member of the Governing Council of the APHA and is currently solicited program chair and section councilor for the APHA's Medical Care Section. He has chaired the disparities program committee for Academy Health. He is a member of the board of directors for the Maryland Citizen's Health Initiative. Dr. Gaskin earned his Ph.D. in health economics at The Johns Hopkins University, a master degree in economics from the Massachusetts Institute of Technology, and a bachelors degree in economics from Brandeis University.

Robert C. Gates, M.P.A., began his career in the County of Los Angeles Chief Administrative Office, where he was principal budget analyst for the public health, hospital, and mental health departments. He left Los Angeles to become chief operating officer for the University of California, Irvine, Medical Center in Orange County. While in Orange County, he was instrumental in creating its paramedic system. Mr. Gates then returned to Los Angeles County and spent 6 years as chief deputy director of the Department of Health Services, guiding the creation of the Los Angeles County Trauma Center system. He was then appointed director of health services for Los Angeles County and served in that capacity for over 11 years. Mr. Gates is currently serving as medical services for indigents project director for the Orange County Health Care Agency.

Marianne Gausche-Hill, M.D., F.A.C.E.P., F.A.A.P., serves as professor of clinical medicine at the David Geffen School of Medicine at the University of California, Los Angeles (UCLA). She is director of EMS and EMS fellowship and director of pediatric emergency medicine fellowship at Harbor-UCLA Medical Center. Dr. Gausche-Hill also serves as director of pediatric emergency medicine at the Little Company of Mary Hospital in Torrance, California. Board certified in both emergency medicine and pediatric emergency medicine, she earned her medical degree and completed her residency at UCLA. Dr. Gausche-Hill is the first emergency physician in the United States to have completed a pediatric emergency fellowship and passed the sub-board examination. She has done extensive research on prehospital pediatric care, authoring *Pediatric Advanced Life Support: Pearls of Wisdom* in 2001 and *Pediatric Airway Management for the Prehospital Professional* in 2004. Her research tracking the results of the use of the windpipe tube method versus the traditional bag-and-pump method as oxygen treatment for pediatric emergencies was published in the *Journal of the American Medical Association* and in *Annals of Emergency Medicine*. In May 1999, her work earned the prestigious Best Clinical Science Presentation award from the Society for Academic Emergency Medicine.

John D. Halamka, M.D., M.S., is chief information officer of the CareGroup Health System, chief information officer and associate dean for educational technology at Harvard Medical School, chair of the New England Health Electronic Data Interchange Network (NEHEN), acting chief executive officer of MA-Share, chief information officer of the Harvard Clinical Research Institute, and a practicing emergency physician. As chief information officer at CareGroup, he is responsible for all clinical, financial, administrative, and academic information technology serving 3,000 doctors, 12,000 employees, and 1 million patients. As chief information officer and associate dean for educational technology at Harvard Medical School, he oversees all educational, research, and administrative computing for 18,000 faculty and 3,000 students. As chair of NEHEN, he oversees administrative data exchange in Massachusetts. As chief executive officer of MA-Share, he oversees the clinical data exchange efforts in Massachusetts. As chair of the Healthcare Information Technology Standards Panel, he coordinates the process of harmonization of electronic standards among all stakeholders nationwide.

Mary M. Jagim, R.N., B.S.N., C.E.N., FAEN, is an experienced emergency/trauma nurse with extensive leadership background in program development and implementation, emergency department management and nursing workforce issues, emergency preparedness, government affairs, and community-based injury prevention. She is currently internal consultant for emergency preparedness and pandemic planning for MeritCare Health System in Fargo, North Dakota. Well versed in current issues affecting emergency/trauma nursing and emergency care, Ms. Jagim has served on the Emergency Nurses Association board of directors, for which she was national president in 2001. She currently serves as chair of the Emergency Nurses Association Foundation, is a member of the faculty for Key Concepts in Emergency Department Management, and is a fellow in the Academy of Emergency Nursing. She also served on the Centers for Disease Control and Prevention's (CDC) National Strategies for Advancing Child Pedestrian Safety Panel to Prevent Pedestrian Injuries and currently is cochair for Advocates for Highway and Auto Safety. Ms. Jagim received her B.S.N. from the University of North Dakota in 1984.

Arthur L. Kellermann, M.D., M.P.H., is professor and chair of the Department of Emergency Medicine at the Emory University School of Medicine and director of the Center for Injury Control at the Rollins School of Public Health at Emory University. His primary research focus is injury prevention and control. He has also conducted landmark research on prehospital cardiac care, use of diagnostic technology in emergency departments, and health care for the poor. His papers have been published in many of the nation's leading medical journals. He is a recipient of the Hal Jayne Academic Excellence Award from the Society for Academic Emergency Medicine, the Excellence in Science Award from the Injury Control and Emergency Health Services Section of the American Public Health Association, and the Scholar/Teacher Award from Emory University. A member of the IOM, Dr. Kellermann served as cochair of the IOM's Committee on the Consequences of Uninsurance from 2001 to 2004.

William N. Kelley, M.D., currently serves as professor of medicine, biochemistry, and biophysics at the University of Pennsylvania School of Medicine. Previously, he served as chief executive officer of the University of Pennsylvania Medical Center and Health System and dean of the School of Medicine from 1989 to February 2000. At the University of Pennsylvania, Dr. Kelley led the development of one of the first academic fully integrated delivery systems in the nation. He also built and implemented the largest health and disease management program in the country, with over 500 physicians and staff and 60 separate clinical sites engaged in implementing the program. Dr. Kelley holds a patent in a frequently used gene transfer technique that has allowed for numerous advances in the application of gene therapy. He received his M.D. from Emory University School of Medicine and completed his residency in internal medicine at Parkland Memorial Hospital in Dallas. After a fellowship with the National Institutes of Health and a teaching fellowship at Harvard Medical School, he began his academic career as assistant professor of medicine at Duke University School of Medicine, moving on to head Duke's Division of Rheumatic and Genetic Diseases before becoming chair of internal medicine at the University of Michigan Medical School.

Peter M. Layde, M.D., M.Sc., is professor and interim director of the Health Policy Institute at the Medical College of Wisconsin. He has been an epidemiologist for over 25 years and an active injury control researcher for over 20 years. He has published extensively on agricultural injuries and methods for injury epidemiology, including early work on the use of case–control studies for homicide and on the epidemiological representativeness of trauma center–based studies. He has been an ad hoc reviewer for the Injury Grant Review Committee for over 10 years and served as a member of that committee from 1997 to 2000. Dr. Layde serves as codirector of the Injury Research Center at the Medical College of Wisconsin and as director of its Research Development and Support Core. He is also principal investigator for the Risk Factors for Medical Injury research project.

Eugene Litvak, Ph.D., is cofounder and director of the Program for the Management of Variability in Health Care Delivery at the Boston University Health Policy Institute. He is also a professor at the Boston University School of Management. He received his doctorate in operations research from the Moscow Institute of Physics and Technology in 1977. In 1990, he joined the faculty of the Harvard Center for Risk Analysis in the Department of Health Policy and Management at the Harvard School of Public Health, where he still teaches as adjunct professor of operations management. Prior to that time he was chief of the Operations Management Group at the Computing Center in Kiev, Ukraine. His research interests include operations management in health care delivery organizations, cost-effective medical decision making, screening for HIV and other infectious diseases, and operations research. He was leading author of cost-effective protocols for screening for HIV and is principal investigator from the United States for an international trial of these protocols, which is supported by the U.S. Agency for International Development. Dr. Litvak was also principal investigator for the Emergency Room Diversion Study, supported by a grant from the Massachusetts Department of Public Health. He serves as a consultant on operations improvement to several major hospitals and is on the faculty of the Institute for Health Care Improvement.

John R. Lumpkin, M.D., M.P.H., is senior vice president and director, Health Care Group at The Robert Wood Johnson Foundation. Dr. Lumpkin joined the Illinois Department of Public Health (IDHP) in1985 as associate director of IDPH's Office of Health Care Regulations, and later became the first African American to hold the position of director. Dr. Lumpkin served 6 years as chair of the National Committee for Vital and Health Statistics, advising the Secretary of the U.S. Department of Health and Human Services on health information policy. He received his medical degree in 1974 from Northwestern University Medical School. He trained in emergency medicine at the University of Chicago and earned his M.P.H. from the University of Illinois at Chicago, School of Public Health. Dr. Lumpkin is past president of the Association of State and Territorial Health Officials, a former member of the board of trustees of the Foundation for Accountability, former commissioner of the Pew Commission on Environmental Health, former board member of the National Forum for Health Care Quality Measurement and Reporting, past board member of the American College of Emergency Physicians, and past president of the Society of Teachers of Emergency Medicine. He has been the recipient of the Bill B. Smiley Award, Alan Donaldson Award, and African American History Maker Award, and was named Public Health Worker of the Year.

Mary Beth Michos, a former R.N., is chief of the Department of Fire and Rescue for Prince William County, Virginia. Prior to assuming the duties of chief in 1994, she had been associated with the Montgomery County Fire and Rescue Service since 1973. Chief Michos is past chair of the International Association of Fire Chiefs' (IAFC) Emergency Medical Services (EMS) Section, is nationally known for her work with the American Heart Association, and currently serves as president of the board of directors of the Greater Washington Regional Heart Association. She is immediate past chair of the board of directors of the National Registry of Emergency Medical Technicians. She was chair of the National Fire Protection Association Task Group on EMS Response to Hazardous Materials Incidents and is a member of the Metro Chiefs Section of IAFC. In 2003 she was recognized with the James O. Page EMS Leadership Award and named Career Fire Chief of the Year.

Fred A. Neis, R.N., M.S., C.H.E., C.E.N., currently serves as a director with H*Works Clinical Operations Team for The Advisory Board Company.

Previously, he served as director of the Emergency Department of Carolinas Medical Center, the flagship hospital for Carolinas HealthCare Systems; as clinical manager of emergency services for Oregon Health and Science University; and earlier as EMS-C program coordinator for the Oregon Department of Human Services. Mr. Neis is also an experienced firefighter, field paramedic, flight nurse, and ED nurse. He earned his B.S.N. and M.S. in nursing administration from the University of Kansas. He also completed paramedic training in 1990 at the University of Iowa Hospitals and Clinics. Mr. Neis is an active member of the Emergency Nurses Association and the American College of Healthcare Executives.

Richard A. Orr, M.D., serves as professor at the University of Pittsburgh School of Medicine, associate director of the Cardiac Intensive Care Unit at the Children's Hospital of Pittsburgh, and medical director of the Children's Hospital Transport Team of Pittsburgh, Pennsylvania. Dr. Orr has devoted much of his career to interfacility transportation problems of infants and children in need of tertiary care. He is a member of many professional organizations and societies and has authored numerous articles regarding the safe and effective air and surface transport of the critically ill and injured pediatric patient. Dr. Orr is also a noted lecturer to the air and ground transport community, both nationally and internationally. He is editor of *Pediatric Transport Medicine*, a unique 700-page book published in 1995. He is the 2001 recipient of the Air Medical Physician Association (AMPA) Distinguished Physician Award and a founding member of AMPA.

Jerry L. Overton, M.A., serves as executive director, Richmond Ambulance Authority, Richmond, Virginia, and has overall responsibility for the Richmond EMS system. His duties extend to planning and administering the high-performance system's design, negotiating and implementing performance-based contracts, maximizing fee-for-service revenues, developing advanced patient care protocols, and employing innovative equipment and treatment modalities. Mr. Overton was previously executive director of the Kansas City, Missouri, EMS system. In addition, he has provided technical assistance to EMS systems throughout the United States and Europe, Russia, Asia, Australia, and Canada. He designed an implementation plan for an emergency medical transport program in Central Bosnia–Herzegovina. Mr. Overton is a faculty member of the Emergency Medical Department of the Medical College of Virginia, Virginia Commonwealth University, and the National EMS Medical Directors Course, National Association of EMS Physicians. He is past president of the American Ambulance Association and serves on the board of directors of the North American Association of Public Utility Models.

John E. Prescott, M.D., is dean of the West Virginia University (WVU) School of Medicine, and received both his B.S. and M.D. degrees at Georgetown University. He completed his residency training in emergency medicine at Brooke Army Medical Center, San Antonio, and was then assigned to Fort Bragg, North Carolina, where he was actively engaged in providing both operational and hospital emergency care in a variety of challenging situations. In 1990 he joined WVU and soon assumed leadership of the Section of Emergency Medicine. During that same year, he founded and became the first director of WVU's Center for Rural Emergency Medicine. In 1993 he became the first chair of WVU's newly established Department of Emergency Medicine. Dr. Prescott is a past recipient of major CDC and private foundation grants. His research and scholarly interests include rural emergency care, injury control and prevention, medical response to disasters and terrorism, and academic and administrative medicine. In 1999 Dr. Prescott became WVU's associate dean for the clinical enterprise and president/chief executive officer of University Health Associates, WVU's physician practice plan. In 2003 he was named senior associate dean; he was appointed dean of the WVU School of Medicine in 2004. He has been a fellow of the American College of Emergency Physicians since 1987 and is the recipient of WVU's Presidential Heroism Award.

Nels D. Sanddal, M.S., REMT-B, is president of the Critical Illness and Trauma Foundation (CIT) in Bozeman, Montana, and is currently on detachment as director of the Rural Emergency Medical Services and Trauma Technical Assistance Center. Mr. Sanddal has been involved in EMS since the 1970s and has held many state, regional, and national positions in organizations furthering EMS causes, including president of the Intermountain Regional EMS for Children Coordinating Council and core faculty for the Development of Trauma Systems Training Programs for the U.S. Department of Transportation. He is a nationally registered EMT-Basic, volunteers with a local fire department, and has been involved with CIT since its inception in 1986. He holds an M.S. in psychology and is currently pursuing a Ph.D. in health services.

C. William Schwab, M.D., F.A.C.S., is professor of surgery and chief of the Division of Traumatology and Surgical Critical Care at the University of Pennsylvania. His surgical practice reflects his expertise in trauma systems, including caring for the severely injured patient and incorporating the most advanced techniques into trauma surgery. He is director of the Firearm and Injury Center at Penn and holds several grants supporting work on reducing firearm and nonfirearm injuries and other repercussions. He has served as a trauma systems consultant to CDC, New York State, and several state health departments. He has established trauma centers and hospital-based aeromedical programs in Virginia, New Jersey, and Pennsylvania. He currently directs a network of three regional trauma centers throughout southeastern Pennsylvania. He has been president of the Eastern Association for the Surgery of Trauma and vice chair of the American College of Surgeons Committee on Trauma and currently serves as president of the American Association for the Surgery of Trauma.

Mark D. Smith, M.D., M.B.A., has led the California HealthCare Foundation in developing research and initiatives aimed at improving California's health care financing and delivery systems since the foundation's formation in 1996. Prior to joining the foundation, he was executive vice president at the Henry J. Kaiser Family Foundation and served as associate director of the AIDS Service and assistant professor of medicine and health policy and management at The Johns Hopkins University. Dr. Smith is a member of the IOM and is on the board of the National Business Group on Health. Previously, he served on the Performance Measurement Committee of the National Committee for Quality Assurance and the editorial board of the *Annals of Internal Medicine*. A board-certified internist, Dr. Smith is a member of the clinical faculty at the University of California, San Francisco, and an attending physician at the AIDS clinic at San Francisco General Hospital.

Daniel W. Spaite, M.D., is currently a medical professor in the Department of Emergency Medicine at the University of Arizona College of Medicine, Emergency Medical Services (EMS) Base Hospital medical director at the University Medical Center in Tucson, and medical director of air medical transport for LifeNet Arizona. He also chairs the Southeastern Arizona Regional EMS Council, serves on the Pima County EMS Council, and is a member of the Southeastern Arizona Regional EMS Medical Directors Committee. In addition, Dr. Spaite has had many national EMS responsibilities, including serving as a site reviewer for the EMS system evaluations being conducted by the National Highway Traffic Safety Administration (NHTSA), chair of the EMS Minimum Data Set Task Force for the American College of Emergency Physicians, a member of the National EMS for Children Advisory Board of the Department of Health and Human Services, and a member of the steering committees for NHTSA's EMS Agenda for the Future and EMS Research Agenda for the Future. Dr. Spaite has authored more than 100 scientific articles and abstracts and has presented his research on cardiac arrest, injury prevention, and analysis and modeling of fire department–based EMS systems at many conferences internationally.

David N. Sundwall, M.D., was nominated by Governor Jon Huntsman Jr. to serve as executive director of the Utah State Department of Health in

January 2005 and was subsequently confirmed for this position by the Utah Senate. In this capacity, he supervises a workforce of almost 1,400 employees and a budget of almost $1.8 billion. Previously, Dr. Sundwall served as president of the American Clinical Laboratory Association (ACLA) from September 1994 until he was appointed senior medical and scientific officer in May 2003. Prior to his position at ACLA, he was vice president and medical director of American Healthcare System (AmHS), at that time the largest coalition of not-for-profit multihospital systems in the country. Dr. Sundwall has extensive experience in federal government and national health policy, including serving as administrator, Health Resources and Services Administration; in the Public Health Service, U.S. Department of Health and Human Services (DHHS); and as assistant surgeon general in the Commissioned Corps of the U.S. Public Health Service (1986–1988). During this period, he had adjunct responsibilities at DHHS, including serving as cochair of the secretary's Task Force on Medical Liability and Malpractice and as the secretary's designee to the National Commission to Prevent Infant Mortality. Dr. Sundwall also served as director, Health and Human Resources Staff (Majority), U.S. Senate Labor and Human Resources Committee (1981–1986). He was in private medical practice in Murray, Utah, from 1973 to 1975. He has held academic appointments at the Uniformed Services University of the Health Sciences, Bethesda, Maryland; Georgetown University School of Medicine, Washington, D.C.; and the University of Utah School of Medicine. He is board certified in internal medicine and family practice. He is licensed to practice medicine in the District of Columbia, is a member of the American Medical Association and the American Academy of Family Physicians, and previously served as volunteer medical staff of Health Care for the Homeless Project.

List of Presentations to the Committee

February 2–4, 2004

Overview of Emergency Care in the U.S. Health System
- Overview of the Emergency Care System
  Arthur L. Kellermann (Emory University School of Medicine)
- Emergency Care Supply and Utilization
  Charlotte S. Yeh (Centers for Medicare and Medicaid Services)
- Rural Issues in Emergency Care
  John E. Prescott (West Virginia University)

Major Emergency Care Issue Areas
- Patient Flow and Emergency Department Crowding
  Brent R. Asplin (University of Minnesota)
- Evolution of the Emergency Department (circa 2004): A Systems Perspective
  Eric B. Larson (Group Health Cooperative)
- Mental Health and Substance Abuse Issues
  Michael H. Allen (University of Colorado Health Sciences Center)
- Workforce Education and Training
  Glenn C. Hamilton (Wright State University School of Medicine)
- Information Technology in Emergency Care
  Larry A. Nathanson (Beth Israel Deaconess Medical Center)

Prehospital Care, Public Health, and Emergency Preparedness
- Emergency Care and Public Health
  Daniel A. Pollock (Centers for Disease Control and Prevention)
- Overview of the Issues Facing Prehospital EMS
  Robert R. Bass (Maryland Institute for Emergency Medical Services Systems)
- Emergency Preparedness
  Joseph F. Waeckerle (University of Missouri Baptist Medical Center)

Research Agenda
- Overview of Research in Emergency Care
  E. John Gallagher (Montefiore Medical Center)
- Research Needs for the Future
  Robin M. Weinick (Agency for Healthcare Research and Quality)

June 9–11, 2004

Overview of Emergency Medical Services for Children
- The EMS-C Program: History and Current Challenges
  Jane Ball (The EMSC National Resource Center)
- The 1993 IOM Report: Promise and Progress
  Megan McHugh (IOM Staff)

Issues in Pediatric Emergency Care
- Pediatric Equipment and Care Management
  Marianne Gausche-Hill (Harbor-UCLA Medical Center)
- Special Problems in Pediatric Medication
  Milap Nahata (Ohio State University Schools of Pharmacy and Medicine)
- Training and Skills Maintenance
  Cynthia Wright-Johnson (Maryland Institute for EMS Systems)
- Emergency Research and Data Issues
  David Jaffe (Washington University in St. Louis)

Pediatric Disaster Preparedness
- *George Foltin (New York University Bellevue Hospital Center)*

Organization and Delivery of Emergency Medical Services
- System-Wide EMS and Trauma Planning and Coordination
  Stephen Hise (National Association of State EMS Directors)
- Fire Perspective on EMS
  John Sinclair (International Association of Fire Chiefs)
- Trauma Systems
  Alasdair Conn (Massachusetts General Hospital)
- Critical Care Transport
  Richard Orr (Children's Hospital of Pittsburgh)

History and Organization of EMS in the United States
- EMS System Overview and History
  Robert Bass (Maryland Institute for Emergency Medical Services Systems)
- Overview of Local EMS Systems
  Mike Williams (Abaris Group)

- Issues Facing Rural Emergency Medical Services
  Fergus Laughridge (Emergency Medical Services, Nevada State Health Division)

Prehospital EMS Issue Areas

- EMS Financing and Reimbursement
  Jerry Overton (Richmond Ambulance Authority)
- EMS Quality Improvement and Patient Safety
  Robert A. Swor (William Beaumont Hospital)
- Overview of the EMS Agenda for the Future
  Ted Delbridge (University of Pittsburgh)
- EMS Data Needs
  Greg Mears (University of North Carolina-Chapel Hill)
- Overview of Current EMS Research
  Ron Maio (University of Michigan)

Agency Reaction Panel

- Health Resources and Services Administration, Maternal and Child Health Bureau
  Dave Heppel (Division of Child, Adolescent, and Family Health) and/or Dan Kavanaugh (EMSC-Program)
- National Highway Traffic Safety Administration
  Drew Dawson (EMS Division)
- Agency for Healthcare Research and Quality
  Robin Weinick (Safety Nets and Low Income Populations and Intramural Research)
- Centers for Disease Control and Prevention, National Center for Injury Prevention and Control
  Rick Hunt (Division of Injury and Disability Outcomes and Programs)
- Health Resources and Services Administration, Office of Rural Health Policy
  Evan Mayfield (U.S. Public Health Service and Public Health Analyst)

June 24–25, 2004

Workforce Issues in the Emergency Department

- Issues Facing the Emergency Care Nursing Workforce
  Mary Jagim (MeritCare Hospital)
  Carl Ray (Bon Secours DePaul Medical Center)
  Kathy Robinson (Pennsylvania Department of Health)

Current Initiatives in Patient Flow
- Patient Flow Initiative Implemented at University of Utah
  Jadie Barrie (University of Utah)
  Pamela Proctor (University of Utah)
- Program for Management of Variability in Health Care Delivery
  Eugene Litvak (Boston University Health Policy Institute)

Luncheon Speaker—Medical Technology in Emergency Medicine
- *Michael Sachs (Sg2)*

September 20–21, 2004

Prehospital EMS Issue Areas
- International EMS Systems
  Jerry Overton (Richmond Ambulance Authority)
- Current Status of Federal Emergency Care Legislation and Funding
  Mark Mioduski (Cornerstone Government Affairs)
- Overview of EMS Workforce Issues
  John Becknell (Consultant)
- EMS System Design and Coordination
  Bob Davis (USA Today)

Reimbursement and Funding of Pediatric Emergency Care Services
- Reimbursement Issues in Pediatric Emergency Care
  *Steven E. Krug (Northwestern University/Children's Memorial
  Hospital)*
- Current Status of Federal Emergency Care Legislation and Funding
  Mark Mioduski (Cornerstone Government Affairs)

Issues Facing Pediatric Emergency Care
- Funding of Children's Hospitals
  Peter Holbrook (Children's National Medical Center)
- Survey on Pediatric Preparedness
  Marianne Gausche-Hill (Harbor-UCLA Medical Center)

October 4–5, 2004

No open sessions held.

March 2–4, 2005

Public Health Perspectives
- Overview of EMS and Trauma System Issues
  William Koenig (Emergency Medical Services Agency, LA County)

- The Hospital Perspective
  Doug Bagley (Riverside County Regional Medical Center)
- The Safety Net and Community Providers Perspective
  John Gressman (San Francisco Community Clinics Consortium)
- Mental Health and Substance Abuse
  Barry Chaitin (University of California—Irvine)
- The Patient Perspective
  Sandy Schuhmann-Atkins (University of California—Irvine)

On-Call Coverage Issues
- Survey of On-Call Coverage in California
  Mark Langdorf (University of California—Irvine)
- Specialty Physician Perspective—Orthopedics
  Nick Halikis (Little Company of Mary Hospital)
- Specialty Physician Perspective—Neurosurgery
  John Kusske (University of California—Irvine)

Issues in Rural Emergency Care
- The Family Practice Perspective
  *Arlene Brown (Southern New Mexico Family Medicine Residency
  and Family Practice Associates of Ruidoso, PC)*
- Telemedicine in Rural Emergency Care
  Jim Marcin (University of California—Davis)

APPENDIX
D

List of Commissioned Papers

1. **The Role of the Emergency Department in the Health Care Delivery System**
   Consultant: Eva Stahl, Brandeis University

2. **Patient Safety and Quality of Care in Emergency Services**
   Consultant: Jim Adams, Northwestern University

3. **Patient Flow in Hospital-Based Emergency Services**
   Consultant: Brad Prenny, Boston University, Health Policy Institute

4. **Models of Organization, Delivery, and Planning for EMS and Trauma Systems**
   Consultant: Tasmeen Singh, Children's National Medical Center

5. **Information Technology in Emergency Care**
   Consultant: Larry Nathanson, Harvard Medical School

6. **Emergency Care in Rural America**
   Consultant: Janet Williams, University of Rochester

7. **The Emergency Care Workforce**
   Consultant: Jean Moore, State University of New York School of Public Health

8. **The Financing of EMS and Hospital-Based Emergency Services**
   Consultants: John McConnell, Oregon Health and Sciences University
   David Gray, Medical University of South Carolina
   Richard Lindrooth, Medical University of South Carolina

9. **The Impact of New Medical Technologies on Emergency Care**
Consultant: Sg2

10. **Mental Health and Substance Abuse in the Emergent Care Setting**
Consultant: Linda Degutis, DrPH, Yale University

11. **Emergency Care Research Funding**
Consultant: Roger Lewis, Harbor-UCLA Medical Center

APPENDIX
E

Recommendations and Responsible Entities from the *Future of Emergency Care* Series

HOSPITAL-BASED EMERGENCY CARE: AT THE BREAKING POINT

	Congress	DHHS	DOT	DHS	DOD	States	Hospitals	EMS Agencies	Private Industry	Professional Organizations	Other
Chapter 2: The Evolving Role of Hospital-Based Emergency Care											
2.1 Congress should establish dedicated funding, separate from Disproportionate Share Hospital payments, to reimburse hospitals that provide significant amounts of uncompensated emergency and trauma care for the financial losses incurred by providing those services.	X	X									
2.1a Congress should initially appropriate $50 million for the purpose, to be administered by the Centers for Medicare and Medicaid Services.											
2.1b The Centers for Medicare and Medicaid Services should establish a working group to determine the allocation of these funds, which should be targeted to providers and localities at greatest risk; the working group should then determine funding needs for subsequent years.											
Chapter 3: Building a 21st-Century Emergency Care System											
3.1 The Department of Health and Human Services and the National Highway Traffic Safety Administration, in partnership with professional organizations, should convene a panel of individuals with multidisciplinary expertise to develop evidence-based categorization systems for emergency medical services, emergency departments, and trauma centers based on adult and pediatric service capabilities.	X	X	X							X	

Recommendation						
3.2 The National Highway Traffic Safety Administration, in partnership with professional organizations, should convene a panel of individuals with multidisciplinary expertise to develop evidence-based model prehospital care protocols for the treatment, triage, and transport of patients.		X				X
3.3 The Department of Health and Human Services should convene a panel of individuals with emergency and trauma care expertise to develop evidence-based indicators of emergency and trauma care system performance.		X				
3.4 The Department of Health and Human Services should adopt regulatory changes to the Emergency Medical Treatment and Active Labor Act and the Health Insurance Portability and Accountability Act so that the original goals of the laws will be preserved, but integrated systems can be further developed.		X				
3.5 Congress should establish a demonstration program, administered by the Health Resources and Services Administration, to promote coordinated, regionalized, and accountable emergency care systems throughout the country, and appropriate $88 million over 5 years to this program.	X	X				

	Congress	DHHS	DOT	DHS	DOD	States	Hospitals	EMS Agencies	Private Industry	Professional Organizations	Other
3.6 Congress should establish a lead agency for emergency and trauma care within 2 years of the release of this report. The lead agency should be housed in the Department of Health and Human Services, and should have primary programmatic responsibility for the full continuum of emergency medical services and emergency and trauma care for adults and children, including medical 9-1-1 and emergency medical dispatch, prehospital emergency medical services (both ground and air), hospital-based emergency and trauma care, and medical-related disaster preparedness. Congress should establish a working group to make recommendations regarding the structure, funding, and responsibilities of the new agency, and develop and monitor the transition. The working group should have representation from federal and state agencies and professional disciplines involved in emergency and trauma care.	X	X									

Chapter 4: Improving the Efficiency of Hospital-Based Emergency Care

	Congress	DHHS	DOT	DHS	DOD	States	Hospitals	EMS Agencies	Private Industry	Professional Organizations	Other
4.1 The Centers for Medicare and Medicaid Services should remove the current restrictions on the medical conditions that are eligible for separate clinical decision unit (CDU) payment.		X					X				
4.2 Hospital chief executive officers should adopt enterprisewide operations management and related strategies to improve the quality and efficiency of emergency care.											

4.3 Training in operations management and related approaches should be promoted by professional associations; accrediting organizations, such as the Joint Commission on Accreditation of Healthcare Organizations and the National Committee for Quality Assurance; and educational institutions that provide training in clinical, health care management, and public health disciplines.

4.4 The Joint Commission on Accreditation of Healthcare Organizations should reinstate strong standards designed to sharply reduce and ultimately eliminate ED crowding, boarding, and diversion.

4.5 Hospitals should end the practices of boarding patients in the emergency department and ambulance diversion, except in the most extreme cases, such as a community mass casualty event. The Centers for Medicare and Medicaid Services should convene a working group that includes experts in emergency care, inpatient critical care, hospital operations management, nursing, and other relevant disciplines to develop boarding and diversion standards, as well as guidelines, measures, and incentives for implementation, monitoring, and enforcement of these standards.

Chapter 5: Technology and Communication

5.1 Hospitals should adopt robust information and communications systems to improve the safety and quality of emergency care and enhance hospital efficiency.

Chapter 6: The Emergency Care Workforce

6.1 Hospitals, physician organizations, and public health agencies should collaborate to regionalize critical specialty care on-call services.

	Congress	DHHS	DOT	DHS	DOD	States	Hospitals	EMS Agencies	Private Industry	Professional Organizations	Other
6.2 Congress should appoint a commission to examine the impact of medical malpractice lawsuits on the declining availability of providers in high-risk emergency and trauma care specialties, and to recommend appropriate state and federal actions to mitigate the adverse impact of these lawsuits and ensure quality of care.	X										
6.3 The American Board of Medical Specialties and its constituent boards should extend eligibility for certification in critical care medicine to all acute care and primary care physicians who complete an accredited critical care fellowship program.										X	X
6.4 The Department of Health and Human Services, the Department of Transportation, and the Department of Homeland Security should jointly undertake a detailed assessment of emergency and trauma workforce capacity, trends, and future needs, and develop strategies to meet these needs in the future.		X	X	X							
6.5 The Department of Health and Human Services, in partnership with professional organizations, should develop national standards for core competencies applicable to physicians, nurses, and other key emergency and trauma professionals, using a national, evidence-based, multidisciplinary process.		X								X	
6.6 States should link rural hospitals with academic health centers to enhance opportunities for professional consultation, telemedicine, patient referral and transport, and continuing professional education.						X	X				

Chapter 7: Disaster Preparedness

7.1 The Department of Homeland Security, the Department of Health and Human Services, the Department of Transportation, and the states should collaborate with the Veterans Health Administration (VHA) to integrate the VHA into civilian disaster planning and management.

7.2 All institutions responsible for the training, continuing education, and credentialing and certification of professionals involved in emergency care (including medicine, nursing, emergency medical services, allied health, public health, and hospital administration) should incorporate disaster preparedness training into their curricula and competency criteria.

7.3 Congress should significantly increase total preparedness funding in fiscal year 2007 for hospital emergency preparedness in the following areas: strengthening and sustaining trauma care systems; enhancing emergency department, trauma center, and inpatient surge capacity; improving emergency medical services' response to explosives; designing evidence-based training programs; enhancing the availability of decontamination showers, standby intensive care unit capacity, negative pressure rooms, and appropriate personal protective equipment; and conducting international collaborative research on the civilian consequences of conventional weapons terrorism.

Chapter 8: Enhancing the Emergency and Trauma Care Research Base

8.1 Academic medical centers should support emergency and trauma care research by providing research time and adequate facilities for promising emergency care and trauma investigators, and by strongly considering the establishment of autonomous departments of emergency medicine.

	Congress	DHHS	DOT	DHS	DOD	States	Hospitals	EMS Agencies	Private Industry	Professional Organizations	Other
8.2 The Secretary of the Department of Health and Human Services should conduct a study to examine the gaps and opportunities in emergency and trauma care research, and recommend a strategy for the optimal organization and funding of the research effort.	X	X	X	X	X						
8.2a This study should include consideration of training of new investigators, development of multicenter research networks, funding of General Clinical Research Centers that specifically include an emergency and trauma care component, involvement of emergency and trauma care researchers in the grant review and research advisory processes, and improved research coordination through a dedicated center or institute.											
8.2b Congress and federal agencies involved in emergency and trauma care research (including the Department of Transportation, the Department of Health and Human Services, the Department of Homeland Security, and the Department of Defense) should implement the study's recommendations.											
8.3 States should ease their restrictions on informed consent to match federal law.	X										
8.4 Congress should modify Federalwide Assurance (FWA) Program regulations to allow the acquisition of limited, linked, patient outcome data without the existence of an FWA.											

EMERGENCY MEDICAL SERVICES AT THE CROSSROADS

	Congress	DHHS	DOT	DHS	DOD	States	Hospitals	EMS Agencies	Private Industry	Professional Organizations	Other
Chapter 3: Building a 21st-Century Emergency Care System											
3.1 The Department of Health and Human Services and the National Highway Traffic Safety Administration, in partnership with professional organizations, should convene a panel of individuals with multidisciplinary expertise to develop evidence-based categorization systems for emergency medical services, emergency departments, and trauma centers based on adult and pediatric service capabilities.		X	X							X	
3.2 The National Highway Traffic Safety Administration, in partnership with professional organizations, should convene a panel of individuals with multidisciplinary expertise to develop evidence-based model prehospital care protocols for the treatment, triage, and transport of patients.			X							X	
3.3 The Department of Health and Human Services should convene a panel of individuals with emergency and trauma care expertise to develop evidence-based indicators of emergency and trauma care system performance.		X									
3.4 Congress should establish a demonstration program, administered by the Health Resources and Services Administration, to promote coordinated, regionalized, and accountable emergency and trauma care systems throughout the country, and appropriate $88 million over 5 years to this program.	X	X									

	Congress	DHHS	DOT	DHS	DOD	States	Hospitals	EMS Agencies	Private Industry	Professional Organizations	Other
3.5 Congress should establish a lead agency for emergency and trauma care within 2 years of the release of this report. This lead agency should be housed in the Department of Health and Human Services, and should have primary programmatic responsibility for the full continuum of emergency medical services and emergency and trauma care for adults and children, including medical 9-1-1 and emergency medical dispatch, prehospital emergency medical services (both ground and air), hospital-based emergency and trauma care, and medical-related disaster preparedness. Congress should establish a working group to make recommendations regarding the structure, funding, and responsibilities of the new agency, and design and monitor the transition to its assumption of the responsibilities outlined above. The working group should include representatives from federal and state agencies and professional disciplines involved in emergency and trauma care.	X	X									
3.6 The Department of Health and Human Services should adopt regulatory changes to the Emergency Medical Treatment and Active Labor Act and the Health Insurance Portability and Accountability Act so that the original goals of the laws will be preserved, but integrated systems can be further developed.		X									
3.7 The Centers for Medicare and Medicaid Services should convene an ad hoc working group with expertise in emergency care, trauma, and emergency medical services systems to evaluate the reimbursement of emergency medical services and make recommendations with regard to including readiness costs and permitting payment without transport.		X									

Chapter 4: Supporting a High-Quality EMS Workforce

Recommendation						
4.1 State governments should adopt a common scope of practice for emergency medical services personnel, with state licensing reciprocity.					X	
4.2 States should require national accreditation of paramedic education programs.					X	
4.3 States should accept national certification as a prerequisite for state licensure and local credentialing of emergency medical services providers.					X	
4.4 The American Board of Emergency Medicine should create a subspecialty certification in emergency medical services.		X				

Chapter 5: Advancing System Infrastructure

Recommendation						
5.1 States should assume regulatory oversight of the medical aspects of air medical services, including communications, dispatch, and transport protocols.					X	
5.2 Hospitals, trauma centers, emergency medical services agencies, public safety departments, emergency management offices, and public health agencies should develop integrated and interoperable communications and data systems.	X		X	X		
5.3 The Department of Health and Human Services should fully involve prehospital emergency medical services leadership in discussions about the design, deployment, and financing of the National Health Information Infrastructure.						X

	Congress	DHHS	DOT	DHS	DOD	States	Hospitals	EMS Agencies	Private Industry	Professional Organizations	Other
Chapter 6: Preparing for Disasters											
6.1 The Department of Health and Human Services, the Department of Transportation, the Department of Homeland Security, and the states should elevate emergency and trauma care to a position of parity with other public safety entities in disaster planning and operations.		X	X	X		X					
6.2 Congress should substantially increase funding for emergency medical services–related disaster preparedness through dedicated funding streams.	X										
6.3 Professional training, continuing education, and credentialing and certification programs for all the relevant professional categories of emergency medical services personnel should incorporate disaster preparedness into their curricula and require the maintenance of competency in these skills.		X	X			X				X	X
Chapter 7: Optimizing Prehospital Care Through Research											
7.1 Federal agencies that fund emergency and trauma care research should target additional funding at prehospital emergency medical services research, with an emphasis on systems and outcomes research.		X	X	X	X						X
7.2 Congress should modify Federalwide Assurance program regulations to allow the acquisition of limited, linked patient outcome data without the existence of a Federalwide Assurance program.	X										

	Congress	DHHS	DOT	DHS	DOD	States	Hospitals	EMS Agencies	Private Industry	Professional Societies	Other
7.3 The Secretary of the Department of Health and Human Services should conduct a study to examine the research gaps and opportunities in emergency and trauma care research, and recommend a strategy for the optimal organization and funding of the research effort. This study should include consideration of the training of new investigators, the development of multicenter research networks, the involvement of emergency medical services researchers in the grant review and research advisory processes, and improved research coordination through a dedicated center or institute. Congress and federal agencies involved in emergency and trauma care research (including the Department of Transportation, the Department of Health and Human Services, the Department of Homeland Security, and the Department of Defense) should implement the study's recommendations.	X	X	X	X	X						

EMERGENCY CARE FOR CHILDREN: GROWING PAINS

Chapter 3: Building a 21st-Century Emergency Care System

	Congress	DHHS	DOT	DHS	DOD	States	Hospitals	EMS Agencies	Private Industry	Professional Societies	Other
3.1 The Department of Health and Human Services and the National Highway Traffic Safety Administration, in partnership with professional organizations, should convene a panel of individuals with multidisciplinary expertise to develop evidence-based categorization systems for emergency medical services, emergency departments, and trauma centers based on adult and pediatric service capabilities.		X	X							X	

268

	Congress	DHHS	DOT	DHS	DOD	States	Hospitals	EMS Agencies	Private Industry	Professional Societies	Other
3.2 The National Highway Traffic Safety Administration, in partnership with professional organizations, should convene a panel of individuals with multidisciplinary expertise to develop evidence-based model prehospital care protocols for the treatment, triage, and transport of patients, including children.			X							X	
3.3 The Department of Health and Human Services should convene a panel of individuals with emergency and trauma care expertise to develop evidence-based indicators of emergency and trauma care system performance, including the performance of pediatric emergency care.		X									
3.4 Congress should establish a demonstration program, administered by the Health Resources and Services Administration, to promote coordinated, regionalized, and accountable emergency care systems throughout the country, and appropriate $88 million over 5 years to this program.	X	X									
3.5 The Department of Health and Human Services should adopt rule changes to the Emergency Medical Treatment and Active Labor Act and the Health Insurance Portability and Accountability Act so that the original goals of the laws are preserved, but integrated systems may further develop.		X									

3.6 Congress should establish a lead agency for emergency and trauma care within 2 years of the release of this report. The lead agency should be housed in the Department of Health and Human Services, and should have primary programmatic responsibility for the full continuum of emergency medical services and emergency and trauma care for adults and children, including medical 9-1-1 and emergency medical dispatch, prehospital emergency medical services (both ground and air), hospital-based emergency and trauma care, and medical-related disaster preparedness. Congress should establish a working group to make recommendations regarding the structure, funding, and responsibilities of the new agency, and design and monitor the transition to its assumption of the responsibilities outlined above. The working group should have representation from federal and state agencies and professional disciplines involved in emergency and trauma care.

3.7 Congress should appropriate $37.5 million per year for the next 5 years to the Emergency Medical Services for Children program.

Chapter 4: Arming the Emergency Care Workforce with Knowledge and Skills

4.1 Every pediatric- and emergency care–related health professional credentialing and certification body should define pediatric emergency care competencies and require practitioners to receive the level of initial and continuing education necessary to achieve and maintain those competencies.

4.2 The Department of Health and Human Services should collaborate with professional organizations to convene a panel of individuals with multidisciplinary expertise to develop, evaluate, and update clinical practice guidelines and standards of care for pediatric emergency care.

	Congress	DHHS	DOT	DHS	DOD	States	Hospitals	EMS Agencies	Private Industry	Professional Societies	Other
4.3 Emergency medical services agencies should appoint a pediatric emergency coordinator, and hospitals should appoint two pediatric emergency coordinators—one a physician—to provide pediatric leadership for the organization.							X	X			
Chapter 5: Improving the Quality of Pediatric Emergency Care											
5.1 The Department of Health and Human Services should fund studies of the efficacy, safety, and health outcomes of medications used for infants, children, and adolescents in emergency care settings in order to improve patient safety.		X									
5.2 The Department of Health and Human Services and the National Highway Traffic Safety Administration should fund the development of medication dosage guidelines, formulations, labeling, and administration techniques for the emergency care setting to maximize effectiveness and safety for infants, children, and adolescents. Emergency medical services agencies and hospitals should incorporate these guidelines, formulations, and techniques into practice.		X	X				X	X			
5.3 Hospitals and emergency medical services agencies should implement evidence-based approaches to reducing errors in emergency and trauma care for children.		X	X				X	X			
5.4 Federal agencies and private industry should fund research on pediatric-specific technologies and equipment used by emergency and trauma care personnel.				X					X		

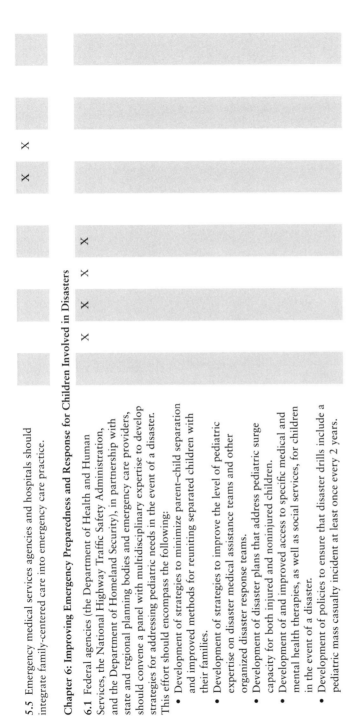

5.5 Emergency medical services agencies and hospitals should integrate family-centered care into emergency care practice.

Chapter 6: Improving Emergency Preparedness and Response for Children Involved in Disasters

6.1 Federal agencies (the Department of Health and Human Services, the National Highway Traffic Safety Administration, and the Department of Homeland Security), in partnership with state and regional planning bodies and emergency care providers, should convene a panel with multidisciplinary expertise to develop strategies for addressing pediatric needs in the event of a disaster. This effort should encompass the following:

- Development of strategies to minimize parent–child separation and improved methods for reuniting separated children with their families.
- Development of strategies to improve the level of pediatric expertise on disaster medical assistance teams and other organized disaster response teams.
- Development of disaster plans that address pediatric surge capacity for both injured and noninjured children.
- Development of and improved access to specific medical and mental health therapies, as well as social services, for children in the event of a disaster.
- Development of policies to ensure that disaster drills include a pediatric mass casualty incident at least once every 2 years.

Chapter 7: Building the Evidence Base for Pediatric Emergency Care

	Congress	DHHS	DOT	DHS	DOD	States	Hospitals	EMS Agencies	Private Industry	Professional Societies	Other
7.1 The Secretary of Health and Human Services should conduct a study to examine the gaps and opportunities in emergency care research, including pediatric emergency care, and recommend a strategy for the optimal organization and funding of the research effort. This study should include consideration of the training of new investigators, development of multicenter research networks, involvement of emergency and trauma care researchers in the grant review and research advisory processes, and improved research coordination through a dedicated center or institute. Congress and federal agencies involved in emergency and trauma care research (including the Department of Transportation, Department of Health and Human Services, Department of Homeland Security, and Department of Defense) should implement the study's recommendations.		X	X	X	X						
7.2 Administrators of state and national trauma registries should include standard pediatric-specific data elements and provide the data to the National Trauma Data Bank. Additionally, the American College of Surgeons should establish a multidisciplinary pediatric specialty committee to continuously evaluate pediatric-specific data elements for the National Trauma Data Bank and identify areas for pediatric research.											X

Index

S